A Colour Atlas of
OCCLUSION & MALOCCLUSION

A Colour Atlas of
OCCLUSION & MALOCCLUSION

Alison P. Howat

PhD, BDS, FDS, RCS, Dip. Orth. RCS
Locum Consultant Orthodontist,
North East Thames Regional Health Authority,
Formerly Lecturer in Children's Dentistry and Orthodontics,
University of Birmingham,
Honorary Senior Registrar in Orthodontics,
West Midlands Regional Health Authority

Nicholas J. Capp

BDS, FDS, RCS, MS (Michigan)
Honorary Senior Clinical Lecturer in Restorative Dentistry,
Institute of Dental Surgery/Eastman Dental Hospital, London,
Restorative Dental Practice, London

N. Vincent J. Barrett

BDS, MS (Texas)
Clinical Assistant in Prosthetic Dentistry,
Guy's Hospital,
Restorative Dental Practice, London

Wolfe Publishing Ltd

Copyright © 1991 A. P. Howat, N. J. Capp and
N. V. J. Barrett
Published by Wolfe Publishing Ltd, 1991
Printed by BPCC Hazell Books Ltd, Aylesbury,
Bucks, England
ISBN 0 7234 1538 2

All rights reserved. No reproduction, copy or
transmission of this publication may be made
without written permission.

No part of this publication may be reproduced,
copied or transmitted save with written permission
or in accordance with the provisions of the
Copyright Act 1956 (as amended), or under the
terms of any licence permitting limited copying
issued by the Copyright Licensing Agency,
33–34 Alfred Place, London, WC1E 7DP.

Any person who does any unauthorised act in
relation to this publication may be liable to
criminal prosecution and civil claims for damages.

A CIP catalogue record for this book is available
from the British Library.

This book is one of the titles in the series of Wolfe
Medical Atlases, a series that brings together the
world's largest systematic published collection of
diagnostic colour photographs.

For a full list of Atlases in the series, plus
forthcoming titles and details of our surgical,
dental and veterinary Atlases, please write to
Wolfe Publishing Ltd, 2–16 Torrington Place,
London, WC1E 7LT, England.

Contents

	Page
Preface	7
Acknowledgements	8

Part I: Mandibular movements and definitions — 9

1. Mandibular movements and positions — 9
   - Border movements in a sagittal plane — 10
   - Border movements in a coronal plane — 12
   - Border movements in a horizontal plane — 15
   - Control of mandibular movements — 15
2. The role of articulators in duplicating movements — 17
   - Classification — 17
   - Cast relators — 17
   - Average-value articulators — 18
   - Semi-adjustable articulators — 18
   - The facebow transfer — 23
   - Interocclusal records — 26
   - Fully-adjustable articulators — 28

Part II: Assessment of the occlusion — 33

3. Restorative assessment — 33
   - Aims of occlusal examination — 33
   - History — 34
   - Examination — 34
4. Restorative special investigations — 53
   - Radiographs — 53
   - Articulated diagnostic casts — 55
   - Conforming to the existing ICP — 55
   - Reorganizing so that RCP = ICP — 59
   - Pantographics — 67
   - Occlusal splint therapy — 69
5. Orthodontic assessment — 73
   - History — 73
   - Examination — 74
6. Orthodontic special investigations — 109
   - General growth and development — 109
   - Instrumental analysis of diagnostic casts — 111
   - ICP–RCP conversion on lateral cephalometric radiograph — 112
7. Complete denture assessment — 113
   - History — 113
   - Examination — 114
   - Special investigations — 120

Part III: Optimizing the occlusion — 121

8. The conformative–reorganized equation — 121
9. Introduction to restoration of the occlusion — 123
   - Occlusal splint therapy — 124

Analysis of diagnostic casts mounted in RP	124
Eliminating the RCP–ICP discrepancy	125
10 The restoration of anterior teeth	129
General considerations in restoring anterior guidance	129
Restoring anterior guidance	133
Occlusal considerations for acid etch-retained bridges	147
Partial denture occlusion when anterior teeth require replacement	150
11 The restoration of posterior teeth	151
General considerations in restoring posterior teeth	151
Indications for gold v porcelain occlusal surfaces	157
The restoration of posterior teeth	161
12 The restoration of anterior and posterior teeth	179
13 Introduction to orthodontic treatment	187
14 Conformative orthodontic treatment	189
Conformative interceptive treatment	189
Conformative definitive treatment	190
15 Reorganized orthodontic treatment	201
Interceptive reorganized orthodontic treatment	201
Definitive reorganized orthodontic management	211
16 Complete denture occlusion	217
Intercuspal position coincident with the retruded position at the established vertical dimension of occlusion	217
Arrangement of artificial teeth	221
Verification and maintenance of occlusal contacts	229
Special considerations	231

Further reading   233
Index   236

Preface

This Atlas provides an illustrated guide to the assessment and treatment of occlusion in the specialties of orthodontics, restorative dentistry and complete denture prosthodontics. A multi-disciplinary approach is adopted because communication between and within different specialties is important and requires the understanding of a common language, describing the elements of both static and functional occlusion.

Many texts introduce the topic of occlusion with a list of definitions. An atlas format has allowed the authors to take advantage of written definition, diagram and clinical illustration to produce greater clarity.

Some texts provide a catalogue approach to describe the various articulator systems. The authors feel that it is more important to provide the reader with a clearly illustrated understanding of mandibular movements and then to describe how closely each class of articulator can reproduce these movements. This approach should enable an informed choice to be made of an appropriate articulator system.

The use of mounted diagnostic casts for the assessment of functional rather than static occlusion is emphasized for all three disciplines.

Treatment aimed at optimizing the occlusion has been described as being either 'conformative' or 'reorganized'. These terms are familiar to restorative dentists but unfamiliar to many orthodontists. Conformative treatment is carried out to an existing, stable intercuspal position (ICP) and produces no alteration to the relationship between the retruded contact position (RCP) and the intercuspal position. Reorganized treatment involves eliminating any discrepancy between the retruded contact and intercuspal positions, creating a new, stable intercuspal position close to the retruded position of the mandible.

Within these definitions, localized orthodontic tooth movement carried out to the existing ICP is conformative. Correction of a Class 2 or Class 3 malocclusion to a Class 1 relationship is also conformative if there is no pre-treatment RCP–ICP discrepancy. In this situation, orthodontic treatment should not produce any alteration in condylar position with the teeth in maximum intercuspation. However, treatment becomes reorganized if an existing RCP–ICP discrepancy is eliminated.

In the edentulous mouth, the loss of natural teeth and proprioceptive feedback from periodontal membranes requires a reorganized approach. The retruded position provides the only relatively stable and reproducible maxillomandibular relation at which a new ICP can be established.

This classification of treatment procedures has several advantages. It emphasizes the importance of producing a functional rather than a static occlusion. To achieve this objective, it is advisable to avoid the introduction of restorations or tooth positions which interfere with mandibular movement or reduce the stability of the intercuspal position. This preventive approach will reduce the likelihood of functional disturbances occurring later on.

The FDI two-digit system of tooth designation has been chosen as it is the most internationally accepted system. The four quadrants of the mouth are described by the first digit of each pair of numbers; in the permanent dentition $\frac{1\ 2}{4\ 3}$, and in the deciduous dentition $\frac{5\ 6}{8\ 7}$. The second digit refers to the individual tooth, for example: 18 17 16 15 14 13 12 11 for the teeth in the right maxillary quadrant in the permanent dentition, and 61 62 63 64 65 for the deciduous teeth in the left maxillary quadrant.

The Atlas is directed at the undergraduate and postgraduate dental student, general practitioners, specialist restorative and orthodontic practitioners, and supporting technical staff. It is also applicable to maxillofacial surgeons involved in orthognathic surgery.

Acknowledgements

The authors are indebted to the Department of Clinical Illustration, Birmingham Dental Hospital; Mr M. Sharland, Birmingham Dental School; the Departments of Medical Photography, Burton-on-Trent District Hospital and Westminster Hospital, London; and Wolfe Medical Publications for their expert help with the preparation of diagrams and for undertaking some of the photography.

Thanks are due to Nadim Kurban, Jean Wilkins and Lindsay Munroe for their assistance in the production of some of the restorative technical work illustrated, and to the staff of the orthodontic laboratories of Birmingham Dental Hospital and Burton-on-Trent District Hospital for the production of the casts and removable appliances.

We are grateful to those colleagues who allowed us to include their photographs: Mr D. Birnie (263, 264), Dr J. Clayton (340, 341), Mr S. Cunnington (419, 420), Professor T. D. Foster (183a, 183b), Mr D. Setchell (94) and Miss K. Warren (16, 111, 534).

A. E. Morgan Publications have kindly allowed republication of pictures 165, 167, 374, 375, 376, 377, 378, 518, 519, previously published in several papers in the *Journal of Restorative Dentistry*. Thanks also to Castlemead Publications for permission to publish an illustration of one of their growth charts (299).

Helpful advice and encouragement have been gratefully received from Dr J. Davenport, Professor T. D. Foster, Mr M. J. Shaw, Mr D. J. Spary, and Miss K. Warren to whom special thanks are given.

Finally, we would like to thank the Quintessence Publishing Company for their permission to use the diagram shown in 534, and Ms Rosemary Watts for the line drawings so skilfully prepared.

Part I Mandibular movements and definitions

Chapter 1 describes mandibular movements and positions. This basic knowledge is essential for the clinician whether the occlusion of one tooth or an entire arch is being altered. Changes in the occlusion produced by orthodontics or restorative dentistry should be in harmony with these movements so that minimal adaptation is required from the patient's masticatory system.

Chapter 2 describes the use of articulators in simulating mandibular movements for the purposes of occlusal diagnosis and in the fabrication of restorations. The use of an appropriate articulator is important as inadequate diagnostic information may be obtained from clinical examination alone. The use of an articulator to fabricate restorations will reduce the amount of chairside adjustment required to make them harmonize, and not interfere with mandibular movements.

Chapter 1: Mandibular movements and positions

The study of occlusion involves the whole masticatory system, and will therefore include not only the static relationship of teeth, but also the functional interrelationship between teeth, periodontal tissues, jaws, temporomandibular joints (TMJs), muscles and nervous system. An understanding of the importance of all the components of the masticatory system in normal function, parafunction and dysfunction is essential.

Functional movements of the mandible occur during speech, mastication and swallowing and take place within three-dimensional limits known as the **border positions** The limits are determined by the morphology of the TMJ components and the associated neuromuscular system. Normal functional movements may frequently extend to these borders, provided there is no limitation from tooth contacts. Border positions and movements have been shown to be relatively stable and reproducible over a period of time, and as such provide valuable reference points for use in diagnostic and treatment procedures.

Parafunctional movements of the mandible are usually habitual and include: tooth to tooth contacts (bruxism and clenching), tooth to soft tissue contacts (lip biting, thumb sucking), soft tissue to soft tissue contacts (abnormal swallowing, jaw posturing), and foreign object to tooth contacts (pencil biting).

Dysfunctional movements of the mandible are abnormal or impaired movements caused either by a derangement of the articular disc of the TMJs or by hyperactivity in the muscles of mastication.

Border movements in a sagittal plane

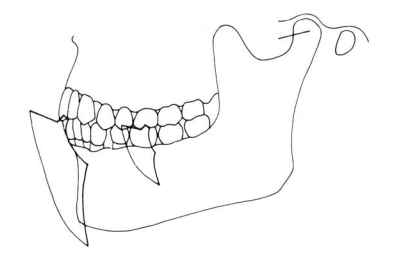

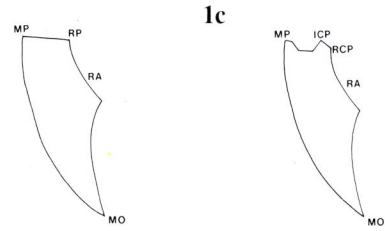

1a–1c Mandibular movements may be studied at condylar or tooth level. Posselt described an envelope of border movement in the sagittal plane which may be represented at incisal, molar, and condylar levels (**1a**). **1b** represents the path of movement when there is no limitation by teeth, and **1c** when anterior tooth contacts influence border movements, when these movements are traced at the tip of the mandibular central incisor.

Key

RP: Retruded position
RA: Retruded axis
RCP: Retruded contact position
ICP: Intercuspal position
MP: Maximum protrusion
MO: Maximum opening

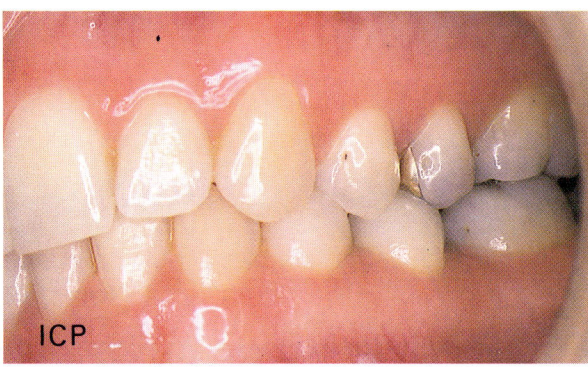

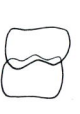

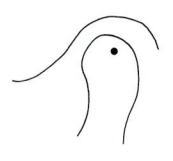

2a, 2b The **intercuspal position** (centric occlusion) is defined as the mandibular position in which there is maximum intercuspation of the teeth. It is a tooth-determined position which is normally the most reproducible relation of mandible to maxilla. It may change when tooth morphology or position is altered, or when teeth are lost.

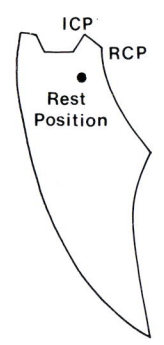

3 When not in function, the mandible is most often held in the **rest position** (R Pos), in which the mandible is open 2–4mm from the intercuspal position. The rest position is used clinically as a reference point for establishing the **vertical dimension of rest** (VDR), defined as a midline measurement of the face between two arbitrary points above and below the mouth with the mandible in the rest position. In clinical practice this so-called position is extremely inconsistent, being affected by many variables such as posture and muscle activity. The **vertical dimension of occlusion** (VDO) is the measurement of the face when the mandible is in the intercuspal position. The separation between VDR and VDO is termed **freeway space** or **interocclusal distance**.

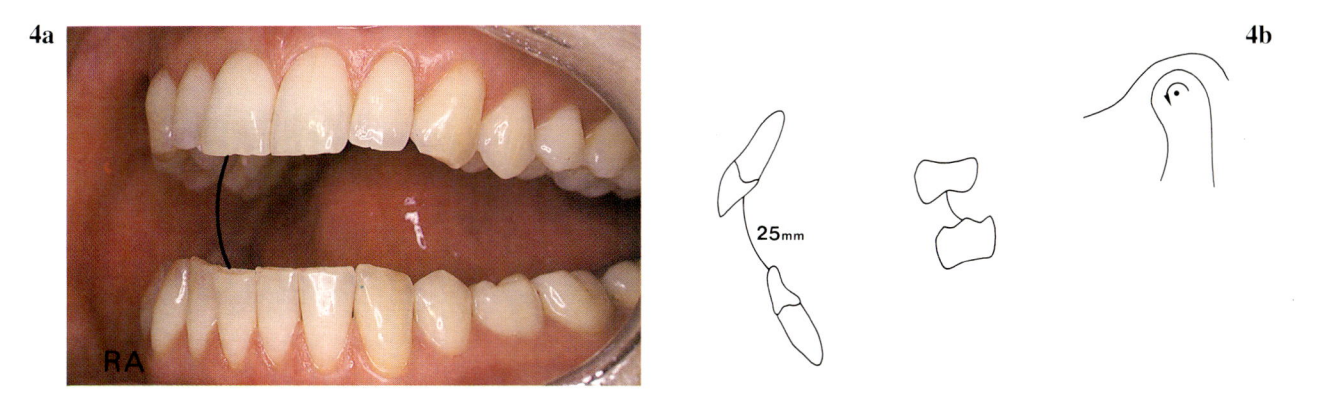

4a, 4b The mandible can hinge about a horizontal axis called the **retruded axis** (terminal hinge axis). This permits an incisal opening of approximately 25 mm with the condyles in the **retruded position** (RP) (centric relation). This is described as the most superior position of the condyles in their respective fossae when joint components and the associated neuromuscular system are in a healthy state.

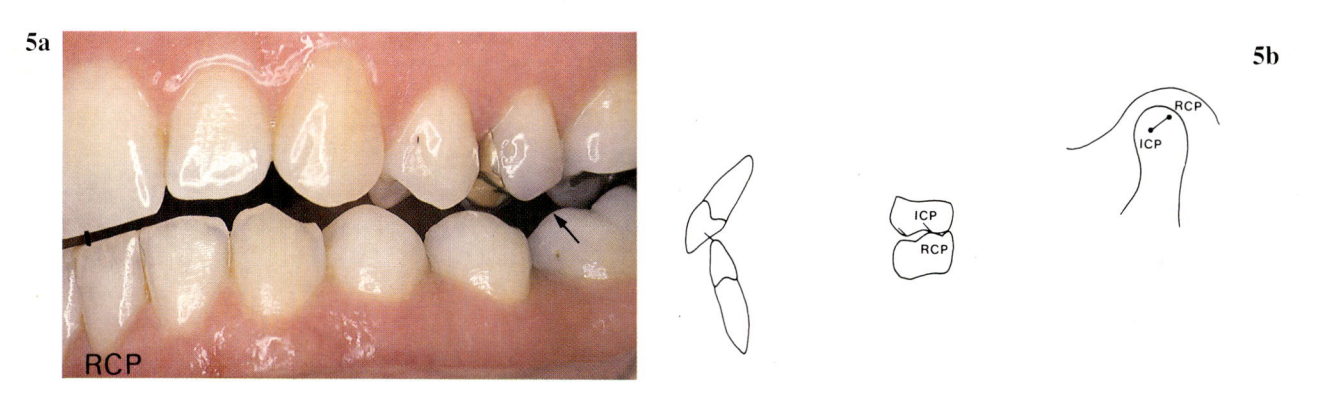

5a, 5b When the mandible closes on the retruded axis, its position when the first tooth contact occurs is referred to as the **retruded contact position** (RCP). Approximately 90 per cent of the population have a discrepancy between the retruded contact position and the intercuspal position. When the intercuspal position is unstable or the patient is edentulous, the only relatively reproducible relation of mandible to maxilla is the retruded position.

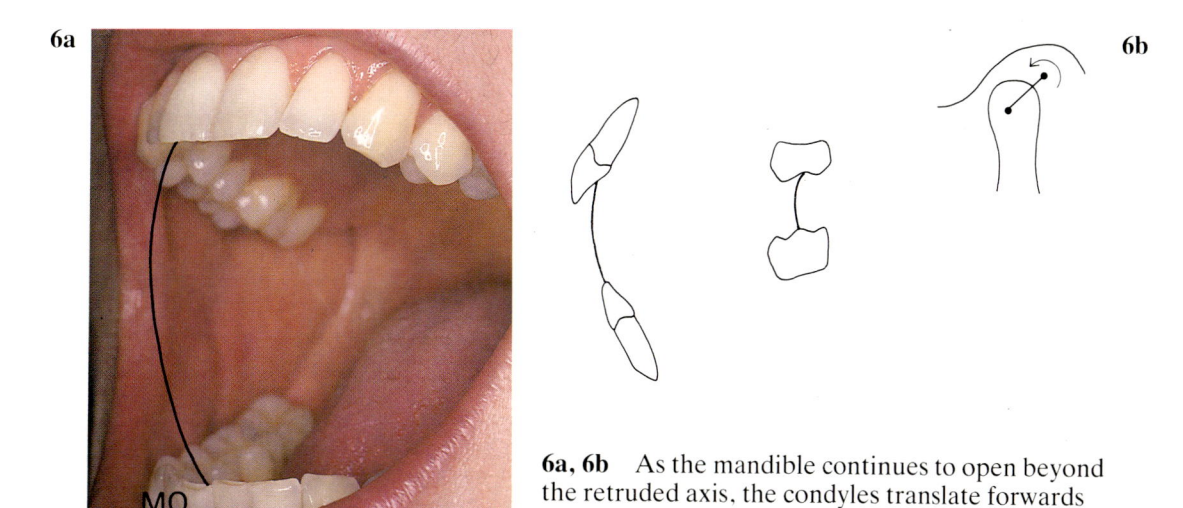

6a, 6b As the mandible continues to open beyond the retruded axis, the condyles translate forwards and downwards to a position of maximum opening.

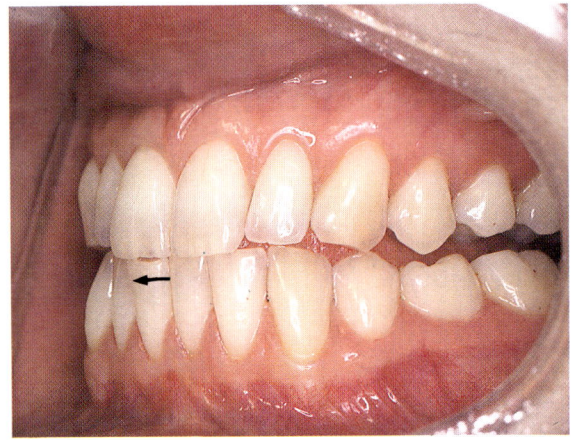

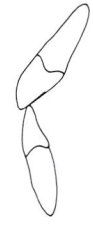

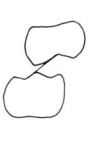

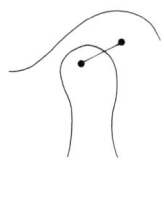

7a, 7b When the anterior teeth are in contact in the intercuspal position, the paths of protrusive and lateral movement are determined by their articulating surfaces. This is called **anterior guidance**. Where there is no anterior tooth contact in the intercuspal position, the path of movement will be influenced by the occlusal surfaces of the posterior teeth and, if no teeth contact, the temporomandibular joints are the sole determinant. In the natural dentition there appears to be little correlation between steepness of the anterior guidance and angle of the protrusive condylar path, although there is an absence of conclusive research in this area.

Border movements in a coronal plane

Condyles

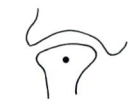

First molars

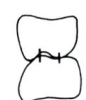

Canines

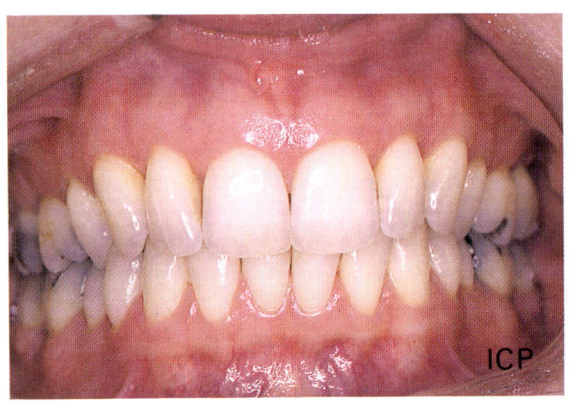

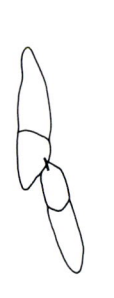

Right   Left

8a, 8b In a normal lateral relationship of the buccal segments, the maxillary palatal and mandibular buccal cusps are called **supporting cusps**. These are primarily involved in maintaining the stability of the intercuspal position. **Non-supporting cusps** are therefore the maxillary buccal cusps and mandibular lingual cusps.

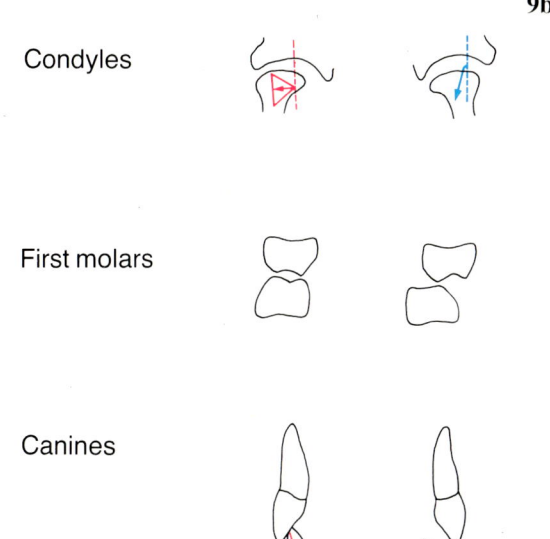

9a, 9b During right lateral movement of the mandible, the right condyle (the condyle on the side towards which movement occurs) is referred to as the **working side condyle**. The left condyle is referred to as the **non-working side** or **balancing side condyle**. During lateral movement, the working side condyle may either rotate, or rotate and move laterally, and also upwards or downwards. This lateral movement is known as **Bennett movement**, which is defined as the bodily shift of the mandible towards the working side during lateral excursion. Bennett movement is thought necessary to permit rotation of the working condyle, because of the restraining influence of the temporomandibular ligament on the working side, the walls of the glenoid fossa and the eccentric shape of the condyle. The timing and extent of Bennett movement varies; if the lateral component occurs early in the movement, it is termed **immediate or early sideshift**. A gradual lateral component is known as **progressive sideshift**.

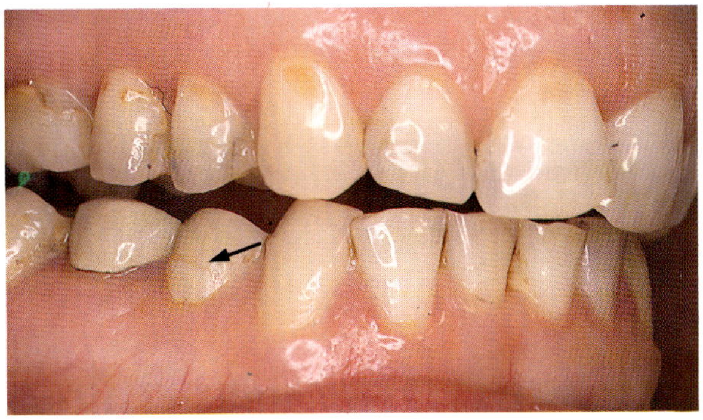

At occlusal level, if there is contact in lateral excursion only between canines on the working side, the term **canine guidance** is used.

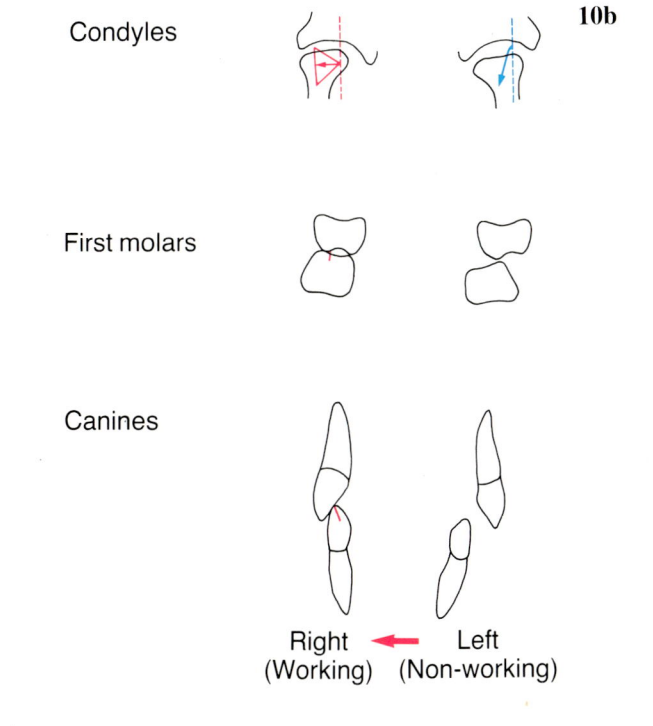

10a, 10b If there is contact on the working side between two or more teeth, the working side guidance is referred to as **group function**. The multiple tooth contacts in group function may involve both anterior and posterior teeth.

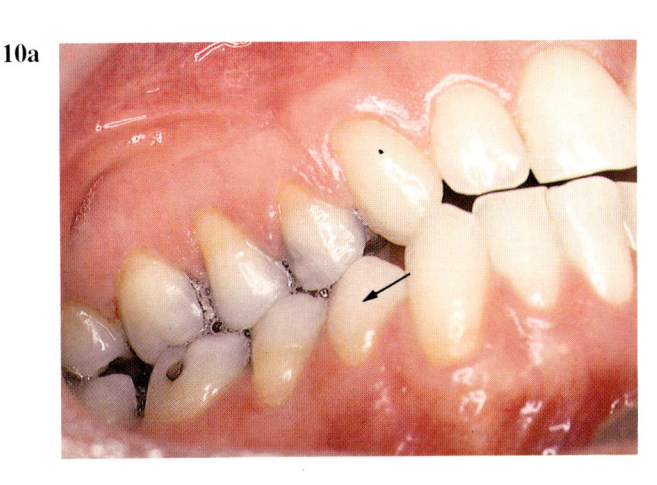

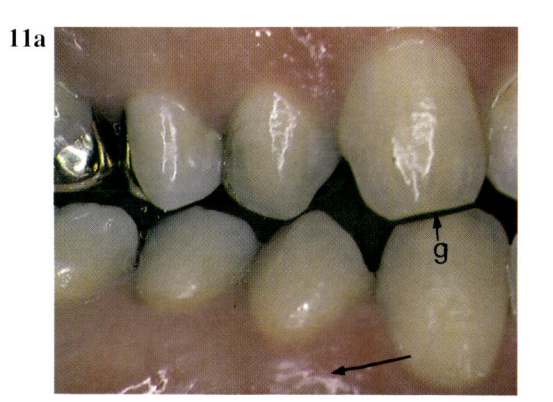

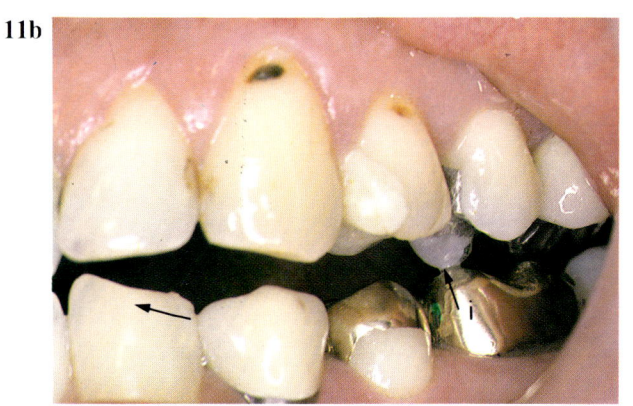

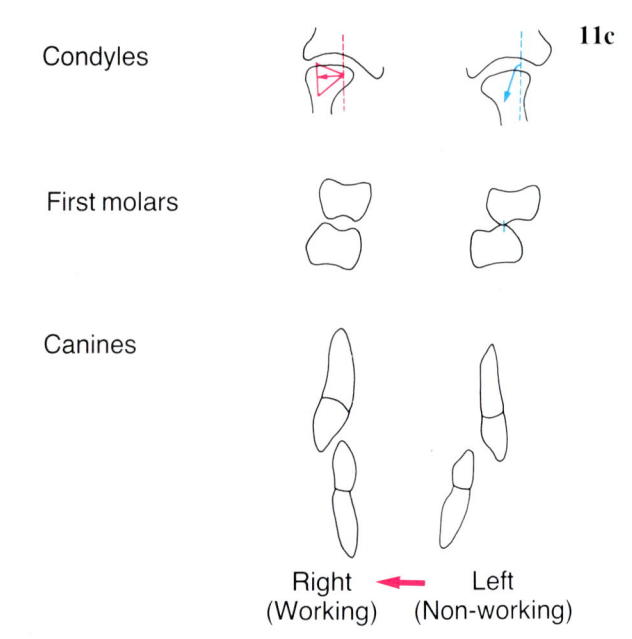

11a–11c Any contact between posterior teeth on the non-working side, which separates the teeth providing working side guidance (g), will deflect the path of lateral movement. These tooth contacts are known as **non-working side interferences** (i).

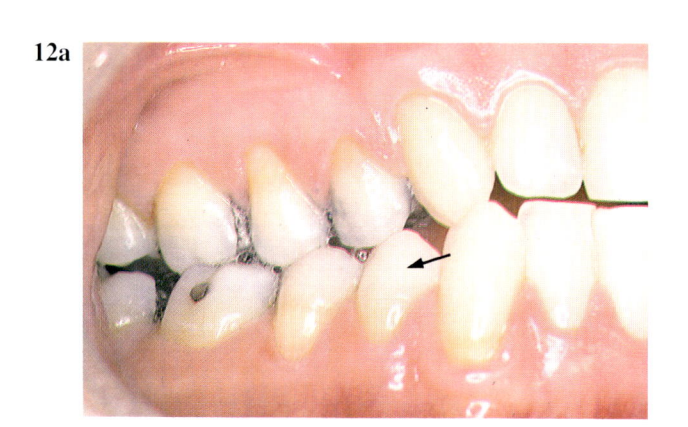

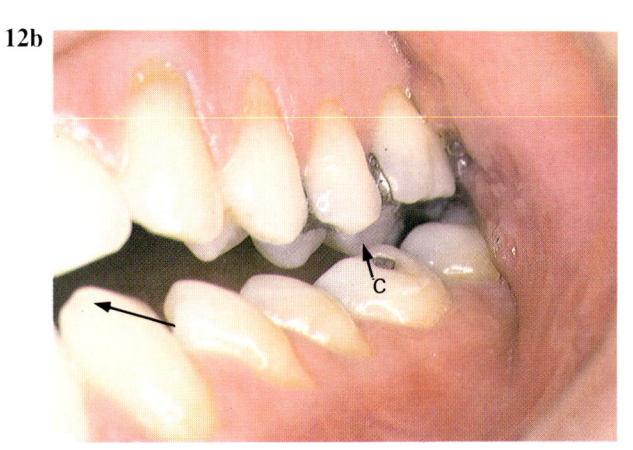

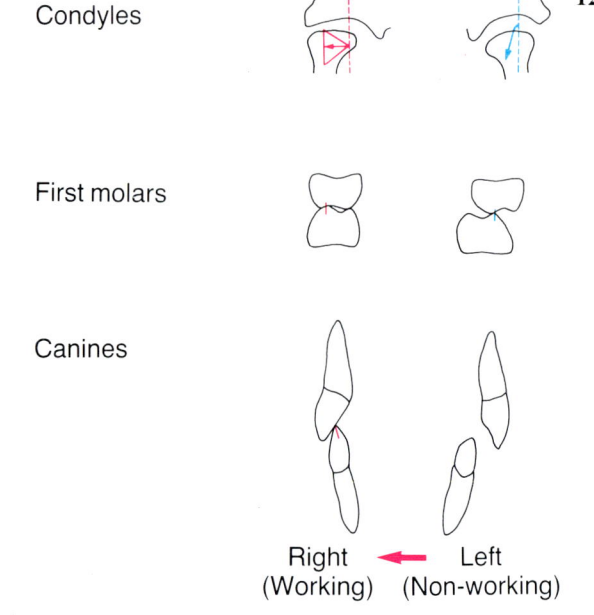

12a–12c However, if tooth contact occurs in lateral excursion on both working and non-working sides, these contacts are referred to as **non-working contacts** (c). The difference between an interference and a contact is important, because an interference will deflect the path of mandibular movement while a contact may not.

Border movements in a horizontal plane

13a, 13b If the working side condyle shifts laterally, it may also move forwards or backwards. The non-working side condyle moves downwards, forwards and inwards. The angle formed between the forward and inward movement of the non-working condyle and a straight forward movement is known as the **Bennett angle (13a)**. The border movements of the mandible in the horizontal plane are often described as a **gothic arch (13b)**, when observed in the incisal area.

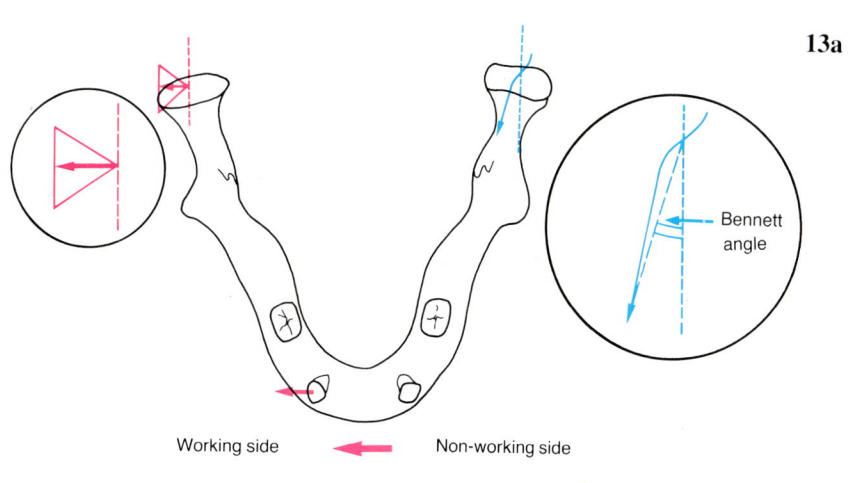

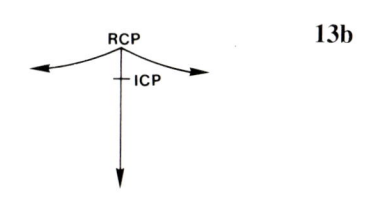

Control of mandibular movements

Patterns of mandibular movement are not only determined by the anatomic constraints of the temporomandibular joints, but also by the physiological action of the muscles as they move the mandible within and up to its border limits.

Sensory receptors in mucosa, periodontal tissues, muscles and temporomandibular joint capsules relay nerve impulses by afferent pathways to the central nervous system. Proprioception from the periodontal ligament receptors is relayed to the mesencephalic nucleus, and sensory information to the sensory nucleus of the trigeminal nerve. Reflex action via the motor nucleus and efferent nerve pathways of the trigeminal nerve leading to muscles of mastication, may be the response to this sensory information. However, regulation from the higher centres of the brain and peripheral stimuli may also influence the response of the muscles. Behavioural stress may affect the activity of the masticatory muscles, usually causing an increase in muscle tension. Any tooth contacts which interfere with the physiologic harmony of muscle function and mandibular movements may produce a similar effect. This increase in muscle activity may manifest itself in several different ways, resulting in increased tooth wear, fractured restorations and teeth, increased tooth mobility and symptoms of mandibular dysfunction. Whether or not any of these signs of occlusal pathology are present depends on the adaptive capacity of the components of the individual's masticatory system. The adaptive capacity of the temporomandibular joints, masticatory muscles, periodontal ligaments and teeth may be reduced by degenerative joint disease, stress, loss of periodontal attachment and weak restorations respectively.

Conclusion

The form of the occlusal surfaces of restorations and complete denture stability are influenced by mandibular movements. Orthodontic treatment may produce a functionally acceptable occlusion only if teeth are moved into positions which accommodate and do not interfere with these movements.

Chapter 2: The role of articulators in duplicating mandibular movements

Articulators are mechanical devices representing the temporomandibular joints, mandible and maxilla, to which casts may be attached and observed in both a static and dynamic relationship. They are useful in diagnosis for analysing a patient's occlusion outside the mouth. Their facility to copy mandibular movements and positions also assists in the fabrication of restorations in the laboratory.

Classification

Articulators have been divided into three main classes:

- Average value.
- Semi-adjustable.
- Fully-adjustable.

This classification is based on their relative abilities in copying mandibular movements. The choice of an articulator will depend upon the clinical application and the knowledge and ability of the operator, and should be based upon a sound knowledge of the advantages and limitations of each type.

In addition, there are simple hinges and other cast relators which may be used for locating casts in one position, but which are not capable of simulating mandibular movements.

Cast relators

14 Simple hinges consist of two rigid bows united by a hinge, and occasionally a screw adjustment to vary the distance between the bows. They permit only a simple hinge opening around a horizontal axis whose distance from the casts is both arbitrarily determined, and also very much less than the distance between the patient's TMJs and teeth. Simple hinges are incapable of simulating any mandibular movements or positions outside ICP and are therefore inadequate for occlusal diagnosis. Their use is reserved for observing static relationships for the construction of single crowns conforming to the existing intercuspal position. The restorations should not be required to contact in the mouth in any position other than ICP, and the patient should possess adequate anterior guidance so that there will be rapid disclusion. Restorations made on this type of instrument may require adjustment in the mouth to remove lateral and protrusive interferences, particularly when there is not a steep anterior guidance.

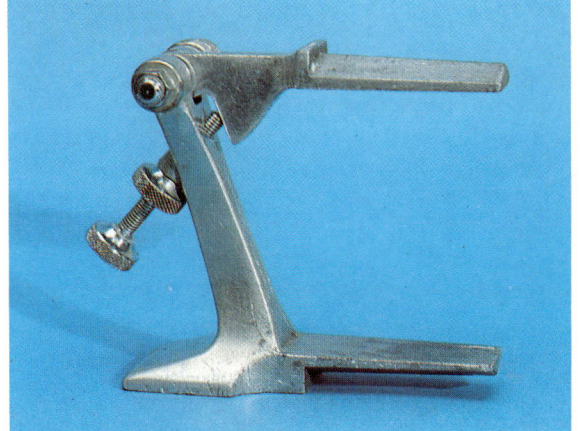

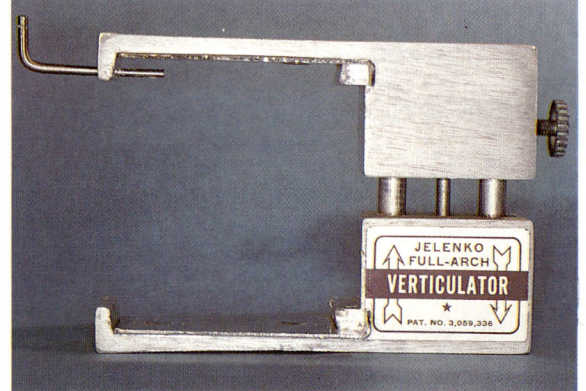

15 **The verticulator** consists of upper and lower members to which casts are attached. The upper member glides up and down metal posts enabling the casts to be brought into ICP contact. Its use is indicated in the same situations as the hinge, but the verticulator is capable of more precise cast location.

Average-value articulators

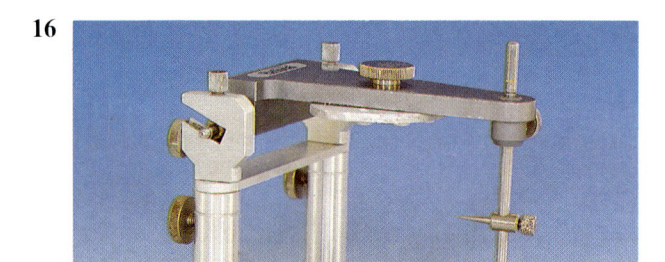

16 **Average-value articulator.** These instruments are capable of lateral and protrusive movements and are of an anatomical size. They do not accept a facebow record; therefore the relationship between the intercondylar axis and casts is arbitrary, and they are incapable of reproducing movements accurately. The angles at which their 'condyles' move are fixed according to average values. These instruments have no real clinical application.
Courtesy of Miss K. Warren.

Semi-adjustable articulators

Semi-adjustable articulators are the most widely used for both diagnostic and treatment procedures. They are designed to be of an anatomical size, their intercondylar distance being similar to that in the average patient, but usually without the capacity for adjustment. They will also accept a facebow record which enables the relationship between the retruded axis and teeth to be transferred from patient to articulator. These two features, together with the capacity to adjust the angle of condylar movement in sagittal and horizontal planes, enable these instruments to provide an approximate simulation of lateral and protrusive mandibular movements.

17a–17c Semi-adjustable articulators may be subdivided into two main types. **Arcon** articulators (**Ar**ticulator–**Con**dyle) such as the Denar MKII (**17a**), Whipmix (**17b**) and Sam (**17c**) more closely represent the anatomical relationship in having their condyles on the lower member and fossae on the upper. The main advantage of this arrangement is that it helps in the understanding of mandibular movement. The ability to remove the upper member of the articulator is of great help in many restorative procedures, such as waxing restorations with the wax-added technique.

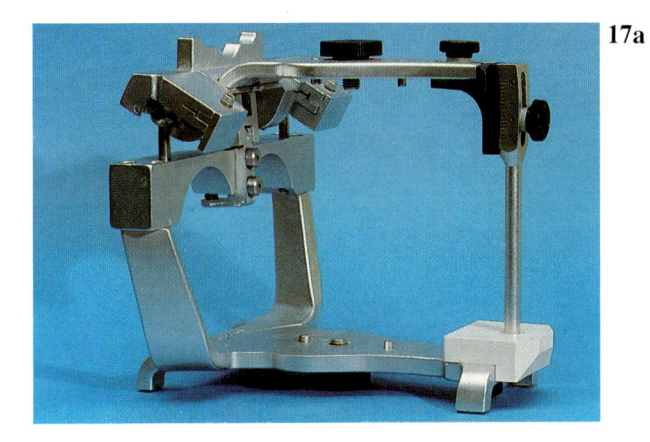

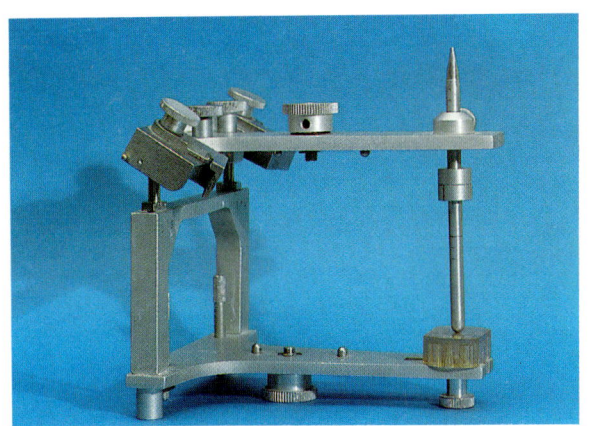

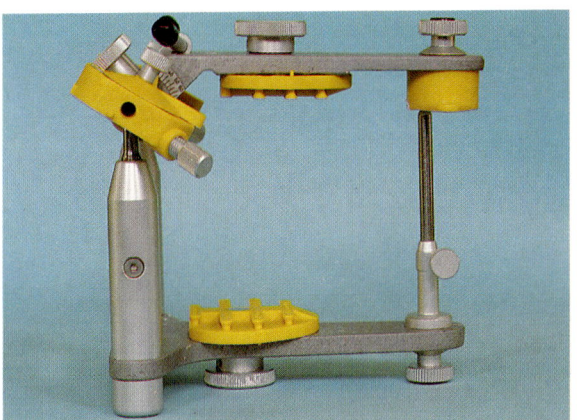

18 Non-arcon articulators such as the Dentatus ARH have their condyles on the upper member. These are locked into condylar tracks making it impossible to lift off the upper member of the articulator. This is helpful when setting denture teeth but is a hindrance for fixed restorative procedures.

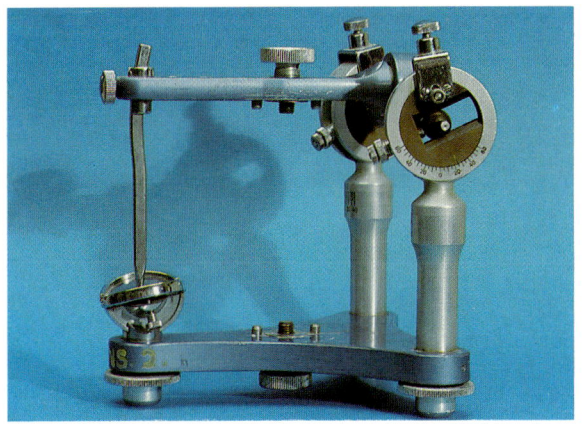

Condylar adjustments in semi-adjustable articulators

These should be made before mounting casts on the articulator. Any attempt to alter the inclination of the fossa walls may change the relationship of the condyle to fossa in the retruded position. This results from lack of precision in the manufacture of some articulators.

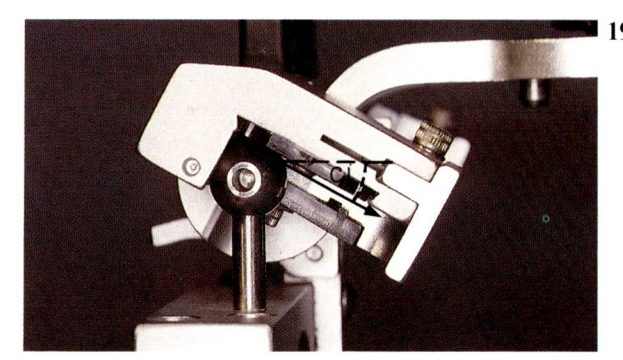

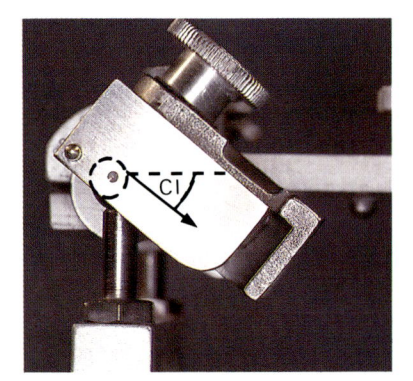

19a–19h Semi-adjustable articulators have an adjustable condylar inclination which will affect the angles of condylar movement during protrusion and the non-working side during lateral movement. Illustrated here are the condylar inclination adjustments of the Denar MKII (**19a, 19b**), Whipmix (**19c, 19d**), the Sam (**19e, 19f**), and the Dentatus (**19g, 19h**); CI = Condylar inclination.

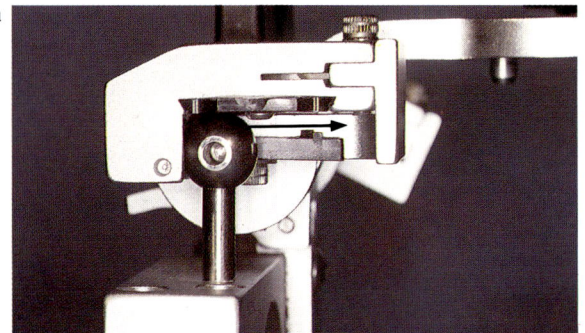

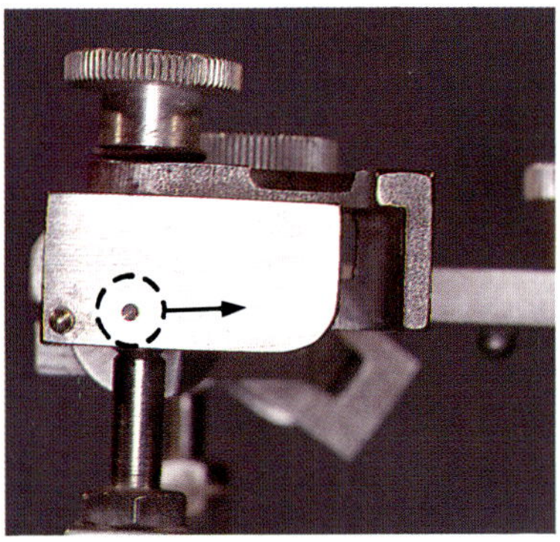

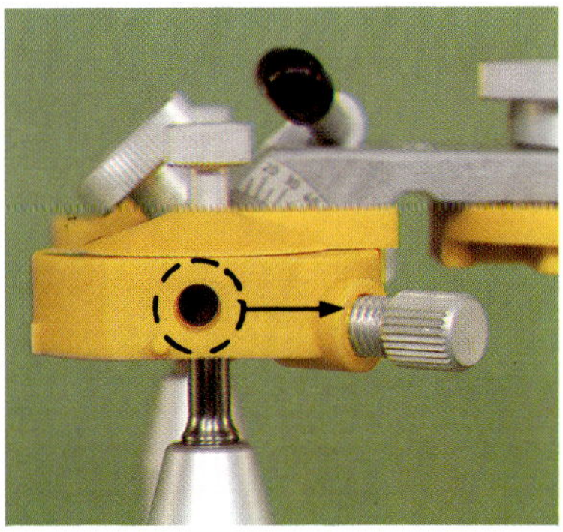

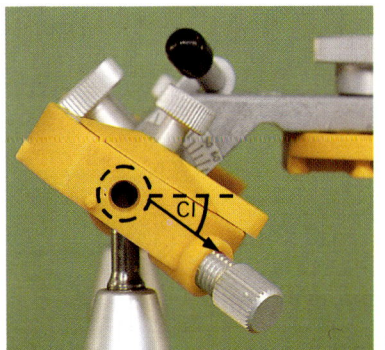

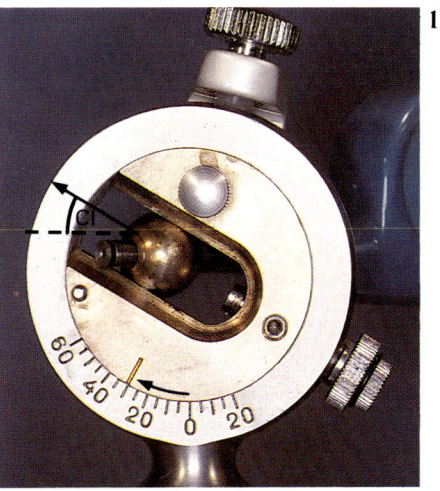

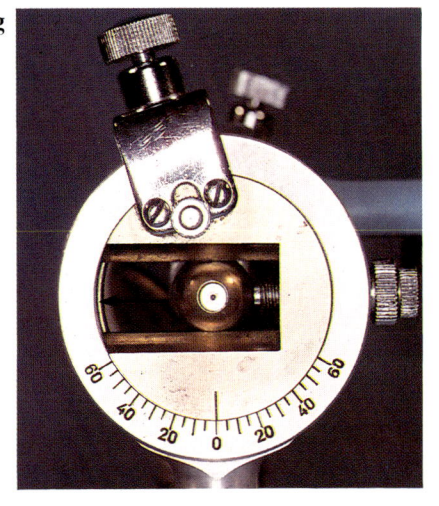

20a–20h These articulators possess an adjustable Bennett angle which will also affect the path of the non-working condyle. The Denar MKII (**20a, 20b**) has an adjustable medial wall whose angulation relative to the sagittal plane may be altered. The Whipmix (**20c, 20d**) and Sam (**20e, 20f**) are very similar. The Dentatus (**20g, 20h**) achieves this by swivelling the entire condylar assembly on its support pillar. BA = Bennett angle; M = Medial wall.

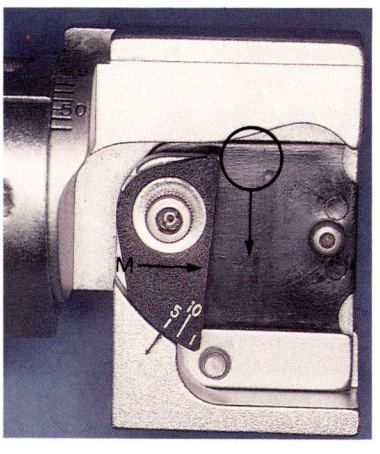

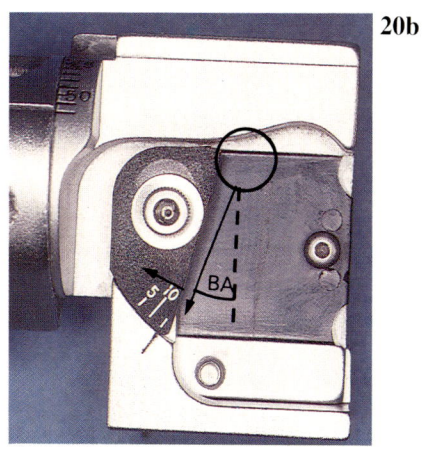

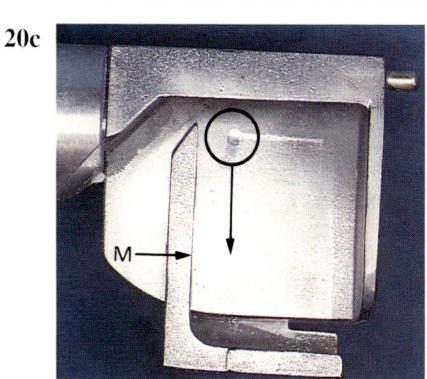

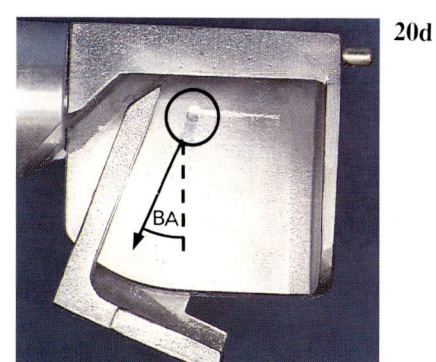

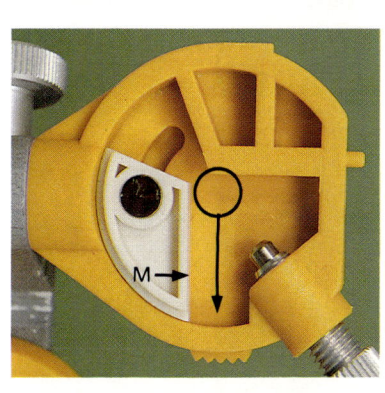

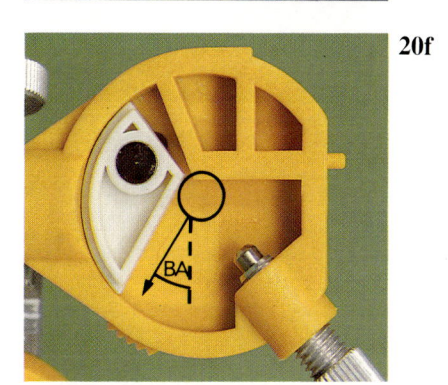

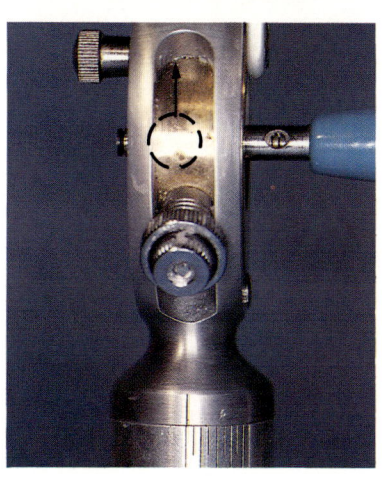

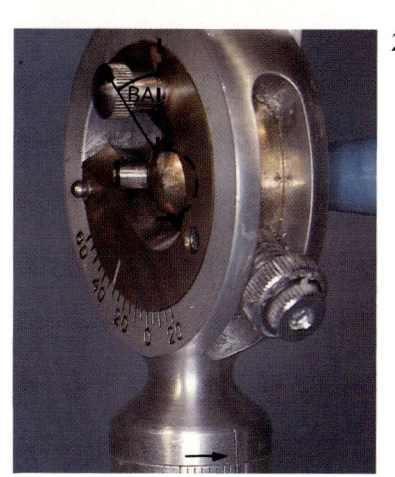

The manufacturers recommend that these adjustments are set using protrusive and lateral checkbites respectively. This procedure is inaccurate for the following reasons: first, the checkbite produces an angle setting formed by the horizontal and a straight line from the retruded position to the point at which the record was taken. Hence checkbites taken at varying degrees of protrusion or lateral movement will produce different values if the patient has a curved path of movement. As over 90 per cent of condylar pathways are curved, this procedure will be inaccurate for most patients. Second, in most semi-adjustable articulators, the working side condyle can only rotate, and there is often no facility for reproducing Bennett movement or sideshift. Consequently, if a patient exhibits any degree of sideshift, a lateral checkbite cannot be made to fit accurately between the casts as a result of the mechanical restraints of the condylar housing. In most situations the condylar inclination and Bennett angle are set using average values. However, when fabricating posterior restorations on a semi-adjustable articulator it is sensible to set the condylar inclination flatter, particularly if the patient has limited anterior guidance. This will result in the production of flatter cusps, more likely to disclude in the mouth.

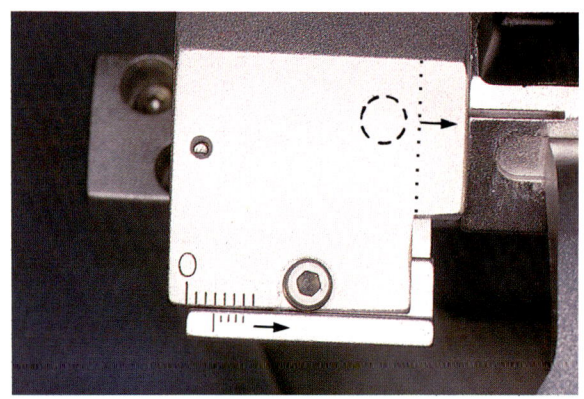

21a, 21b Some semi-adjustable articulators have the capacity for further adjustment. The Denar MKII (**21a**) possesses an adjustment for immediate sideshift which allows the medial wall of the fossa to be moved medially, permitting some early sideshift during lateral movement. Once again this adjustment is usually made on an arbitrary basis. However, when waxing posterior restorations to a wide centric, it may be set to allow the articulator to shift sideways until the guidance teeth contact and provide disclusion. The intercondylar distance on the Whipmix (**21b**) may be altered according to the three settings, small(S), medium(M) and large(L). These are measured directly from the facebow.

22a, 22b Semi-adjustable articulators may be obtained with two types of anterior guidance table. The first is an adjustable metal table with flat surfaces (**22a**), whilst the second is plastic and is designed for custom-moulding with acrylic resin (**22b**). The purpose of this table is to help guide lateral and protrusive movements. As the configuration of its surface should mimic the palatal guidance surfaces of the maxillary anterior teeth, which are concave, the metal table is of little use.

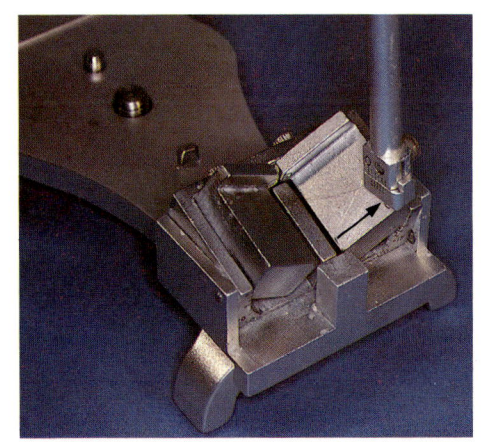

The records needed for mounting casts on a semi-adjustable articulator include the facebow transfer and interocclusal records.

The facebow transfer

23 **A facebow** is a caliper-like device which records the relationship between the retruded axis and the maxillary teeth, and enables this relationship to be transferred to the articulator. As well as enabling a more accurate duplication of lateral movements, this permits casts to be mounted at an increased vertical dimension of occlusion, then closed together to identify and study the occlusal contacts.

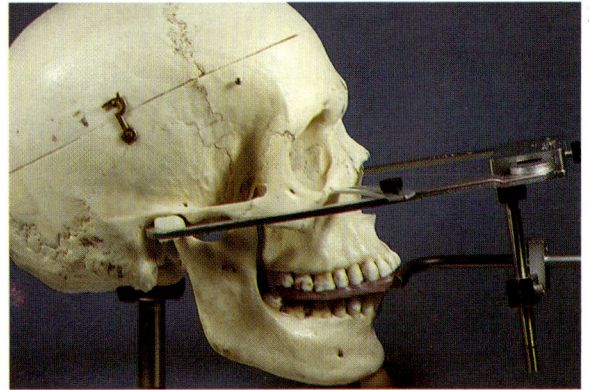

There are two types of facebow: the kinematic or hinge axis facebow, and the average axis facebow.

The kinematic or hinge axis facebow

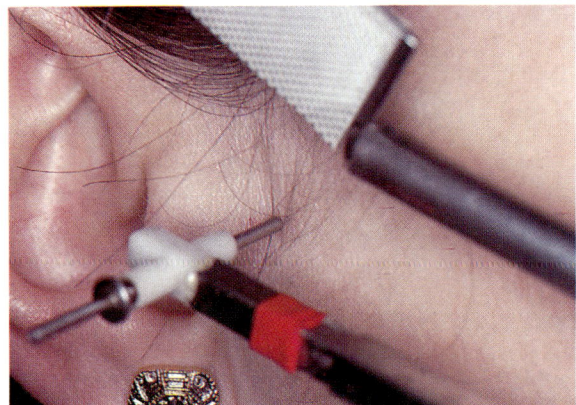

24a, 24b   The kinematic or hinge axis facebow consists of two bows attached to the mandibular and maxillary arches. The maxillary bow supports two vertical metal tables which are positioned over the condyles (**24a**). The mandibular bow has two horizontal metal styli whose pointed tips are aligned with a dot on paper applied to the tables. The patient is manipulated into the retruded position and opened and closed on the retruded axis so that the condyles are only rotating and not translating. The movement of the tips of the styli relative to the dots on the paper is noted, and their position adjusted until they lie over the retruded axis. Ink is applied to the tips of both styli which are then used to mark the patient's skin (**24b**), identifying the position of the horizontal axis. This hinge axis locating instrument is then removed from the patient.

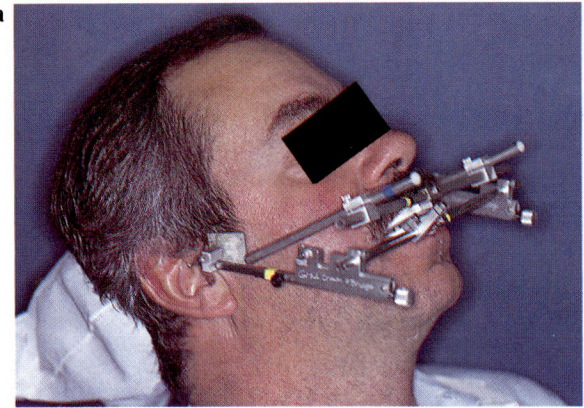

A facebow transfer is then carried out using these two marks as the posterior reference points. To transfer this relationship accurately a third point of reference is needed. This is positioned on the front of the face, the exact location depending on the individual articulator and facebow system used.

The average axis facebow

Hinge axis location is a demanding and time-consuming procedure. Facebow systems have been developed which use average posterior reference points based on reproducibly measurable anatomical landmarks in the region of the intercondylar axis. Their use enables a facebow transfer to be accomplished without any clinically significant loss of accuracy in the movements produced by the articulator. The only situation in which significant errors will occur is when occlusal vertical dimension is altered on the articulator, as the opening or closing movement will not take place on an arc around the true axis. This is of no significance when mounting diagnostic casts, but is important when mounting working casts for the fabrication of restorations.

25a, 25b The Denar system uses a self-centring bow using the external auditory meatae as posterior reference points (**25a**) and a point 42 mm above the tip of the upper right lateral incisor as the anterior reference point (**25b**). The use of this average posterior reference point has been shown to be more accurate than other average points marked on the face.

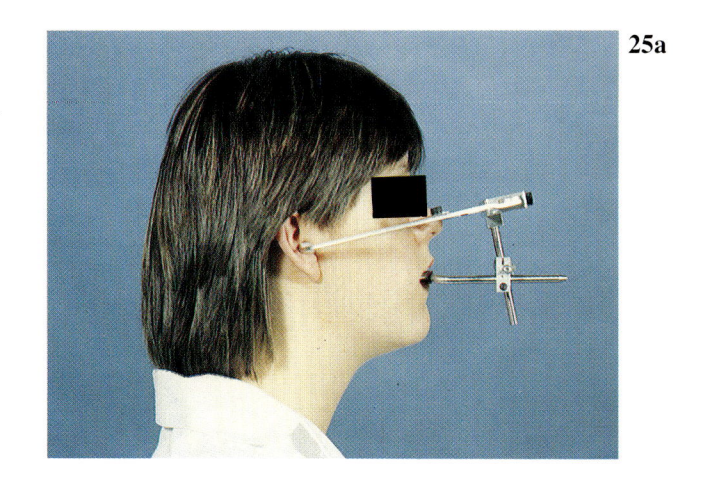

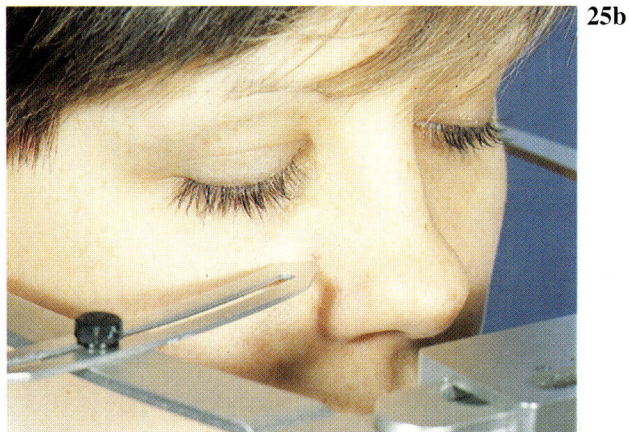

26 After completion of the clinical procedures, the bitefork assembly can be disconnected from the facebow and related to the articulator with a mounting jig which replaces the incisal table. The maxillary cast is then attached to the upper member of the articulator.

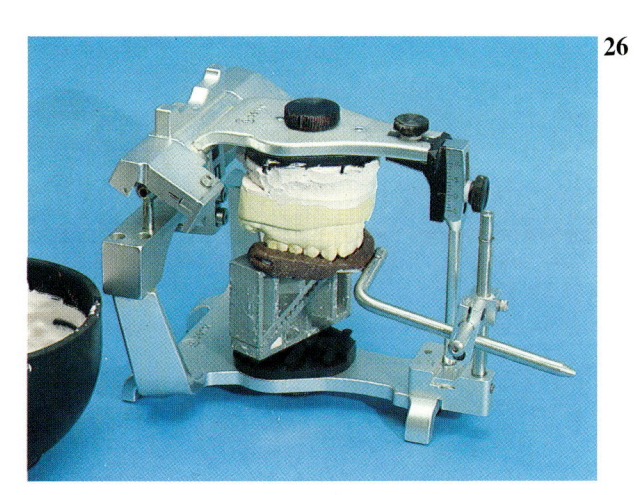

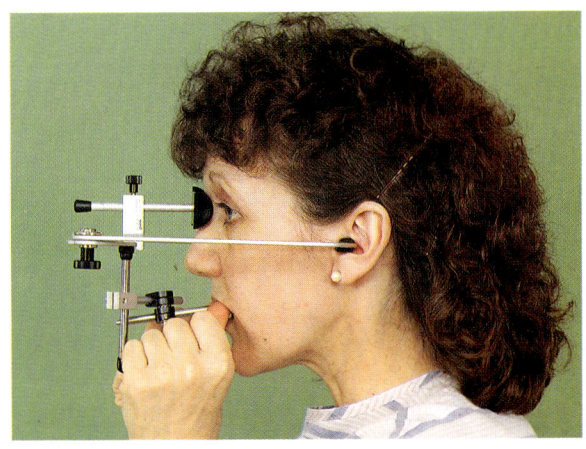

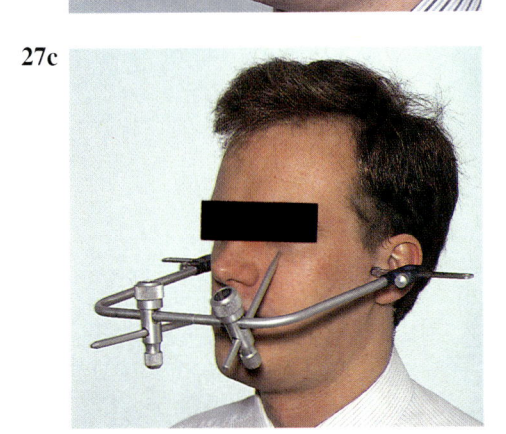

27a–27c The Whipmix (**27a**) and Sam (**27b**) systems also use the external auditory meati as posterior reference points. However, in contrast to the Denar, they use the nasion for the anterior reference point. Also, the whole facebow has to be transferred to the articulator rather than just a small part of it. The Dentatus system (**27c**) is more cumbersome and less accurate, using posterior reference points 13mm in front of the posterior part of the tragus of the ear on a line from the tragus to the outer canthus of the eye. The anterior reference point is the left infra-orbital margin.

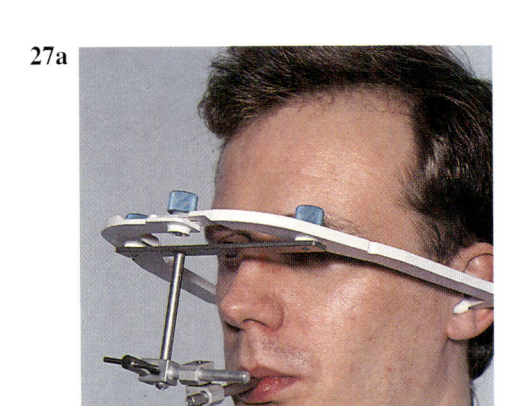

Interocclusal records

For diagnosis, the mandibular cast should be mounted at a point on the retruded axis before tooth contact occurs, using an interocclusal record to relate it to the maxillary cast. This is necessary to prevent an RCP contact from deflecting the mandible away from the retruded axis.

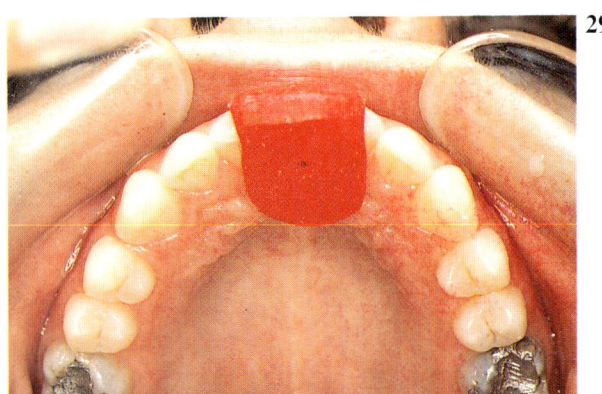

28, 29 An anterior jig or stop is made directly in the mouth from acrylic resin. It provides a flat surface against which one mandibular incisor occludes in the retruded position. It separates the posterior teeth by 2–3mm and, as a result of breaking the feedback from periodontal membrane receptors, helps to relax the masticatory muscles, facilitating location of the retruded axis.

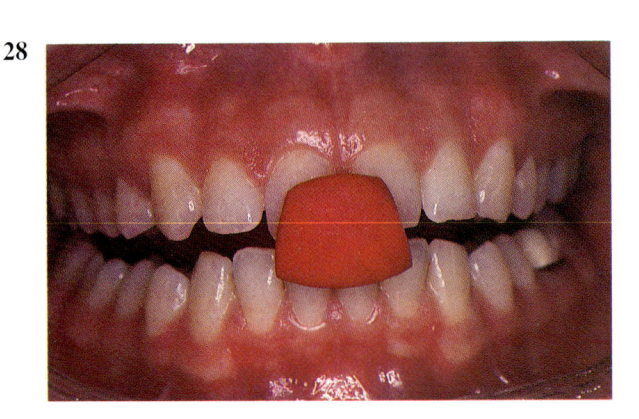

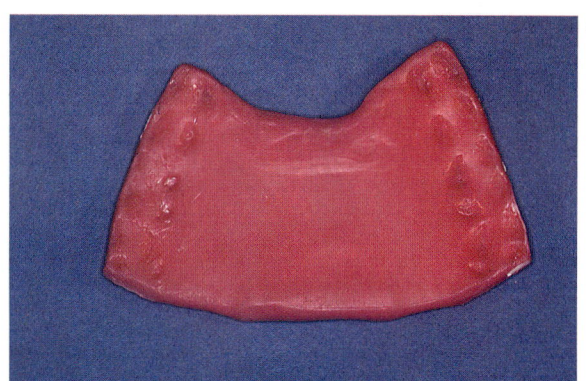

30, 31 A wax record is made on the maxillary cast from extra-hard baseplate wax. It extends from the first premolars to the distal aspect of the second molars, touching only the teeth and avoiding all contact with the soft tissues. Its thickness is adjusted so that with the jig in place and the record seated on the maxillary teeth, no part of the wax touches the lower teeth.

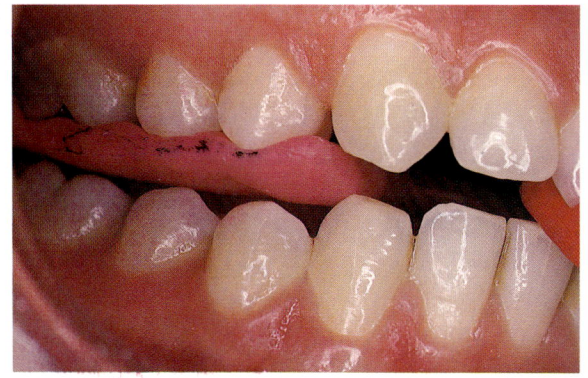

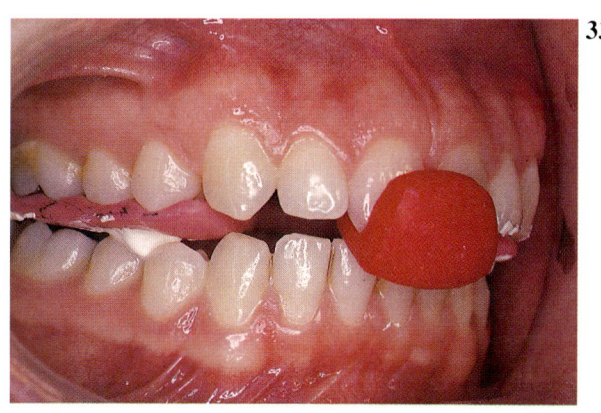

32, 33 Zinc oxide–eugenol paste is applied to the underside of the record in four places and the mandible is guided into the retruded position using bimanual manipulation.

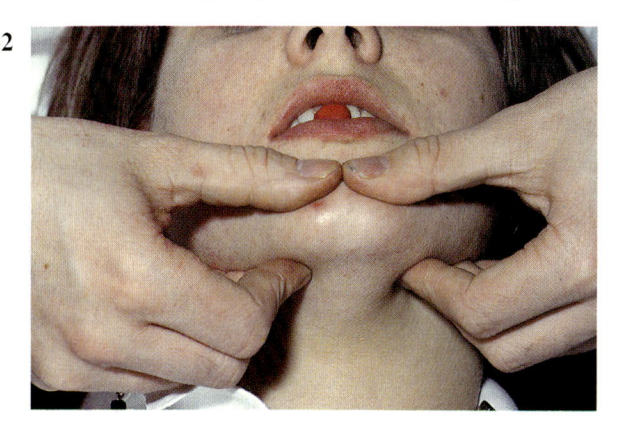

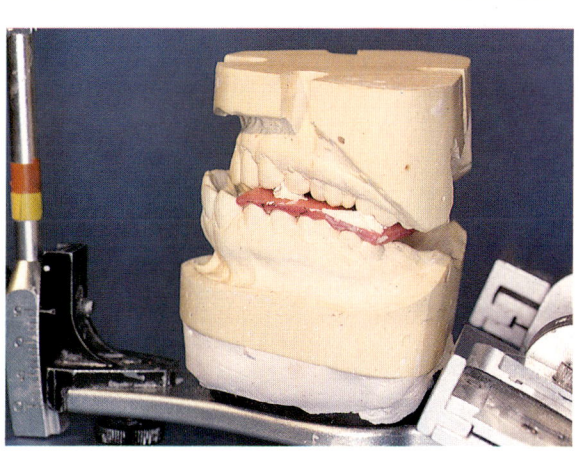

34 Once the paste has set, the record is removed from the mouth and placed on the maxillary cast. The mandibular cast is then seated into the paste indentations and attached to the lower member of the articulator.

Many techniques have been described for taking a retruded record, the technique illustrated here being one of the more accurate and consistent.

It is sometimes advantageous to take three records and to check their consistency using a Denar Vericheck, or a split cast technique.

The techniques for making an interocclusal record to mount working casts are described in Part III.

Applications and limitations of semi-adjustable articulators

Semi-adjustable articulators are widely used for diagnostic and treatment procedures in both fixed and removable prosthodontics. Their limitations in providing only an approximation of true mandibular movements are acceptable when there is adequate anterior guidance. When guidance is reduced it becomes more critical to use an instrument which mirrors the movements more exactly, so that occlusal anatomy may be reproduced in the laboratory to create stable ICP contacts and yet disclude in other positions.

If restorations are made on a semi-adjustable articulator, the occlusal adjustment in lateral excursion needed when they are tried in the mouth becomes progressively less acceptable the greater the number of units being restored. Also, a positive error may be eliminated by grinding, whereas a negative one may require the restoration to be remade.

Semi-adjustable articulators are the instruments of choice for diagnosis and treatment in both orthodontics and complete denture prosthodontics.

Fully-adjustable articulators

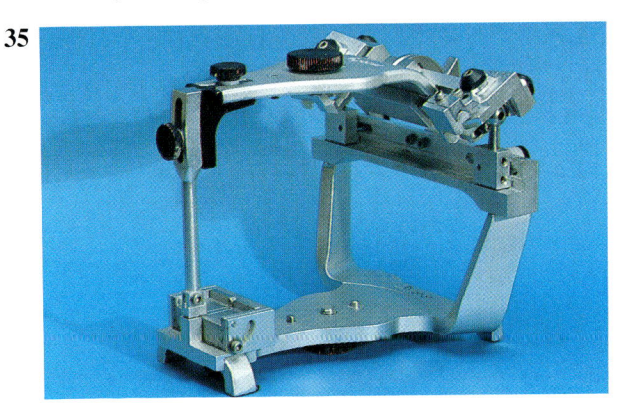

35 These instruments may be calibrated to duplicate the border movements of the mandible with a high degree of accuracy. The example shown is a Denar 5A.

36a, 36b A pantograph (**36a**) is used to record graphic representations of border movements on pressure-sensitive paper (**36b**).

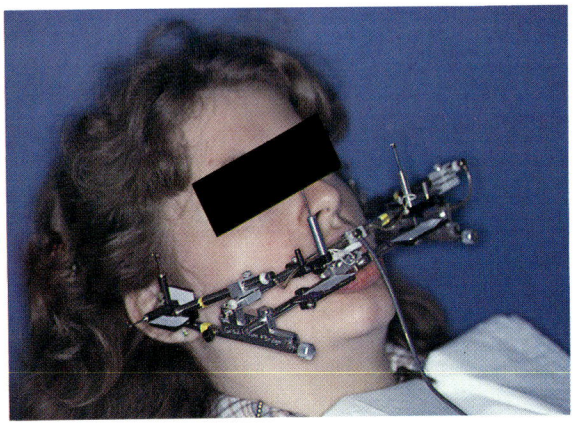

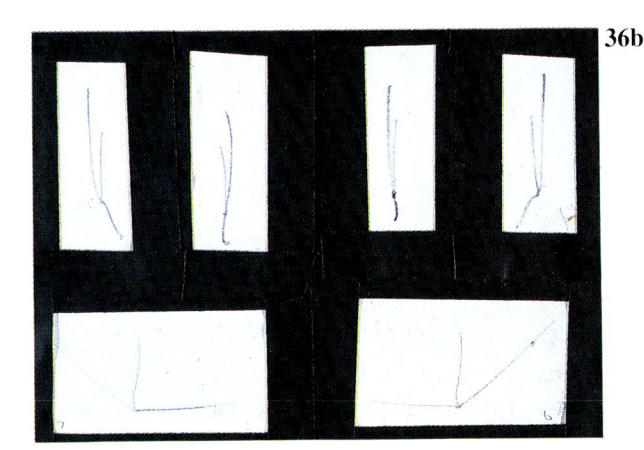

37 After taking a set of six tracings, two anterior and four in the condylar region, the pantograph is transferred to the fully-adjustable articulator which may then be adjusted to follow the same movements.

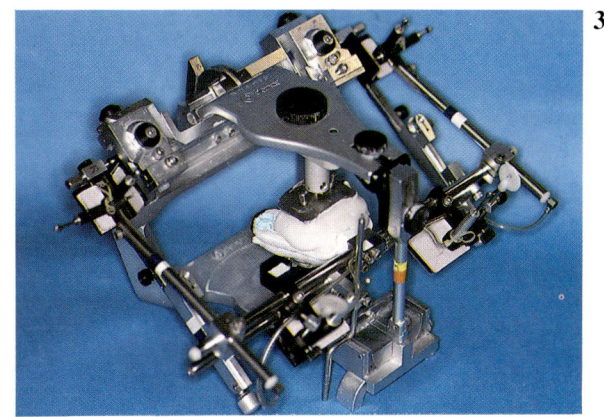

38a, 38b Setting an articulator accurately from pantographic tracings requires a high degree of expertise. The Denar pantronic computerized pantograph (**38a**) eliminates the need for this transfer by producing a numerical print-out (**38b**) of all the condylar determinants which can then be set directly.

Once the articulator has been set from the pantographic records, diagnostic or working casts are mounted in the usual way with face-bow and interocclusal records.

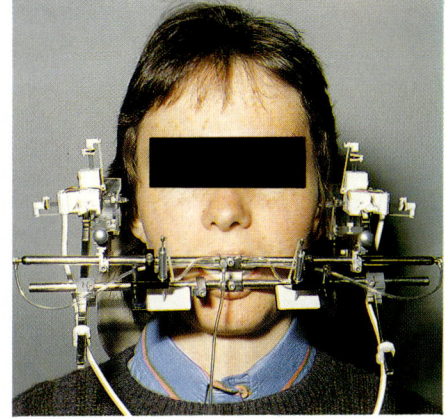

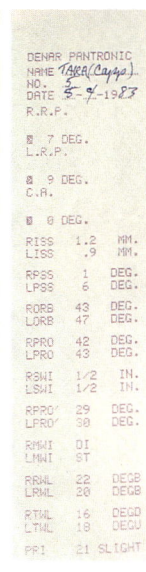

Condylar adjustments in fully-adjustable articulators

The features of a fully-adjustable articulator which enable it to duplicate mandibular movements accurately and which are set from pantographic tracings are illustrated in **39** to **48**.

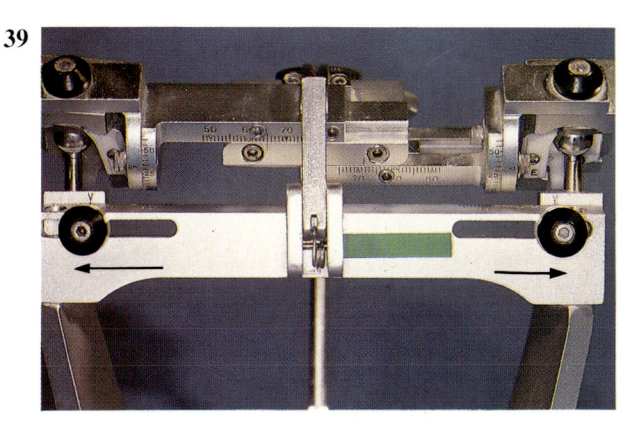

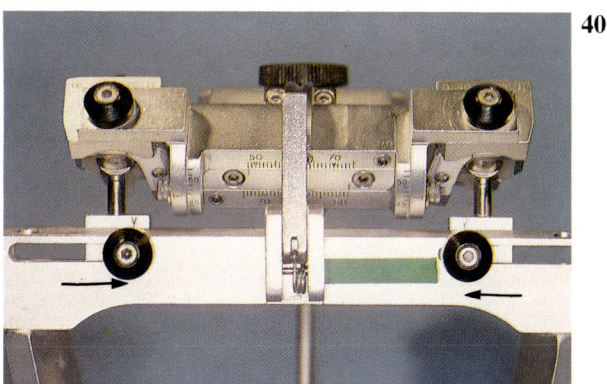

39, 40 An adjustable intercondylar distance which will determine the position of the vertical axes about which lateral movement occurs.

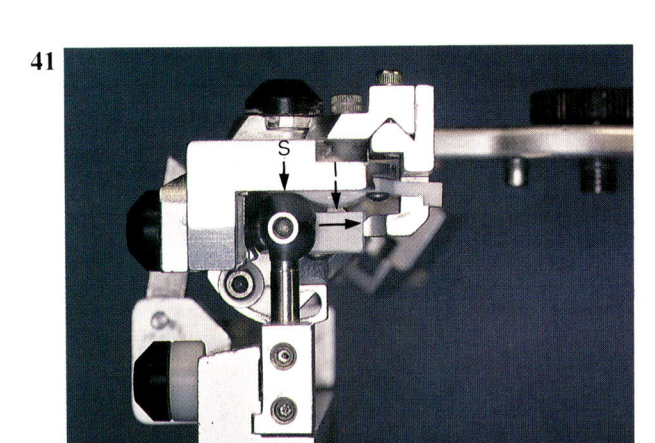

41, 42 The superior fossa wall may receive curved inserts and be adjusted in an anteroposterior direction to duplicate movement on protrusion, and of the non-working condyle moving downwards forwards and medially.

S = Superior wall
I = Insert
M = Medial wall
BA = Bennett angle

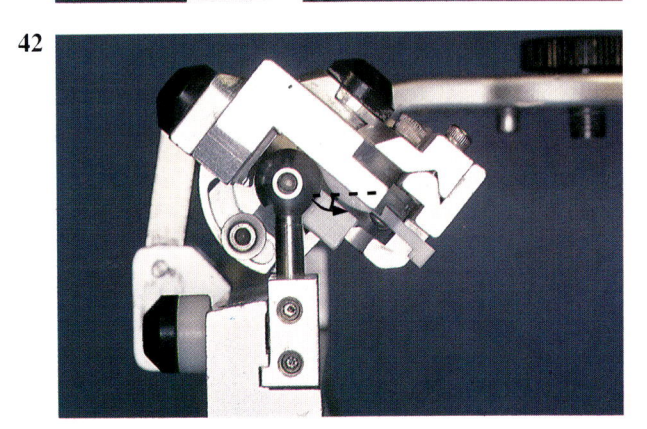

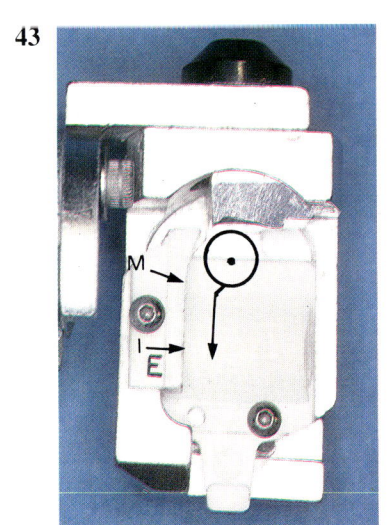

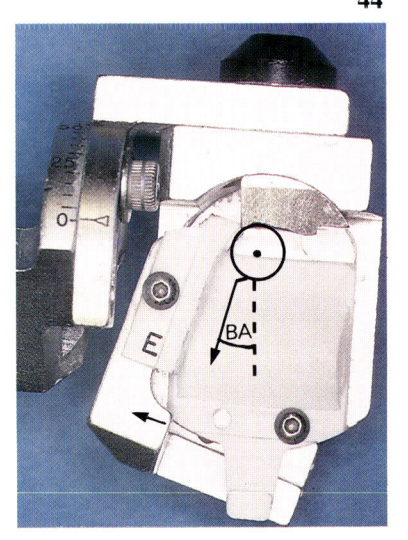

43, 44 The inclination of the medial wall may be adjusted relative to the sagittal plane to vary the Bennett angle. It may also receive curved inserts so that the movements of the non-working condyle may be copied closely. If the inserts do not allow the movements to be copied exactly, they may be custom ground or altered by adding acrylic resin.

45, 46 The movements of the working condyle in rotating and moving laterally may be copied. The superior wall may be tilted in the coronal plane to allow the working condyle to move sideways and up or down.

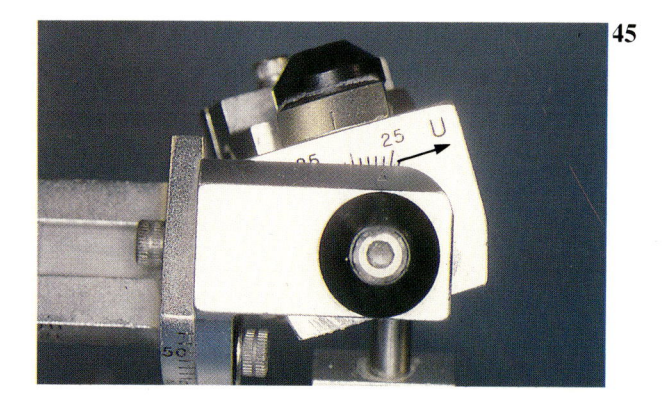

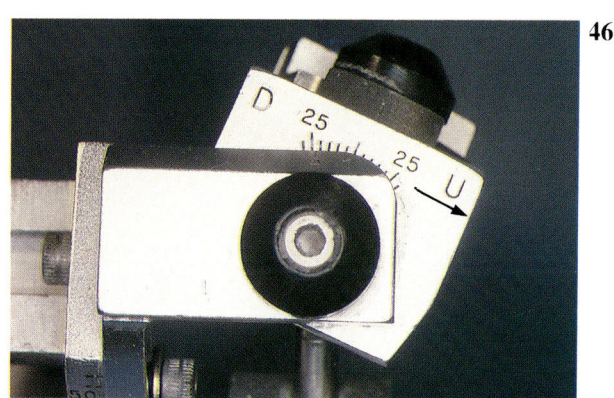

47, 48 The posterior wall (P) can be adjusted to allow the working condyle to move laterally and forwards or backwards.

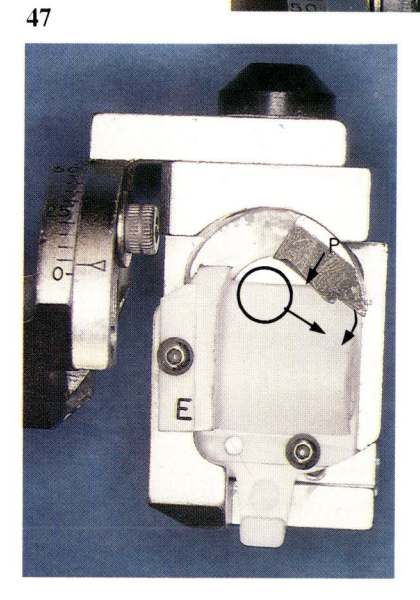

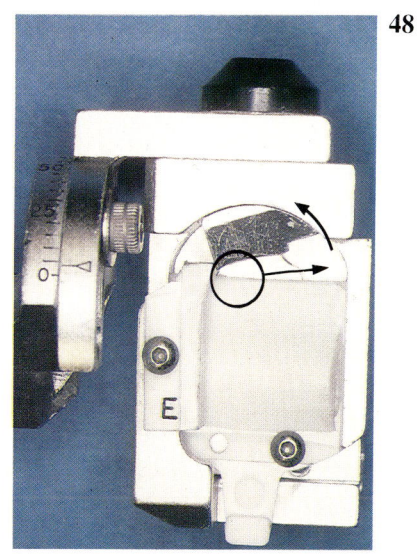

Applications of fully-adjustable articulators

Fully-adjustable articulators are indicated when restoring opposing teeth in complex cases, with minimal anterior guidance or group function. They enable the cusps and grooves to be positioned correctly with respect to the direction of lateral and protrusive movements and will greatly reduce the amount of occlusal adjustment required when restorations are tried in the mouth.

Conclusion

A semi-adjustable articulator is the instrument of choice for orthodontic diagnosis and for the fabrication of complete dentures. It is also the most useful for diagnosis and treatment in most restorative cases. There are occasions when both a simple cast relator and a fully-adjustable articulator and pantograph are helpful. Average value articulators used without a facebow transfer are of little use.

Part II   Assessment of the occlusion

This part of the Atlas deals with the assessment of a patient's occlusion before undertaking restorative dentistry in the dentate patient, orthodontics, or the treatment of the edentulous patient. Each type of assessment has its own particular features based on the requirements of the clinical procedures subsequently used to alter the occlusion.

Chapter 3:   Restorative assessment

Thorough history taking and clinical examination are essential parts of the diagnostic process. However, restorative treatment planning cannot be based entirely on intra-oral examination, as it is impossible to accurately detect, mark and quantify occlusal contacts, relationships and interferences in the mouth. Access and visibility are limited and the presence of saliva and shiny surfaces on wear facets and restorative materials makes the use of articulating paper to mark contacts unreliable. A patient's neuromuscular system may habitually guide the mandible away from interferences, making their detection difficult. Further investigations, including radiographs, articulated diagnostic casts, occlusal splint therapy and, in selected cases, a pantographic survey, provide the additional information required.

Aims of occlusal examination

The aims of an occlusal examination are:

- **To establish baseline measurements** against which any future changes may be detected and quantified.
- **To detect any signs and symptoms of occlusal problems**. If undetected, existing problems may progress, leading to further breakdown in a patient's occlusion. If left uncorrected, they may adversely affect the prognosis of any restorative dentistry carried out.
- **To decide between a conformative or reorganized approach**. Most restorations are made to conform to a patient's existing intercuspal position, provided this position is stable and the patient does not demonstrate any occlusal problems. If any such problems are present, or if a large number of teeth require restoring or replacing, restorative dentistry becomes much more complicated. It is advisable to reorganize the occlusion, creating a new and stable intercuspal position as close to the retruded position of the mandible as possible.

In this chapter the diagnostic stages necessary to formulate a restorative treatment plan are outlined. These include:

- History taking.
- Clinical examination.
- Special investigations.

Not all aspects of the diagnostic process are described: only those areas with direct relevance to the occlusion are highlighted.

History

History taking is important, not only for the facts obtained, but also because it gives an opportunity to assess the patient's personality. The following details should be ascertained:

Present complaint

- Pain associated with the muscles of mastication and TMJs.
- Pain and/or limitation on mandibular movement.
- Facial pain not related to movement.
- Clicking or crepitus from the TMJs.
- Repeated failure or uncementation of restorations.
- Teeth moving.
- Teeth wearing down.
- Awareness of bruxing, clenching or other parafunctional habits.
- Pain in individual teeth.
- Difficulties in chewing.

Dental history

- Previous dental treatment.
- Prolonged operative procedures.
- Expectations of treatment.
- Recent changes in occlusion.

Medical history

- Use of major and minor tranquillizers.
- Rheumatoid arthritis.
- Trauma to the head and neck.
- Any medical conditions contraindicating extensive treatment.
- In addition to these specific points, a full medical questionnaire should be taken.

General

- Personality and stress levels.
- Diet and acid intake.
- Occupation.
- Suitability for lengthy and complex treatment.

Examination

Examination should be both extra-oral and intra-oral, being carried out both visually and by tactile means. It should seek to discover whether a patient's occlusion demonstrates the following desirable features:

- Posterior occlusal stability.
- Satisfactory anterior guidance.
- Absence of non-working side interferences.
- Absence of mandibular dysfunction.

Extra-oral examination

This concentrates on the TMJs and muscles of mastication, both at rest and in function.

The temporomandibular joints

49 Standing behind the patient, both joints are palpated anterior to the external auditory meatae. The patient is asked to open and close the mouth widely and perform left and right lateral excursions. The following signs and symptoms are noted: tenderness to palpation, pain on movement, restricted or jerky movement, deviation to one side on opening. Abnormal, restricted or painful movement may be caused by hyperactivity in the masticatory muscles, which occurs in mandibular dysfunction. It is usually unilateral and should be distinguished from bilateral facial pain that is not related to function, for which aetiology is often psychogenic.

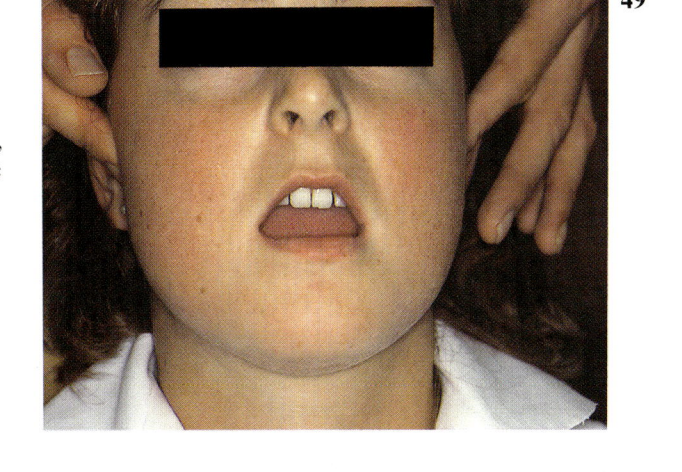

50 Abnormalities in joint function may also be caused by displacement of the articular disc, usually in an anterior and medial direction. This poses an obstruction to smooth joint function and creates an abnormal retruded condylar position. It is clinically evident as a click which occurs on opening, closing or both, dependent upon the severity of disc displacement. It may ultimately progress to a 'closed lock' in which the forward translation of the condyle is obstructed and only hinge movement is possible. Degeneration of the articulator surfaces of the joint leading to perforation of the disc may be felt as crepitus, or heard as a grating sound. It is important that mandibular dysfunction is eliminated and all joint components and associated muscles restored to health and normal function before carrying out any extensive restorative dentistry.

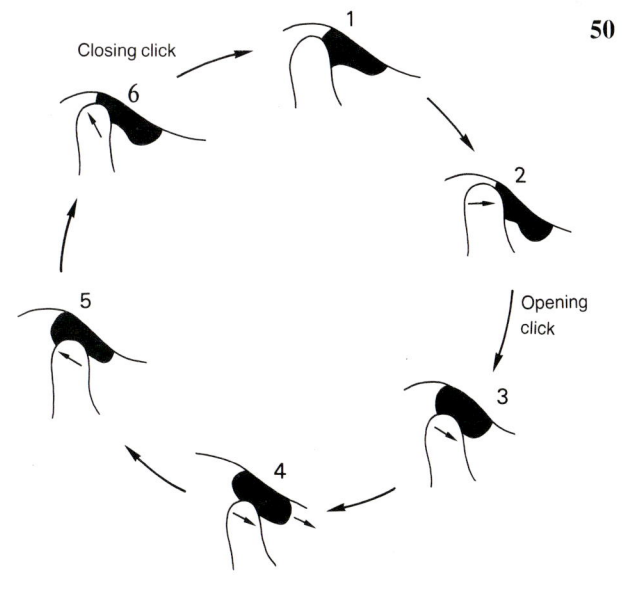

The muscles of mastication

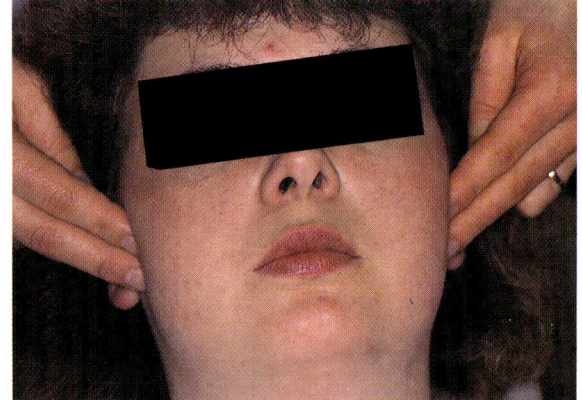

51a, 51b Prolonged muscle hyperactivity often leads to hypertrophy which may be unilateral or bilateral. This is usually observed in patients with bruxing or clenching habits who exert high occlusal forces on restorations, making them more likely to fail. The masseter (**51a**), temporalis (**51b**) and other masticatory and facial muscles are observed for enlargement and then palpated bilaterally at rest and in function. Any tenderness present may be caused by hyperactivity, differences in response between the two sides being noted. Muscle palpation is often inconclusive because it is possible to elicit a painful response from an associated anatomical structure. The patient's response may also be subjective, and the precise location of the tender area impossible to define.

Intra-oral examination

This should include an assessment of the mucosa and soft tissues, teeth and supporting structures for caries, periodontal, periapical and other pathology. Palpation of both medial and lateral pterygoid muscles intra-orally has been advocated for tenderness indicative of muscle hyperactivity. Muscle palpation is of limited diagnostic value for the reasons already stated.

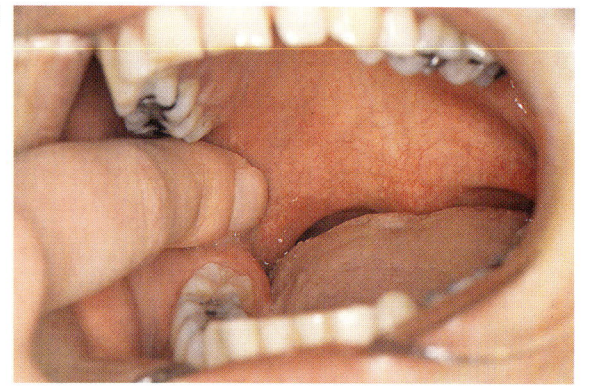

52 It is anatomically impossible to palpate the lateral pterygoid muscle because of inadequate access in the region of the hamular notch. Attempted palpation of the medial pterygoid muscle on the medial aspect of the ramus of the mandible is likely to prove uncomfortable for the patient, irrespective of the presence of hyperactivity in the muscle itself.

Marking occlusal contacts

53a–53c The accurate marking of tooth contacts during examination is important. Articulating paper should be as thin as possible, so that it marks only the small points of true contact. Thick paper will mark a large area surrounding the point of contact, making accurate assessment and adjustment of the occlusion impossible. To illustrate this, ICP contacts have been marked using three different papers of varying thickness: **53a** ash thin blue (200μ); **53b** detex red (70μ); **53c** GHM occlusion foil (19μ).

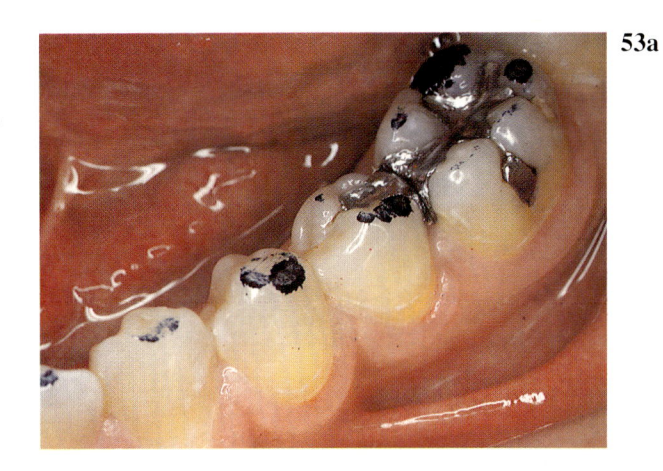

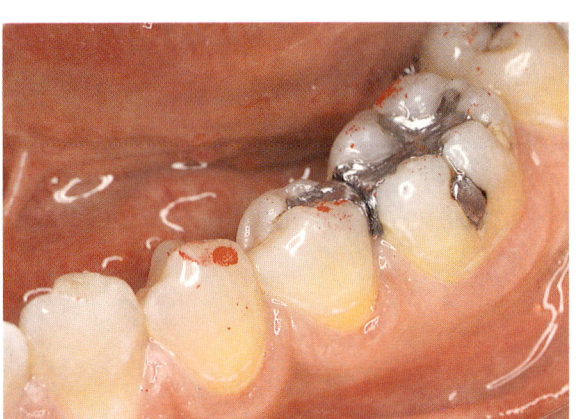

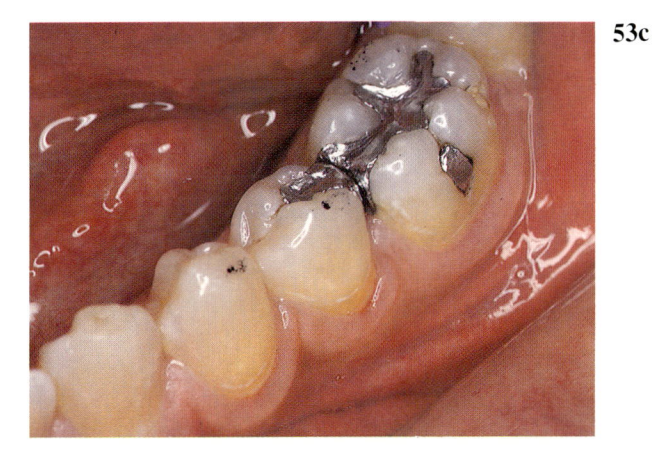

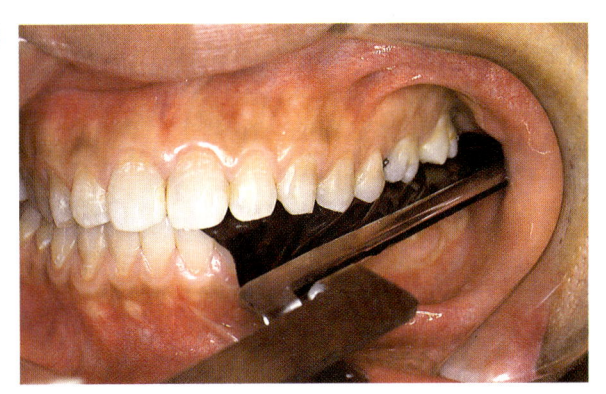

54 To mark contacts, the teeth and paper are dried and GHM occlusion foil held in Miller's forceps is placed between the teeth.

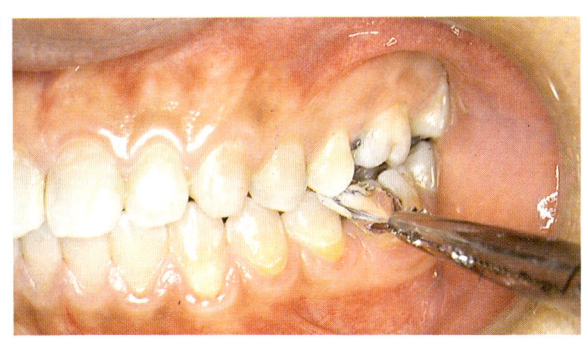

55 Shimstock foil, 12µ in thickness, is used to verify contacts. Teeth or restorations in tight contact will hold shimstock, whereas areas not in contact will allow the foil to be withdrawn from between them. The use of thin foil and paper is also important because some patients are able to detect thicknesses of less than 15µ between their teeth, indicating the level of occlusal accuracy required.

A detailed examination of a patient's occlusion should involve the following:

(**i**) Intercuspal position and posterior occlusal stability.
(**ii**) Signs and symptoms of loss of posterior stability.
(**iii**) Other causes of tooth surface loss.
(**iv**) Discrepancy between RCP and ICP.
(**v**) Anterior guidance.
(**vi**) Assessment of vertical dimension.
(**vii**) Irregularities in the occlusal plane.

(i) Intercuspal position and posterior occlusal stability

56 An occlusal examination begins with an assessment of the intercuspal position to ascertain whether the patient possesses adequate posterior occlusal stability. This may be defined as a simultaneous, even contact between sufficient posterior teeth to direct occlusal forces axially, stabilizing the positions of both the teeth and the TMJs. The number of posterior teeth necessary to meet these requirements varies, and must be assessed for each individual patient, based on the presence or absence of clinical signs of loss of stability. Adequate posterior occlusal stability serves to spread occlusal forces over a wide area, preventing damage to individual components of the masticatory system, usually the teeth.

Proximal tooth contacts play an important role in maintaining teeth in a stable position, particularly if the ICP contacts are not ideally placed to achieve axial loading. Edentulous spaces should usually be restored to prevent drifting and tilting of adjacent teeth.

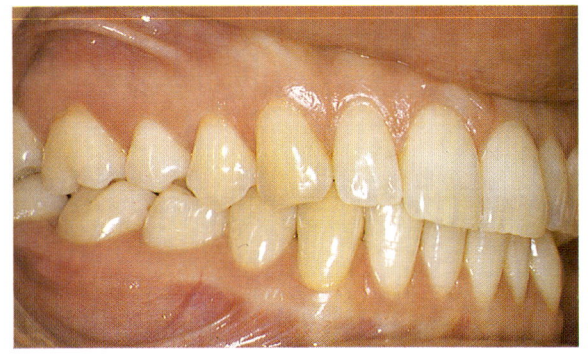

57a, 57b Direction of occlusal forces axially may be achieved by two types of intercuspal contact between opposing teeth: contact between opposing inclined planes (**57a**) or between the tip of a supporting cusp and an opposing fossa (**57b**).

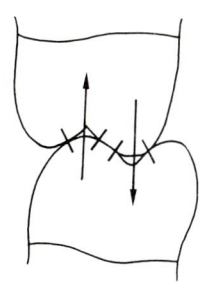

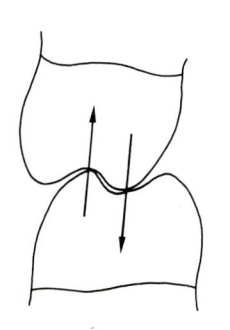

58, 59 To examine ICP contacts, articulating paper is placed between the teeth and the patient is asked to tap the teeth together. ICP contacts in the natural dentition often occur between cusp tips and fossae, as in this patient. It is unusual to observe ideal contact, as teeth are often malaligned or have their occlusal surfaces altered by restorations. This patient's ICP contacts are reasonably stable.

Posterior stability is best maintained by preventive dentistry, thus avoiding unnecessary loss, or the need for extensive restoration of teeth. Most edentulous spaces should be restored to prevent unwanted tooth movement and restorations of all types should be shaped correctly.

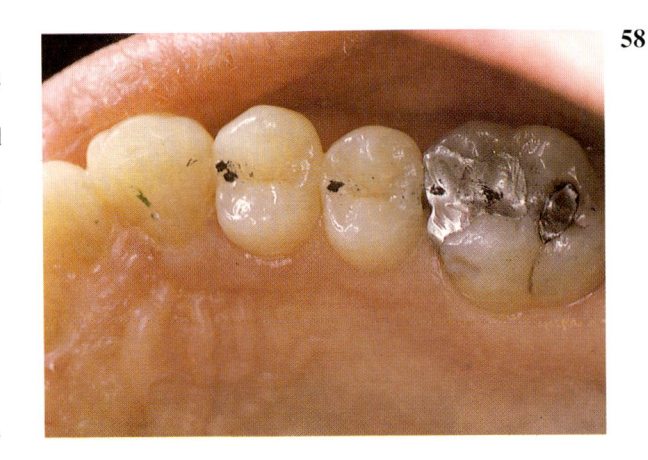

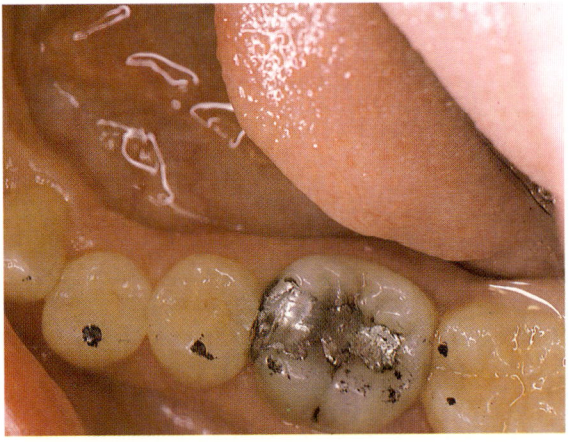

60, 61 To achieve stable ICP contacts, restorative materials must be manipulated to reproduce well defined occlusal anatomy with correctly formed and adequately steep cusps, ridges and grooves.

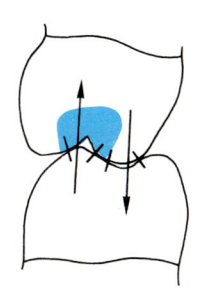

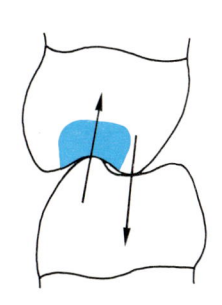

39

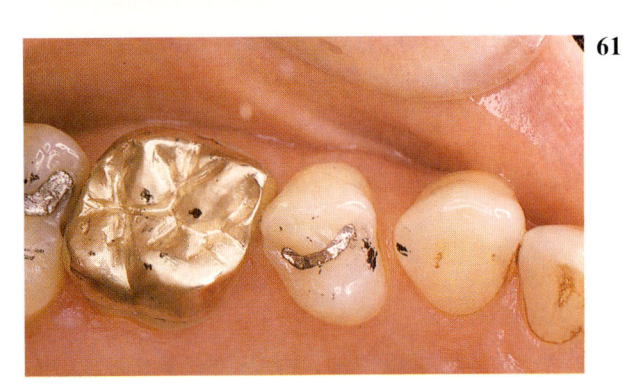

Many patients are able to maintain stability despite tooth loss and the placement of occlusally imperfect restorations. This results from the adaptive capacity of the teeth, periodontal ligaments, neuromuscular system and TMJs:

The teeth may wear very slowly when opposed by other natural teeth.

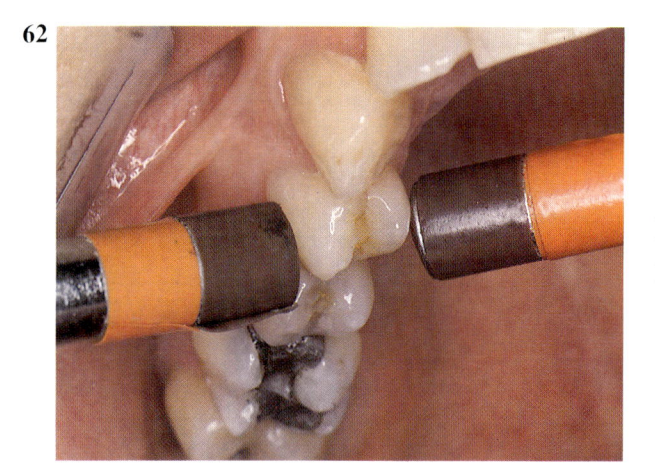

62, 63 The periodontal membrane widens in response to increased lateral force, leading to a clinical increase in tooth mobility. In the absence of periodontal inflammation this is self-limiting, allowing the tooth to move out of the way of the applied force. A periodontal and occlusal examination should determine whether increased tooth mobility is caused by excess occlusal force, loss of periodontal attachment, or both.

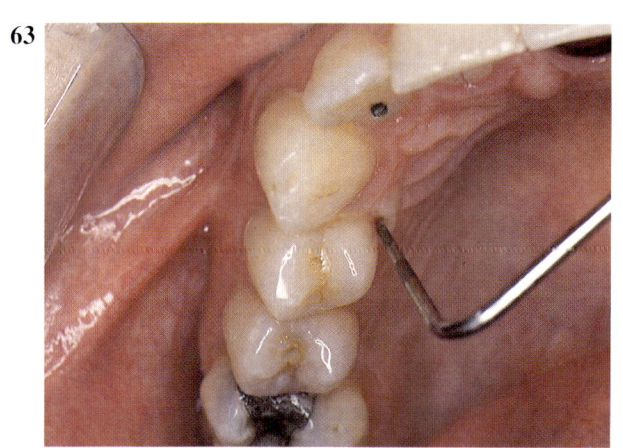

The neuromuscular system possesses an adaptive capacity, enabling it to maintain ICP, despite tooth loss, wear and the placement of inadequate restorations. It develops habitual paths of closure and lateral movement, enabling it to guide the mandible away from interferences and bring the teeth together in ICP.

The condyles may alter their positions relative to the other joint components, to enable the teeth to occlude evenly despite changes in occlusal morphology. Over a period of many years remodelling of the joint components will occur to accommodate gradual changes in the occlusion.

If a patient's occlusion shows adequate posterior occlusal stability, restorations are usually made conformatively. Care is taken to maintain stable occlusal contacts which conform to the pre-treatment intercuspal position.

(ii) The signs and symptoms of loss of posterior stability

Posterior stability may be lost because of tooth loss or the placement of restorations which fail to restore stable occlusal contacts in patients who cannot adapt to these changes. The diagnosis of loss of stability is based on the occurrence of one or more clinical signs and symptoms that indicate the need to reorganize a patient's occlusion, creating a new intercuspal position as close to the retruded position as possible. This new jaw relation should be established before restorations are made. Conformative dentistry carried out in such situations may fail as a result of excessive occlusal forces created by an unstable ICP. The retruded position of the mandible is used because it is the only relatively reproducible relationship of mandible to maxilla outside ICP which has proved physiologically acceptable.

Loss of posterior stability may result in:

- Increased tooth wear.
- Mechanical failure of teeth or restorations.
- Hypermobility and drifting.
- Mandibular dysfunction.

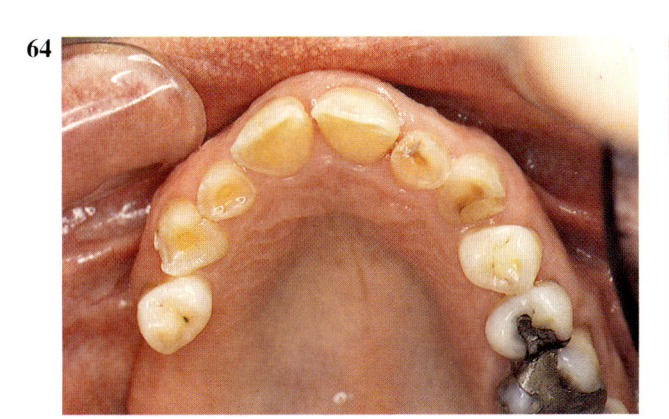

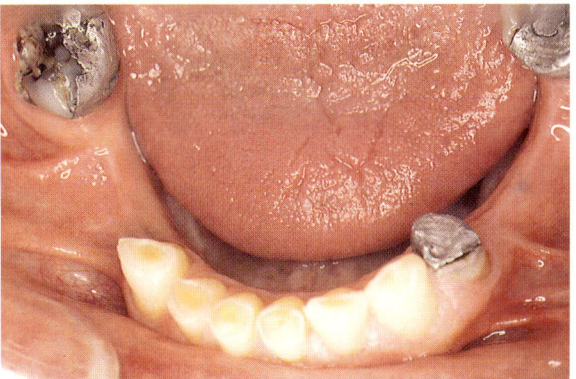

64, 65 This patient has severely worn anterior teeth resulting from an unstable posterior occlusion after the loss of most of the posterior teeth.

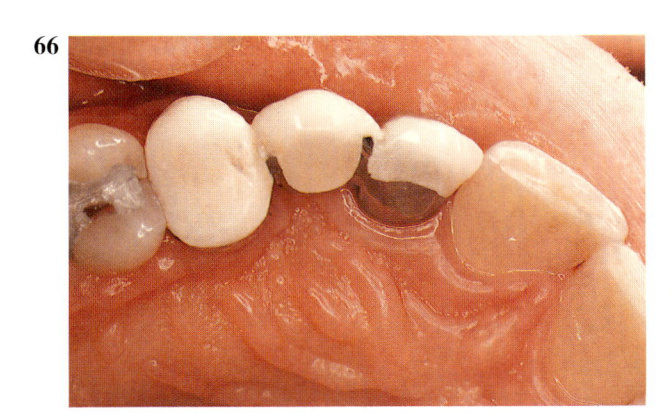

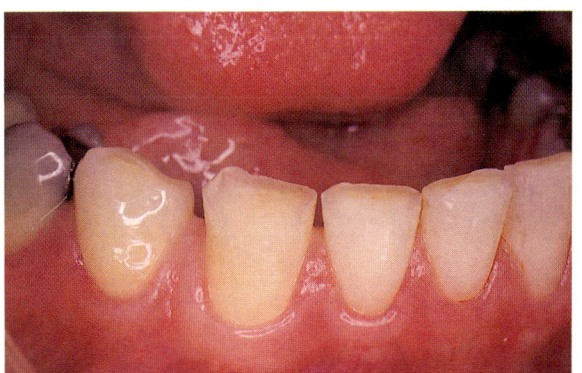

66, 67 The use of porcelain occlusal surfaces opposing natural teeth often contributes to increased wear of the teeth. This is particularly true on surfaces capable of rubbing together and in the mouths of bruxers. This patient exhibits localized wear without any overall loss of stability. However, stability may be lost as a result of increased wear, if most of the teeth in one area are restored in this way.

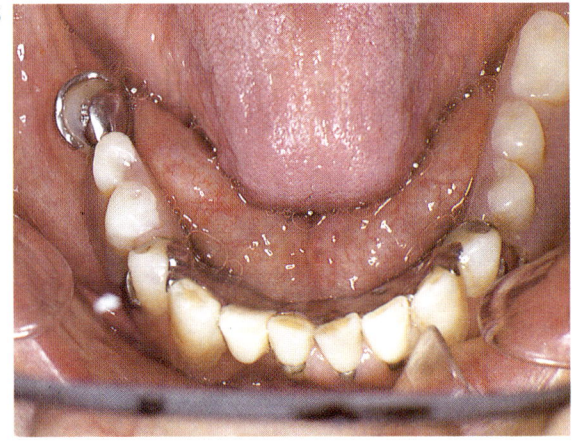

68 The acrylic resin teeth used in partial dentures wear out of ICP contact and then fail to support the posterior occlusion. This may lead either to the loss of ICP contacts or to over-eruption of opposing teeth which maintain contact as the denture teeth wear away.

An unstable posterior occlusion results in excessive occlusal force being applied to both anterior and posterior teeth. This may result in mechanical failure, particularly in patients with parafunctional habits. Restorations may fracture as a result of an unstable posterior occlusion. Remaking them without first reorganizing the occlusion and creating a stable ICP, will lead to repeated failures.

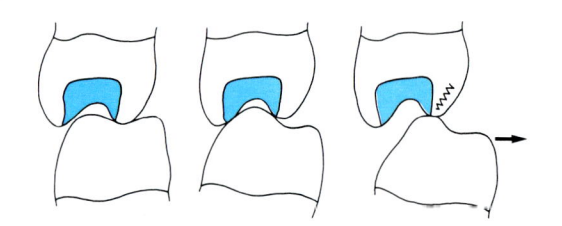

69 Under-contouring restorations results in unstable ICP contacts which may cause tooth movement and tilting. If this involves many of the posterior teeth, loss of stability will occur which may manifest itself as any of the clinical signs described. It also increases the likelihood of lateral interferences occurring.

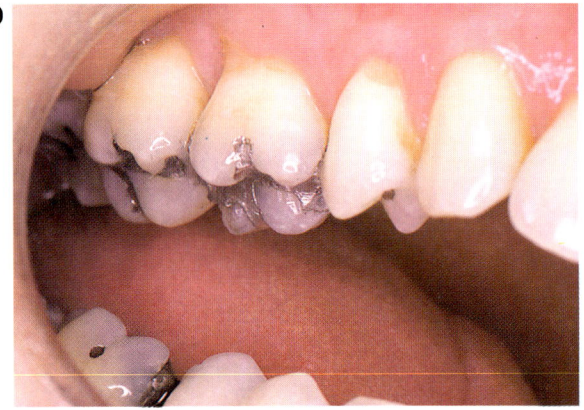

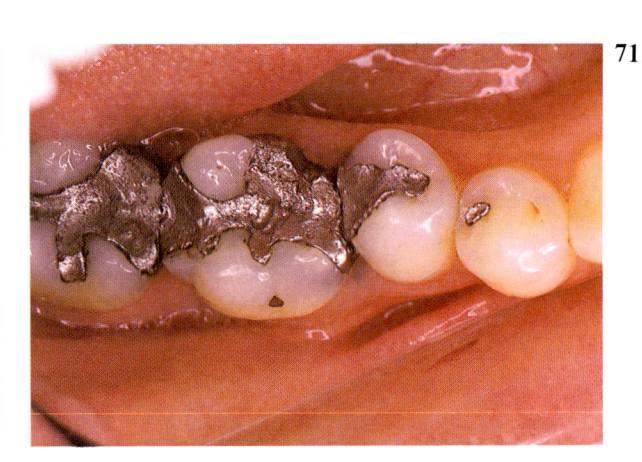

70, 71 This large amalgam is one of several in this patient's mouth which have been under-contoured, resulting in tipping and over-eruption of the opposing teeth, loss of stability and fracture of the restoration.

72, 73 A loss of posterior stability which creates a forward component of force combined with periodontal inflammation may lead to the anterior migration of teeth. This patient presented complaining of an increasing diastema between her maxillary central incisors. Examination revealed an unstable posterior occlusion and periodontal disease around the maxillary anterior teeth.

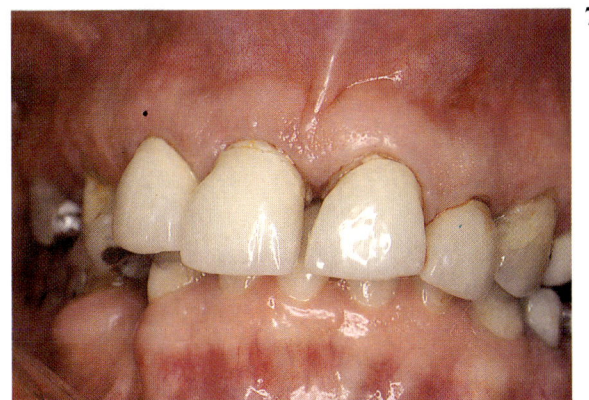

Loss of posterior stability may lead to mandibular dysfunction in susceptible patients. This generally occurs when the TMJs and the associated neuromuscular system cannot adapt to changes in the occlusion. This is most common when occlusal changes are dramatic or occur rapidly, often due to the insertion of an interfering restoration, as well as in patients with reduced adaptive capacity, common in periods of stress-induced muscle hyperactivity.

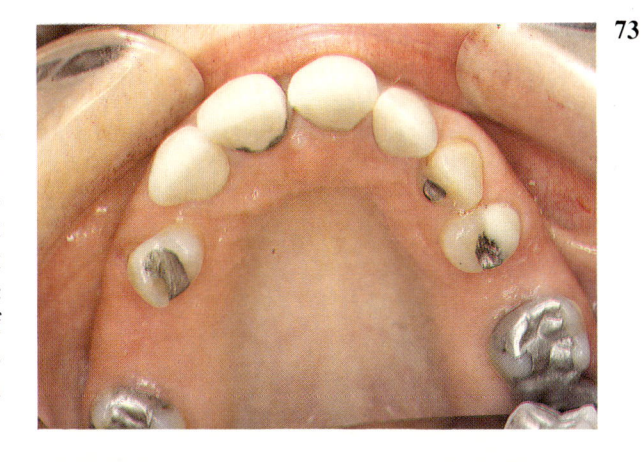

74 This patient presented with acute dysfunction two weeks after placement of these composite resin restorations. The extensive use of composite resins for restoring occlusal surfaces is inadvisable, owing to the difficulties of manipulation and of producing the correct occlusal anatomy and contacts. Composite resin is also an abrasive material which may wear opposing teeth. This patient lost posterior stability in the space of two days when all her amalgam fillings were replaced with poorly contoured composite resin restorations. In addition to the considerable alteration in occlusal morphology of the teeth, the condyles repositioned, further destabilizing ICP.

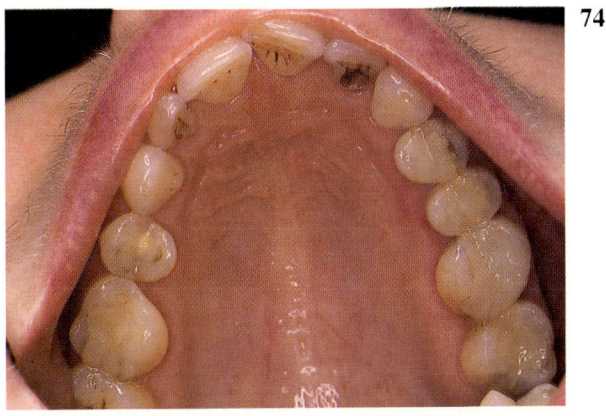

75 This patient presented with dysfunction, one month after cementation of these poorly contoured porcelain-fused-to-metal restorations. Poor occlusal anatomy prevented the restoration of stable ICP contacts; only 21, 22, 23 contacted in ICP. The condyles and muscles were unable to adapt and bring the other teeth into contact.

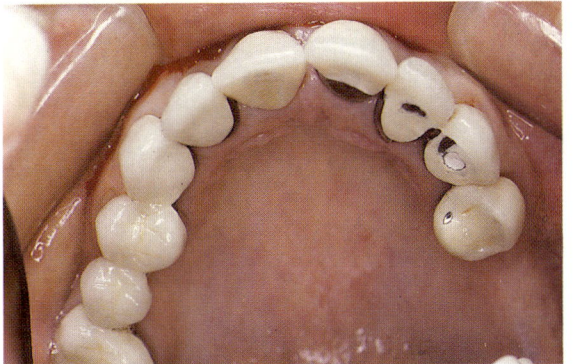

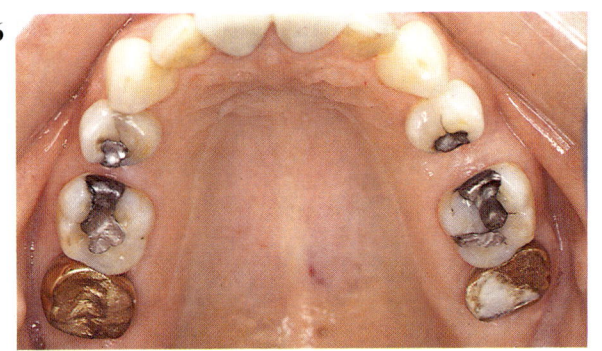

76 These gold crowns have poor occlusal anatomy and provide no occlusal stability; their placement precipitated condylar repositioning and dysfunctional symptoms. Adequate ICP contacts play an important part in maintaining the stability of the condylar position.

77, 78 Other iatrogenic factors include the prolonged use of partial coverage occlusal splints. This patient had worn a posterior onlay splint for nine months which caused the posterior teeth to be intruded and the anterior teeth to over-erupt. There is no posterior contact without the splint in place and the mandibular dysfunction, which the splint was intended to treat, is now more severe.

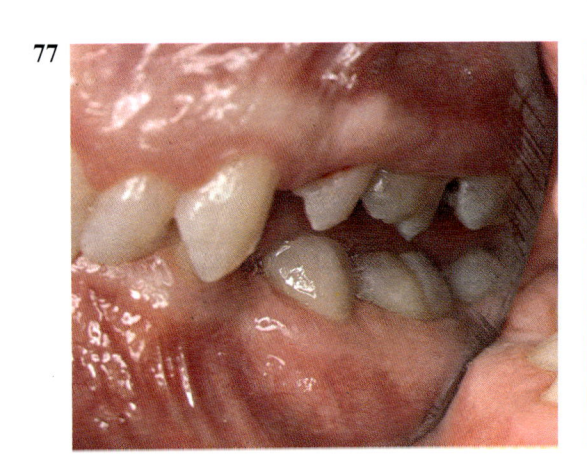

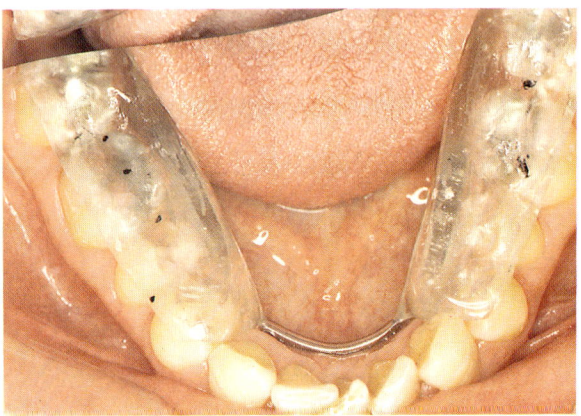

(iii) Other causes of tooth surface loss

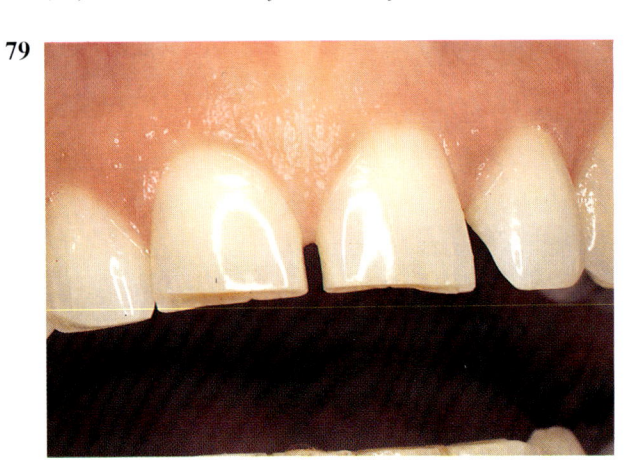

79 Bruxing or tooth grinding is usually stress related and results in increased wear of the affected teeth. They exhibit flattened wear facets which fit precisely against the opposing teeth in the mandibular position in which the bruxing occurs. There is some evidence that bruxing may be aggravated by interferences between the teeth which cause an increase in muscle hyperactivity. However, it is unrealistic to believe that adjustment of the occlusion will cure the habit in the presence of a dominant stress factor. Bruxers are capable of exerting high occlusal forces and spend more time with their teeth together, placing extra demands on any restorations.

80 Erosion by acid, usually from dietary components or regurgitated from the stomach, may lead to extensive loss of enamel and dentine. This may result in a loss of posterior stability if many teeth are badly affected. The eroded surfaces usually have a cupped-out appearance which distinguishes them from the flat facets found in bruxers. Identification of the aetiology is important in order to prevent the condition worsening.

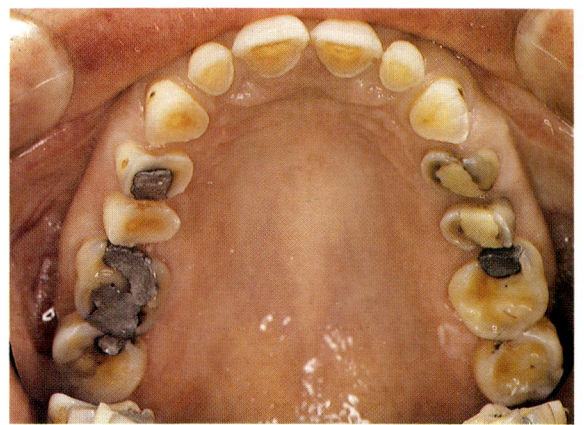

(iv) The discrepancy between RCP and ICP

It is necessary to examine the discrepancy between RCP and ICP for the following reasons:

Simple restorations should not alter the RCP–ICP slide. The alteration of a susceptible patient's occlusion in this way may lead to muscle hyperactivity causing bruxing, clenching and TMJ and muscle problems. These in turn may lead to the mechanical failure of restorations.

The slide needs to be identified and eliminated when reorganizing the occlusion. This is usually carried out when:

- Restoration of posterior occlusal stability by occlusal adjustment or restoring teeth is needed.
- When treating mandibular dysfunction.
- Prior to multi-unit restorations.
- Placing the mandible in retruded creates space for restorations.

81 A potential distal bridge abutment is often the site of the retruded contact, particularly when it is a mesially tipped lower molar. It is essential that any non-working or retruded contacts present are removed and the ICP checked for stability before tooth preparation is begun. If the patient is missing several teeth or has worn occlusal surfaces, the removal of the occlusal surface of a distal molar may remove posterior stability in ICP. The condyles may then reposition because their position is no longer stabilized by adequate ICP contacts. If this occurs after tooth preparation, the prepared tooth may move closer to its antagonist resulting in the restoration being high on try-in.

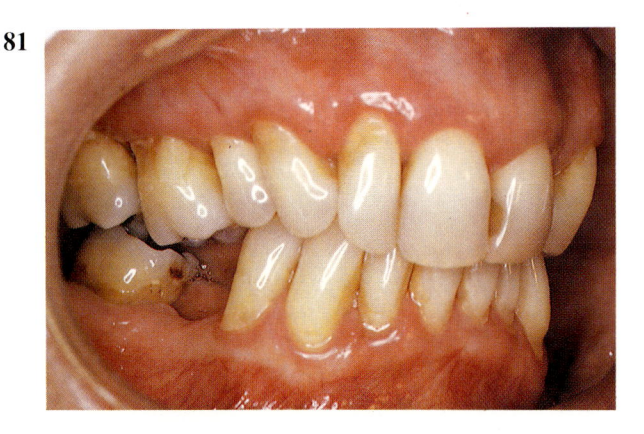

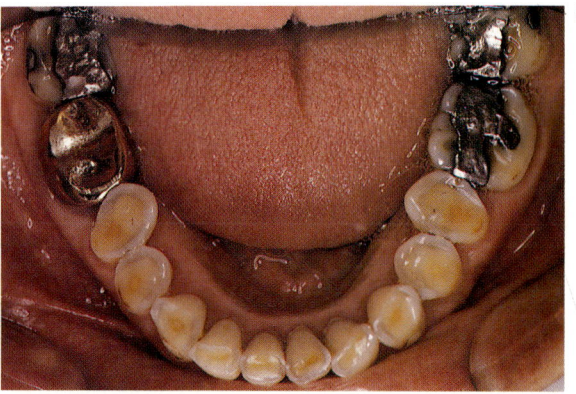

82 This patient requires full-mouth restorations. Any attempt to restore these teeth conformatively one segment at a time would result in flat restorations of a similar contour to the original teeth. This would preclude the establishment of the good cuspal anatomy necessary to achieve stable contacts.

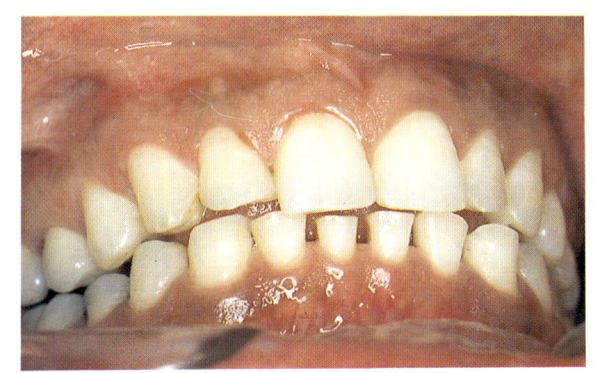

83 This patient has a large horizontal discrepancy between RCP and ICP. Placing the mandible in retruded creates space for the restoration of worn anterior teeth. If restoration of the posterior teeth only was required, it would be more sensible to make the restorations conformatively to maintain the anterior tooth contact in ICP, and hence the anterior guidance.

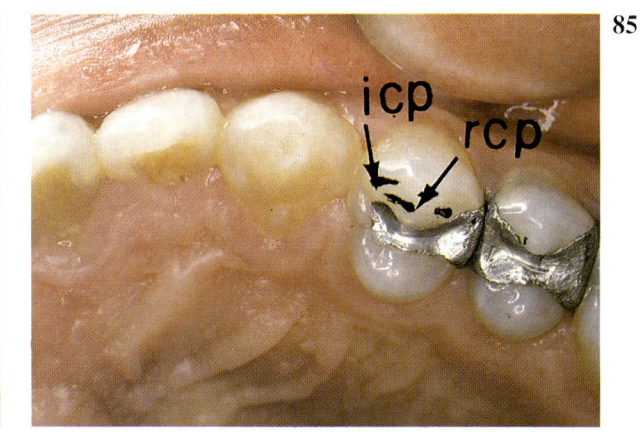

84, 85 To locate and mark the RCP–ICP slide, the articulating paper is held between the patient's teeth by the assistant. The mandible is manipulated bimanually and the patient asked to close to the point of first contact, and then to squeeze into ICP. The slide is usually located on the mesial inclines of the maxillary cusps and on the distal inclines of the mandibular cusps. In this patient it has occurred between the left first premolars.

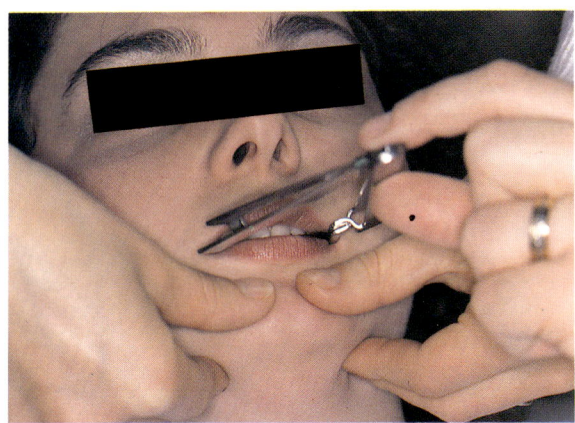

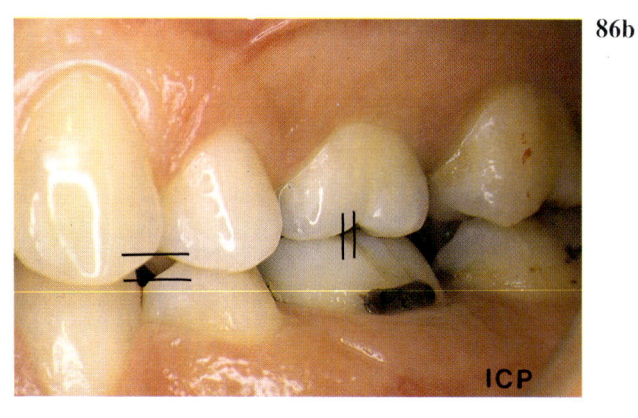

86a–87b The presence of any slide between RCP (**86a, 87a**) and ICP (**86b, 87b**) is noted, along with its size and relative components in horizontal and vertical planes and in a lateral direction. The type of slide expressed in these dimensions is of diagnostic importance, and as it is best observed on diagnostic casts, its significance will be discussed later.

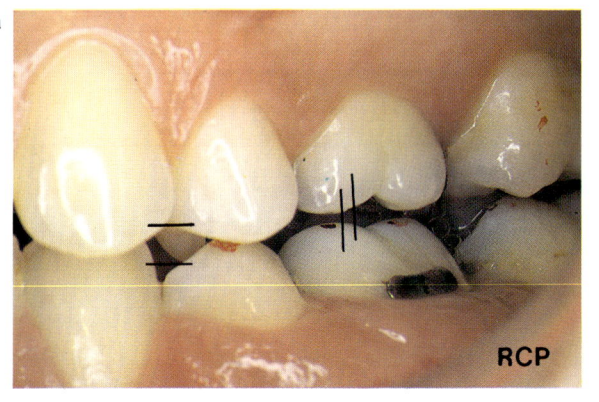

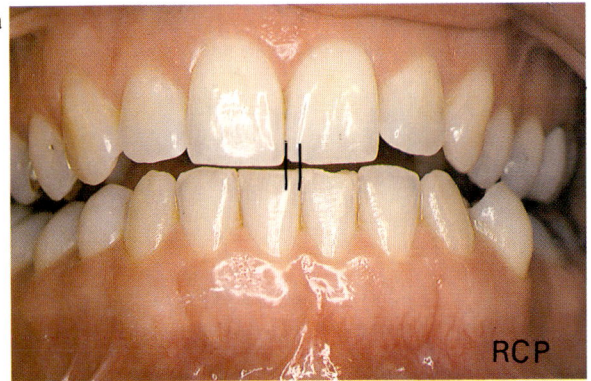

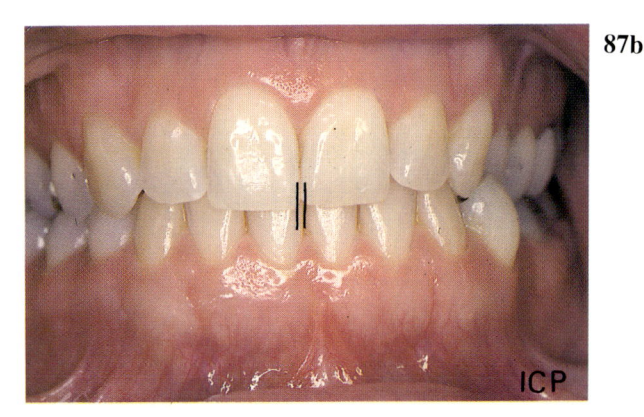

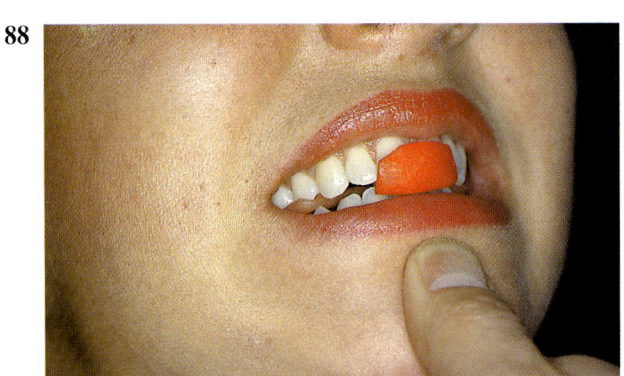

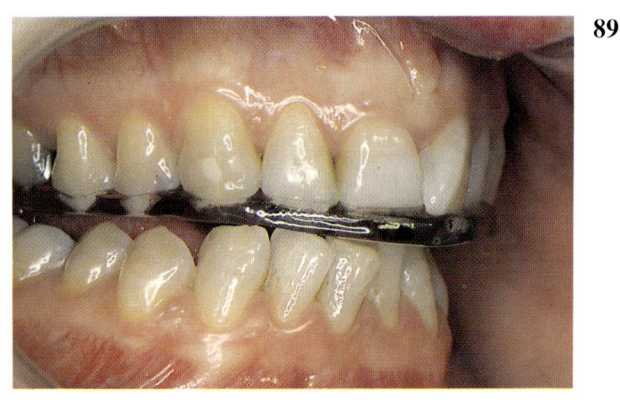

88 In patients with tense musculature, difficulty will be experienced in recording this position. Muscle relaxation can be achieved by fabricating an acrylic resin anterior jig to separate the posterior teeth by 2–3mm, to be worn for several minutes prior to the examination. It works by breaking the proprioceptive feedback responsible for habitual closure into ICP.

89 Patients with severe muscle hyperactivity may require a period of occlusal splint therapy before an accurate recording can be taken. This will be described in greater detail later on.

(v) Anterior guidance

90 The relationship between the patient's anterior teeth in ICP should be examined. Ideally, there should be contact between the maxillary and mandibular incisors and canines. When the patient performs a protrusive or lateral excursion, contact between these teeth should immediately disclude the posteriors. This arrangement is desirable to reduce potentially harmful lateral forces on the posterior teeth. In restorative dentistry, clinical experience has demonstrated the importance of anterior guidance in removing lateral tooth contacts and interferences which may, in susceptible patients, cause muscle hyperactivity, generating excessive forces on weakened teeth, restorations and the TMJs.

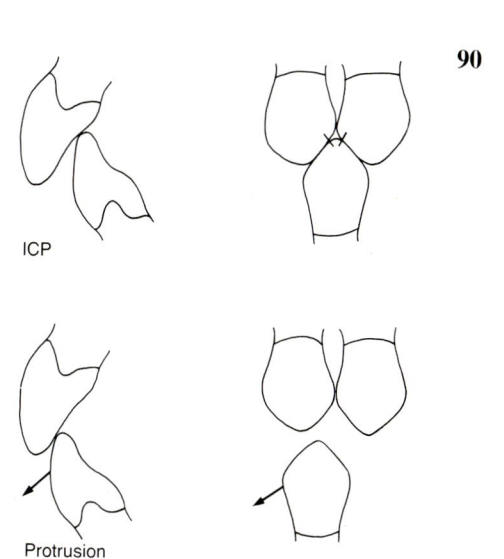

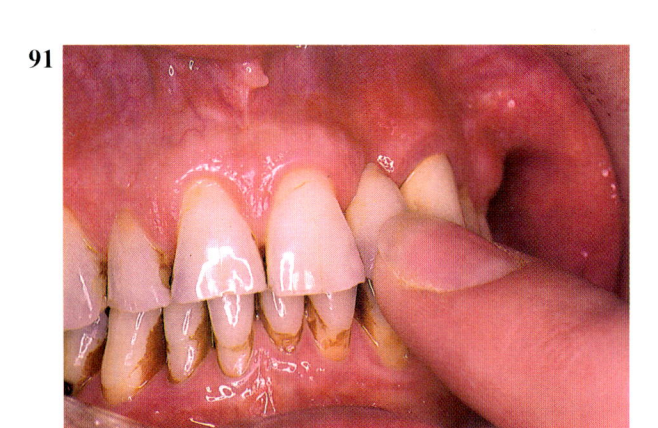

91 Anterior teeth are well equipped to fulfil this function, provided restorations placed on them are correctly shaped and the patient's posterior occlusion is stable. The clinical signs of loss of posterior occlusal stability having been described, the presence of fremitus on tapping in ICP should also be noted as an indication of the lack of posterior support.

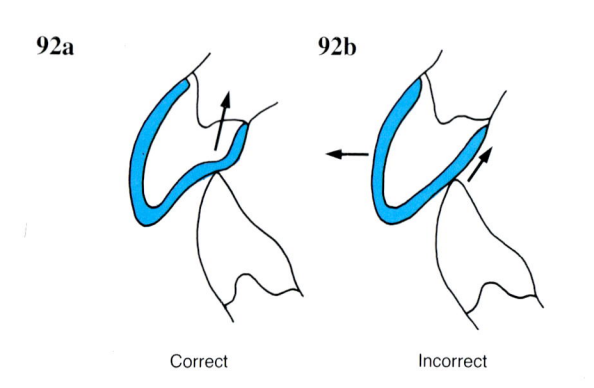

92a, 92b It is important when restoring anterior teeth to reproduce not only their smooth, concave palatal surfaces, against which the lower anterior teeth articulate, but also a flat cingulum area to provide a stable ICP contact with the lower tooth to direct occlusal forces axially. This configuration will not only provide correct guidance, but will also aid in stabilizing anterior tooth position (**92a**). Incorrect tooth preparation will lead to palatal over-contouring of restorations, resulting in an unfavourable load distribution in the anterior teeth (**92b**).

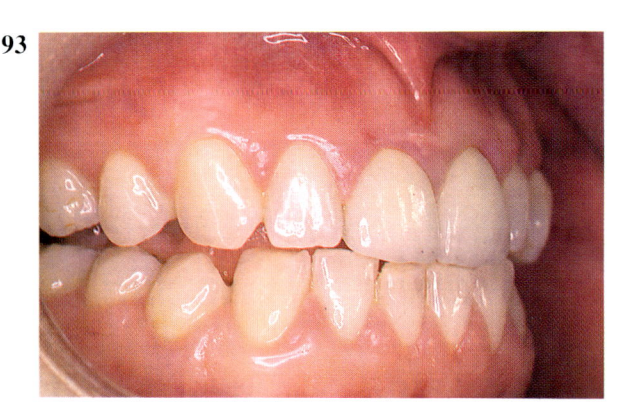

93 In a protrusive movement, guidance should be provided by the strongest anterior teeth, usually the central incisors. If one tooth is weakened by restorations it should be removed from contact, except in ICP.

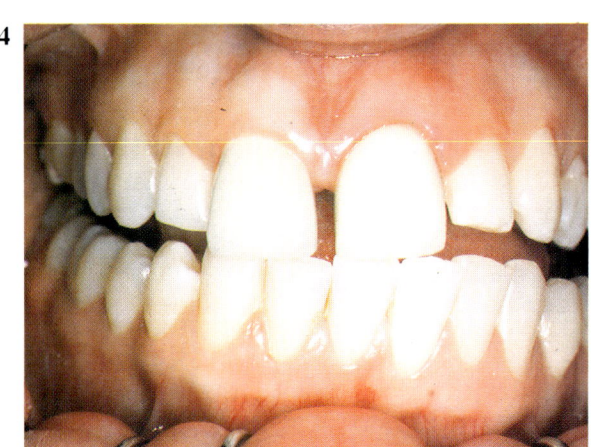

If the palatal surfaces of maxillar anterior teeth are restored improperly, then one or more of the following problems may be observed; excessive wear of a restoration or opposing tooth, decementation of the restoration, fracture of a porcelain facing, hypermobility or drifting, fracture of solder joints in bridgework, pain in the teeth on biting, or hypersensitivity to cold stimuli.

94 This patient's maxillary central incisors were restored with porcelain-fused-to-metal crowns with excessively bulbous palatal surfaces. Within two months the teeth had drifted labially, opening up a diastema due to the excess forces produced. When the crowns were replaced with correctly contoured provisional restorations, the teeth quickly returned to their original positions.
Courtesy of Mr D. Setchell.

95a, 95b In a lateral movement it is desirable for tooth contacts on the working side to disclude those on the non-working side. The patient is guided into left and right lateral excursions and a note made of the teeth that contact on the working side, and of whether the patient has canine guidance (**95a**) or group function (**95b**).

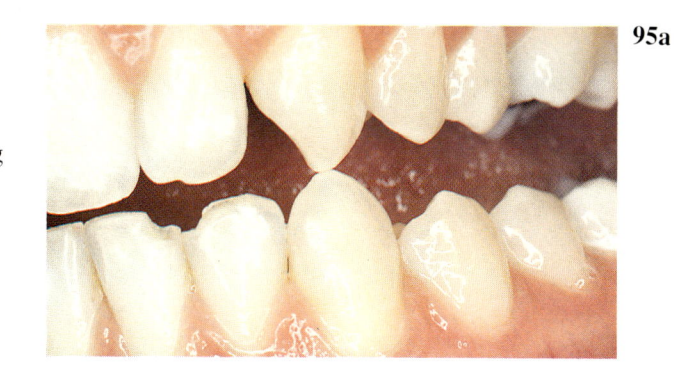

95a

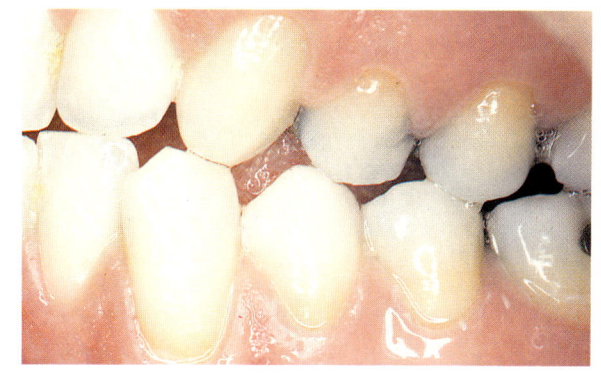

95b

96, 97 It is also useful to use articulating paper to mark the articulating surfaces of the teeth on the working side. Intercuspal contacts are marked in black and working side contacts in red on 23, 24, 26, 33, 34 and 36, indicating group function. In natural dentition the type of guidance is less important; however, when restoring these surfaces a choice usually has to be made between one of the two schemes.

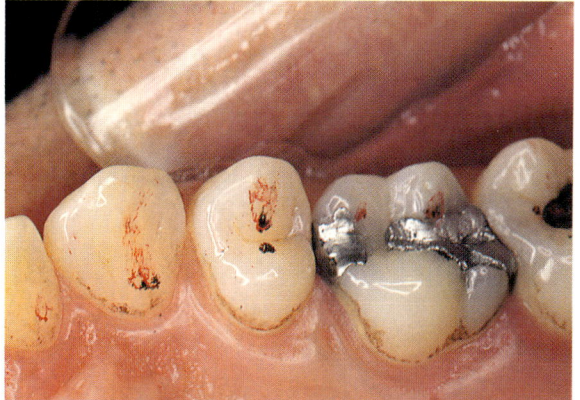

96

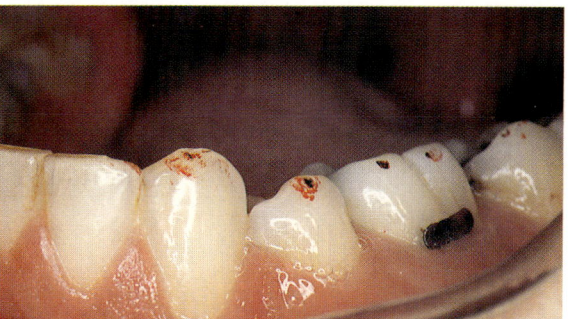

97

The presence of anterior tooth contact in ICP which provides immediate disclusion is of diagnostic importance. Its existence means that posterior restorations will be required to reproduce stable ICP contacts and disclude in all other mandibular positions, which simplifies technical procedures.

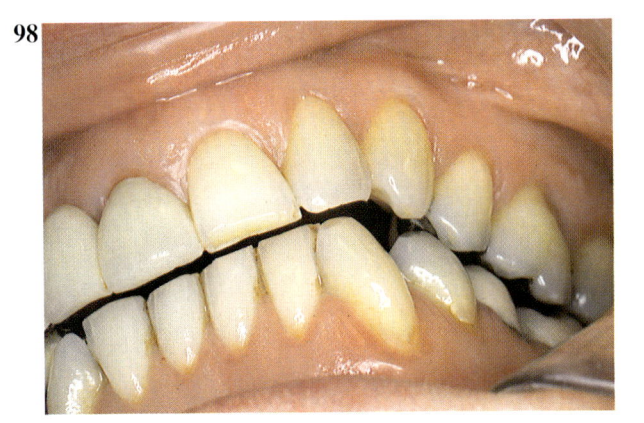

98, 99 If a patient lacks anterior tooth contact in ICP so that they either have to protrude or move laterally before the guidance teeth touch, and then disclude, they are said to have a long or wide centric. This anterior relationship makes the fabrication of posterior restorations more demanding, as it is necessary to make sure that all the posterior teeth move over each other smoothly and simultaneously until the guidance surfaces touch and disclude them. This requires flat fossa areas over which the supporting cusps can move smoothly until they disclude.

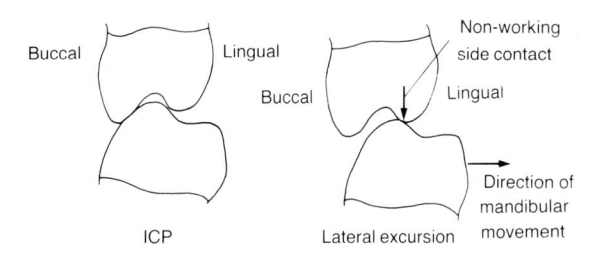

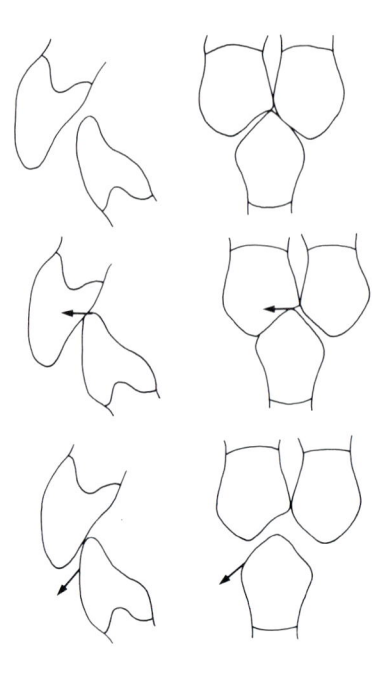

100 Bucco-lingual section through first molars

100, 101 Contacts or interferences occurring on the non-working side are also examined. These usually occur between the lingually facing inclines of lower buccal cusps and buccally facing inclines of maxillary palatal cusps.

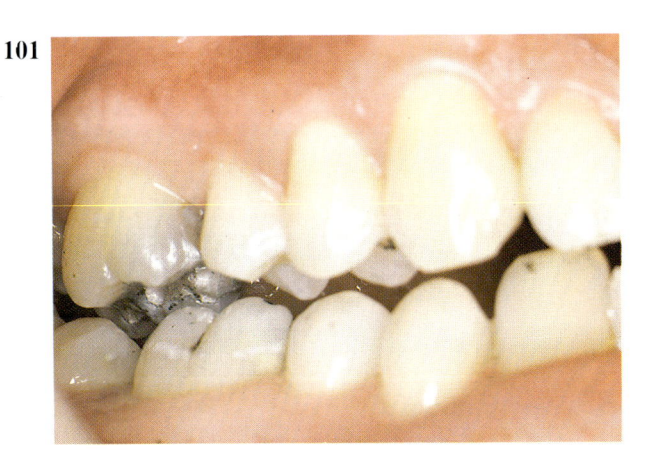

102 It is neccessary to mark both ICP and non-working side contacts, so that if it becomes necessary to adjust the latter, the ICP contacts are not inadvertently removed, resulting in reduced posterior stability.

There is evidence that non-working interferences may lead to muscle hyperactivity in susceptible patients, which may cause bruxing, clenching, TMJ problems and the mechanical failure of restorations due to the large forces generated.

There is no justification for their routine prophylactic removal but, if any of these signs are present, non-working contacts should be adjusted. It is also advisable to remove non-working contacts on teeth prior to carrying out restorative dentistry to reduce the chance of excessive occlusal forces on the new restorations.

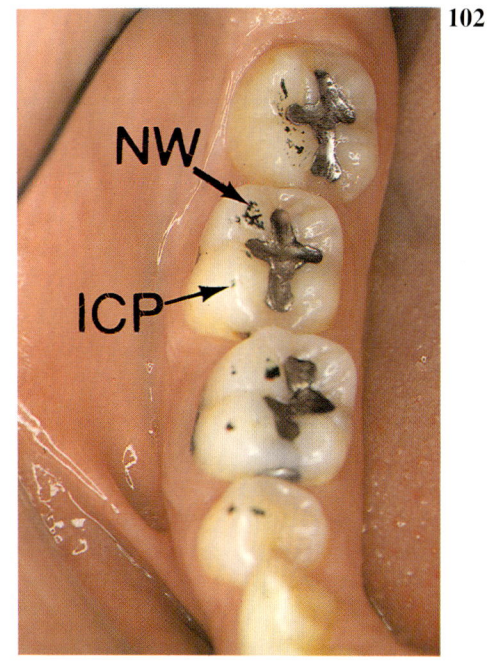

103, 104 It is essential to examine non-working side contacts and interferences and anterior guidance together. If a patient does not demonstrate adequate guidance it may be impossible to separate the non-working side. Restoration of the anterior guidance should be considered if posterior restorations are planned. This patient's posterior teeth were restored producing an ICP with no anterior tooth contact and guidance. Repeated attempts were made to eliminate a non-working side contact on 17, 47 without success.

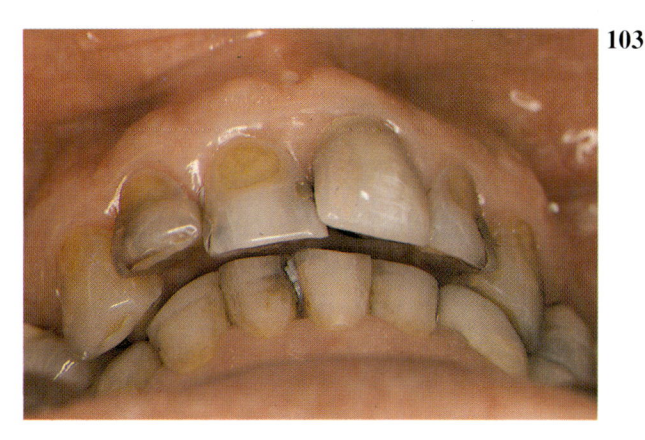

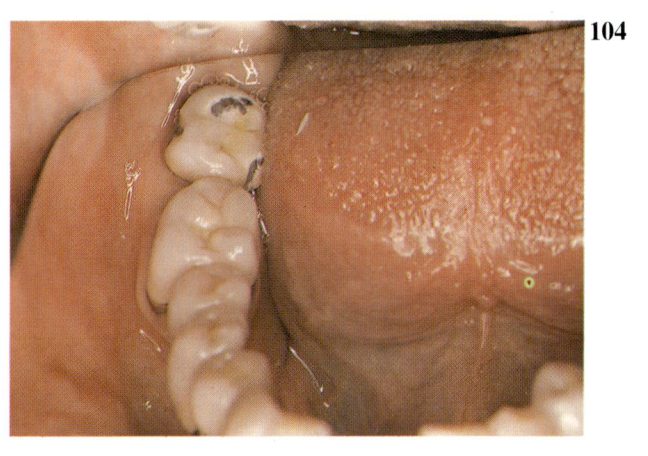

(vi) Assessment of vertical dimension

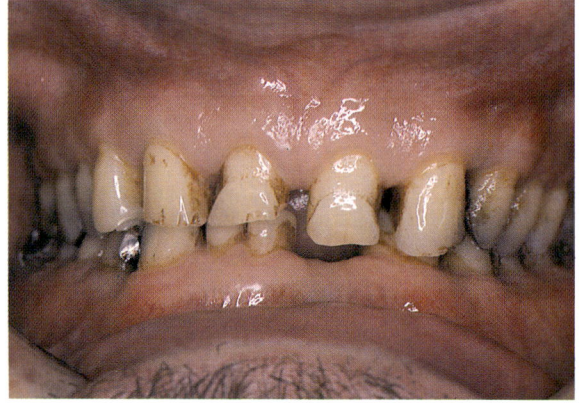

105 The accurate assessment of rest position and interocclusal clearance is extremely difficult. In a dentate patient, restorations are used to increase the occlusal vertical dimension for the following reasons:

- To increase the length of worn teeth to improve appearance.
- To increase the occlusal vertical dimension to improve facial profile.
- To create occlusal space for restorations without the necessity for occlusal reduction, thus preserving maximum preparation height for resistance and retention form. It also increases the vertical space available for solder joints, increasing their strength while maintaining open and cleansable embrasures.

The increase in occlusal vertical dimension is based upon aesthetic and space requirements, being initially determined using diagnostic casts, and tried out for patient acceptance in provisional restorations. This makes accurate assessment of the rest vertical dimension during the initial examination procedures unnecessary. Dentate patients are able to tolerate considerable increases in occlusal vertical dimension owing to neuromuscular adaptation mediated via periodontal proprioceptors.

(vii) Irregularities in the occlusal plane

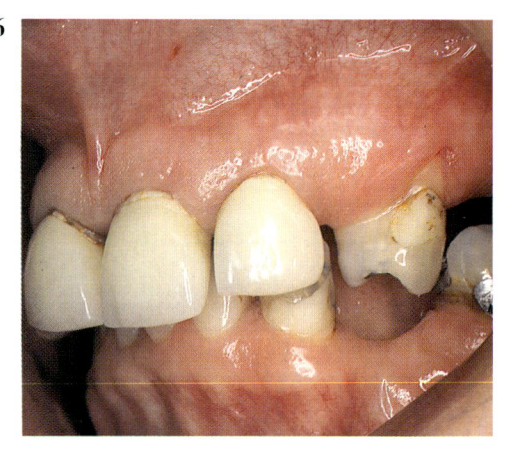

106 Any gross irregularities in the occlusal plane are noted, as they increase the likelihood of lateral and protrusive interferences. Treatment planning should include measures to flatten the occlusal plane.

Conclusion

Clinical assessment of the occlusion may not provide a true picture, as discrepancies and interferences may be hidden by the neuromuscular adaptation of mandibular movements. The belief that, 'The mouth is the best articulator', is untrue and detailed occlusal analysis requires mounted diagnostic casts.

Chapter 4: Restorative special investigations

Clinical examination of the occlusion alone seldom provides adequate information for the diagnosis of occlusal pathology and treatment planning. In most situations further investigations are required, which include where appropriate:

- Radiographs.
- Articulated diagnostic casts.
- Pantographics.
- Occlusal splint therapy.

Radiographs

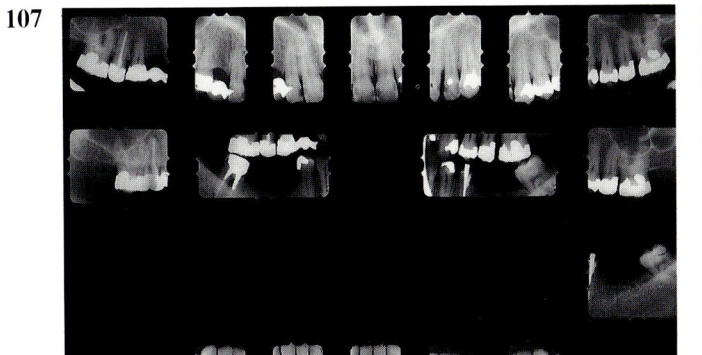

107, 108 Treatment planning requires a full-mouth set of long cone periapical radiographs which provide accurate and well-defined views of the teeth and supporting tissues.

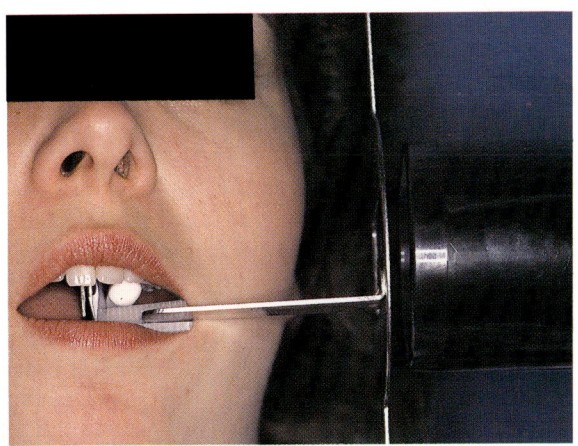

109 A paralleling technique with a long cone X-ray tube and film holder provides accurate, undistorted and reproducible views.

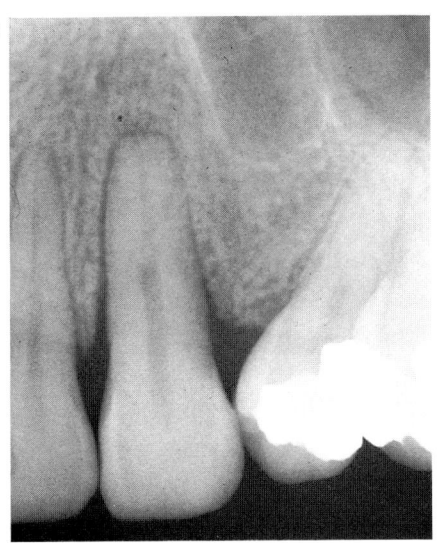

110 Excess occlusal forces leading to clinical hypermobility create a widened periodontal ligament space and may also cause root resorption. This may occur with or without the loss of periodontal attachment and is a physiological adaptation to increased loading.

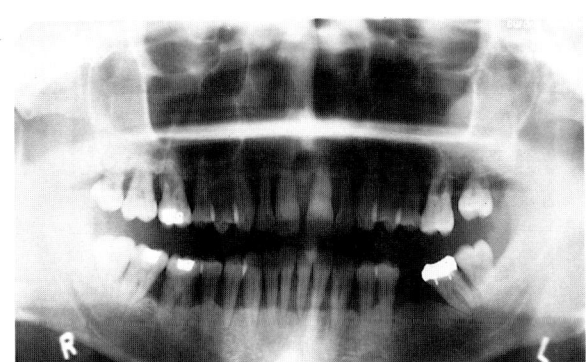

111 Pan-oral radiographs provide poor definition, making detailed examination of the teeth and supporting structures difficult. They are also inadequate as TMJ radiographs because only the lateral third of each condyle is visible, and the fossa is obscured by superimposition of the zygomatic arch. They are useful for general screening and in the detection of gross pathology.
Courtesy of Miss K. Warren.

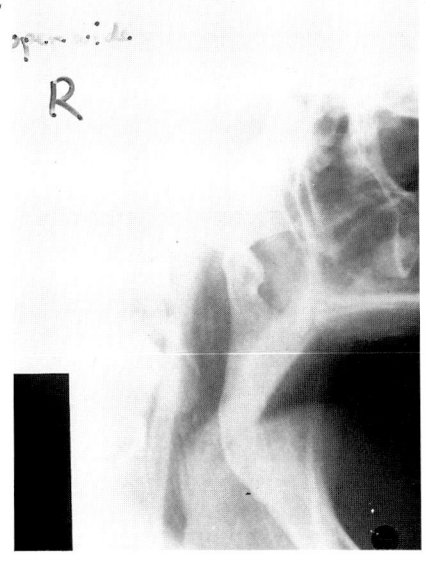

112 Radiographic examination of the TMJs is seldom indicated. Hard tissue views like the transpharyngeal and transcranial show the lateral third of the condyle only, and reveal only gross alterations in shape or form of the bony surfaces. Tomography enables a serial examination of the whole joint to be made, whilst contrast radiography (arthrography) reveals the soft tissues and enables the position of the disc to be shown. Such radiographs are indicated in patients with long-standing joint problems who have not responded to conservative treatment like occlusal splint therapy. They are relatively unreproducible, and do not show whether the condyle is correctly positioned in the fossa unless there is a major subluxation or dislocation. They do not provide a baseline from which to monitor condylar repositioning during splint therapy. Arthrography may reveal displacement of the disc, confirming a diagnosis based on clinical signs and symptoms. It is, however, a difficult and invasive procedure and not widely available.

Articulated diagnostic casts

Articulated diagnostic casts may be used for occlusal analysis, trial tooth adjustment and preparation, diagnostic waxing, shells for provisional restorations, fabrication of custom trays, fabrication of occlusal splints and prediction of orthodontic and orthognathic surgery results.

Only those applications pertinent to management of the occlusion are discussed:

Occlusal analysis

The analysis of articulated diagnostic casts is an essential part of restorative treatment planning. Not only do they allow the occlusion to be examined more easily than in the mouth, but they also permit trial adjustment and diagnostic waxing to be performed. These diagnostic procedures enable the restorative dentist to ascertain whether the treatment plan is feasible, and will demonstrate occlusal problems which may be encountered in carrying it out, prior to starting treatment. The treatment plan can then be altered to avoid these pitfalls.

It is necessary to decide early on in the diagnostic process whether restorations are to be made in a conformative or reorganized manner. The choice is based on the following criteria:

Indications for conforming

- A small number of units being restored.
- The patient possesses a stable posterior occlusion.
- The absence of other occlusal pathology such as mandibular dysfunction.
- The teeth to be restored do not provide the RCP contact.
- The presence of a large horizontal discrepancy between RCP and ICP so that reorganizing would lose anterior guidance.
- There is no need to create space in the anterior region to restore worn teeth.

Indications for reorganizing

- A large number of units being restored.
- A lack of posterior occlusal stability.
- The presence of mandibular dysfunction.
- The teeth to be restored provide the RCP contact.
- A large vertical discrepancy between RCP and ICP such that reorganizing would maintain anterior tooth contact and guidance.
- There is a need to create space in the anterior region to restore worn teeth.

A number of patient cases are presented which illustrate the uses of diagnostic casts in making this decision.

Conforming to the existing ICP

Most of the occlusal problems encountered when making restorations to conform to the existing ICP are due to:

- Uneven opposing occlusal surfaces.
- A lack of anterior guidance.

Uneven opposing occlusal surfaces

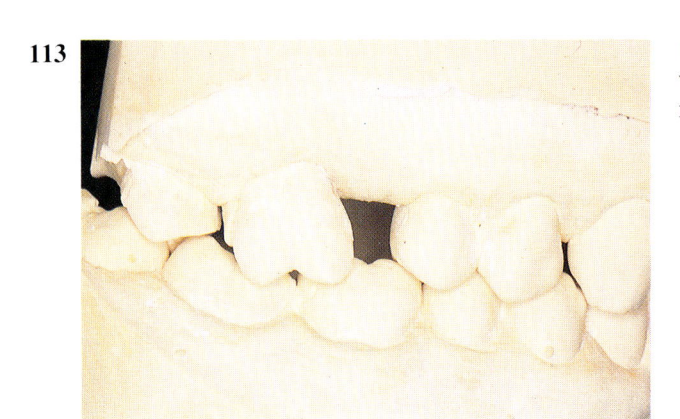

113 This patient required restoration of 17, 18 with crowns. The ICP was stable and the space mesial to 16, did not need restoring.

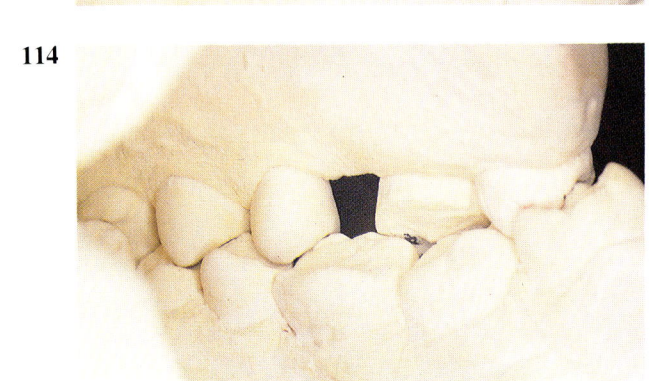

114 A lingual view, not possible clinically, confirmed that inadequate restoration of both teeth had reduced the number of stable ICP contacts and led to the over-eruption and tipping of both molar segments. The intended crowns should restore stable ICP contacts and disclude in lateral excursion.

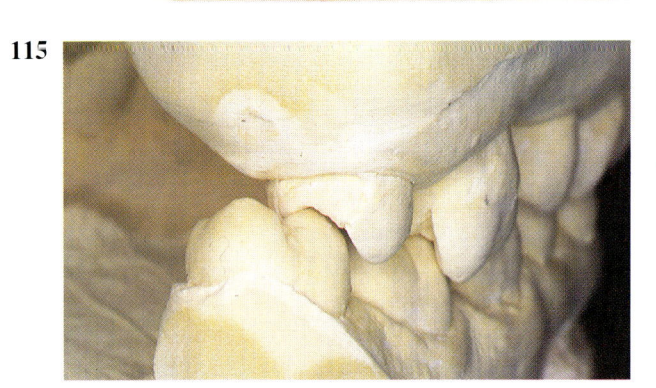

115, 116 Having examined the static cast relations, it is important to examine the dynamic relationship. Tipping of the second molars had resulted in an excessive vertical overlap of the buccal cusps. This caused a working side interference which may lead to fracture of the weakened cusp.

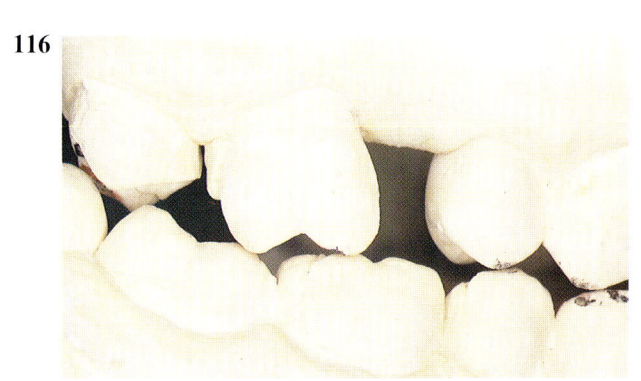

117 The third molar had tipped and the prominent palatal cusp formed a non-working side interference in left lateral excursion. This may lead to a fracture of the weakened cusp or trigger a parafunctional habit. This interference passed through the ICP contact on the palatal cusp tip, making it impossible to eliminate by adjustment alone without eliminating the ICP contact, leading to further over-eruption and recreation of the interference.

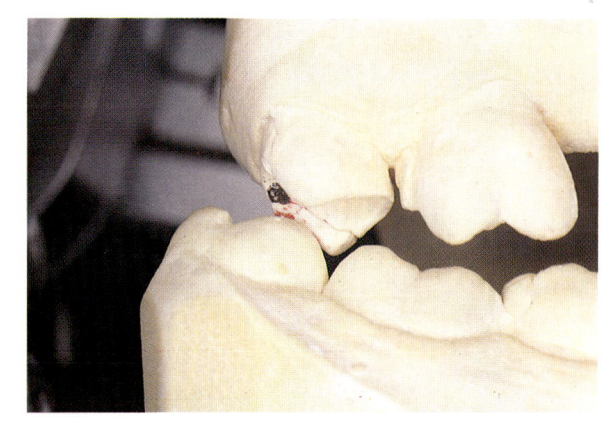

118 Both maxillary molars required full coverage restorations, to protect them against fracture, made conformatively. It was important that the new restorations did not reproduce the interferences present on the teeth. To achieve this it was necessary to flatten the occlusal plane; firstly during occlusal reduction when extra tooth structure was removed from the buccal cusps of 17,18 and much less from the palatal cusps which were already out of contact in ICP. Secondly, by modifying the opposing occlusal surfaces so that the shortened maxillary cusps provided stable ICP contacts, yet discluded in lateral excursion. The buccal cusps of the lower molars were shortened and the central fossa of 48, which had been restored with an overcarved amalgam, was built up in wax.

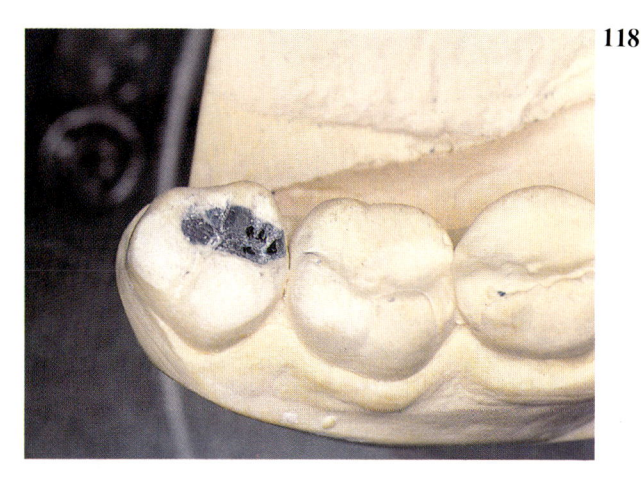

119 After correct occlusal reduction of 17,18 on the casts, the occlusal surfaces were diagnostically waxed to ascertain that the desired contacts could be achieved.

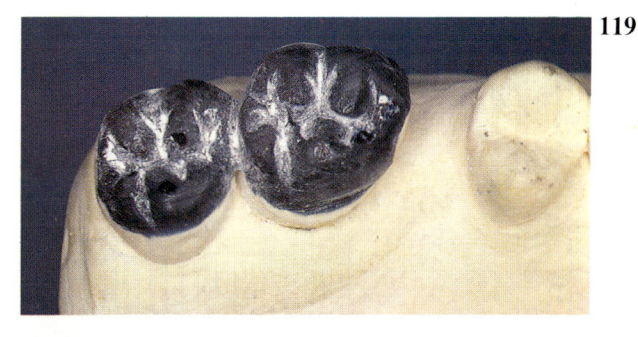

120 Flattening the occlusal plane enabled both teeth to disclude in lateral excursion. A clinically predictable result could now be achieved through modification of the opposing occlusion followed by correct preparation of 17,18. This provided the technician with adequate space to wax the restorations correctly.

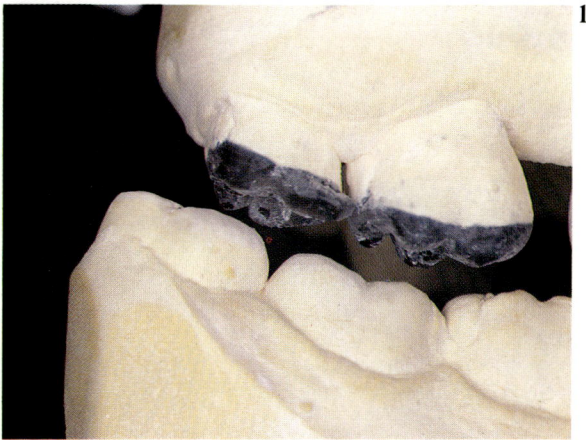

57

A lack of anterior guidance

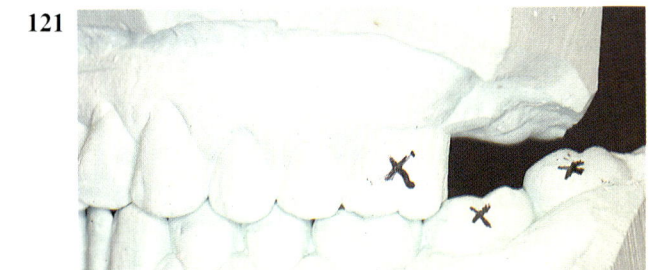

121, 122 It is impossible to provide posterior disclusion without adequate anterior guidance. The three molars marked were destined for extraction. The maxillary first molar was to be replaced with a pontic cantilevered from crowns on 24,25, the bridge being made conformatively. In ICP the anterior teeth were in contact but only just had sufficient vertical overlap to disclude the proposed pontic which had been diagnostically waxed.

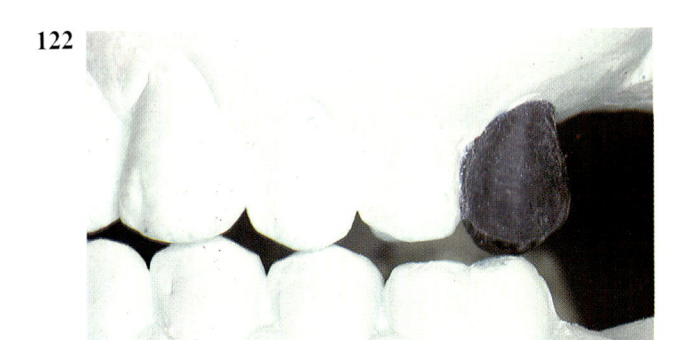

123 Diagnostic casts revealed the difficulties in making a posterior bridge for this patient. The second molar had severely tipped, its distal portion interfering in lateral and protrusive movements. The Class III incisor relation made this more likely. The diagnostic wax-up revealed whether adequate disclusion of the proposed bridge could be achieved by heavy reduction of the distal aspect of 48 in order to flatten the occlusal plane.

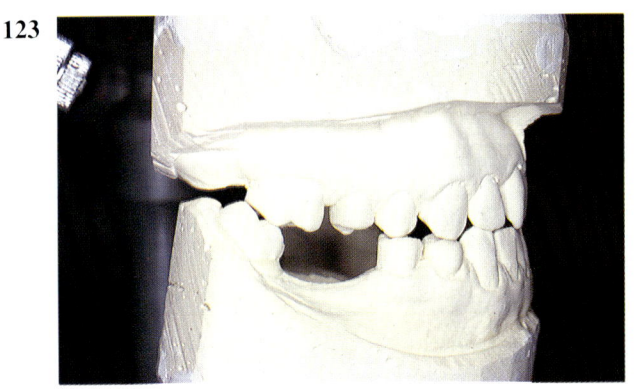

124 A complete lack of anterior tooth contact necessitates disclusion in lateral excursion by the posterior teeth. If these teeth require restoring, care must be taken to reproduce the guidance they provide.

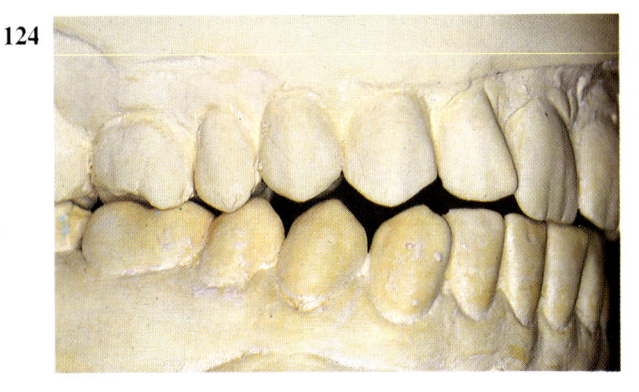

125 Restoration of anterior teeth in the presence of a stable posterior occlusion is usually carried out conformatively. It allows the anterior guidance to be modified to overcome some of the difficulties mentioned and make the subsequent restoration of posterior teeth easier. A diagnostic wax-up helps to predict both occlusal and aesthetic results.

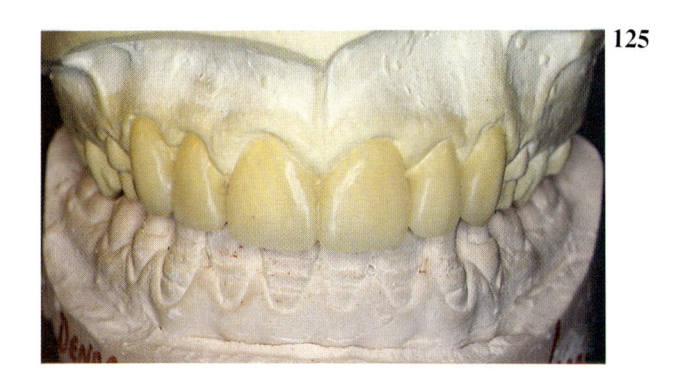

Reorganizing so that RCP = ICP

126a, 126b The presence of any discrepancy between RCP and ICP is noted along with its vertical, horizontal and lateral dimensions (**126a**). This is of great diagnostic value. A large vertical, small horizontal discrepancy (Vh) can be easily eliminated by conservative adjustment ending with anterior tooth contact in ICP and immediate disclusion. The condyles remain in RP and merely rotate, the arc of closure produced bringing both anterior and posterior teeth into even contact in ICP, once the initial RCP contacts have been eliminated (**126b**).

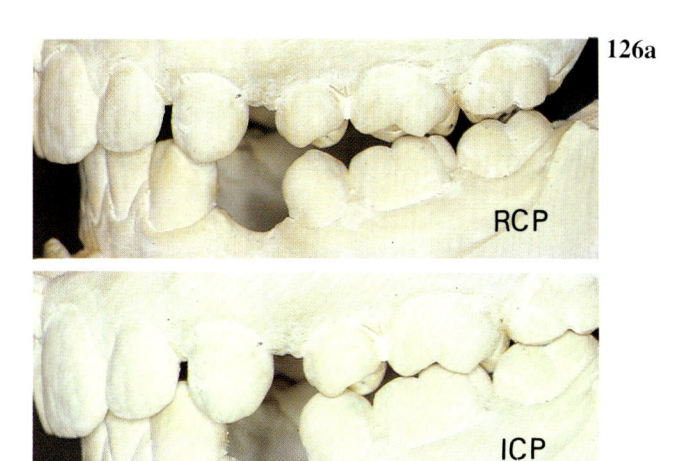

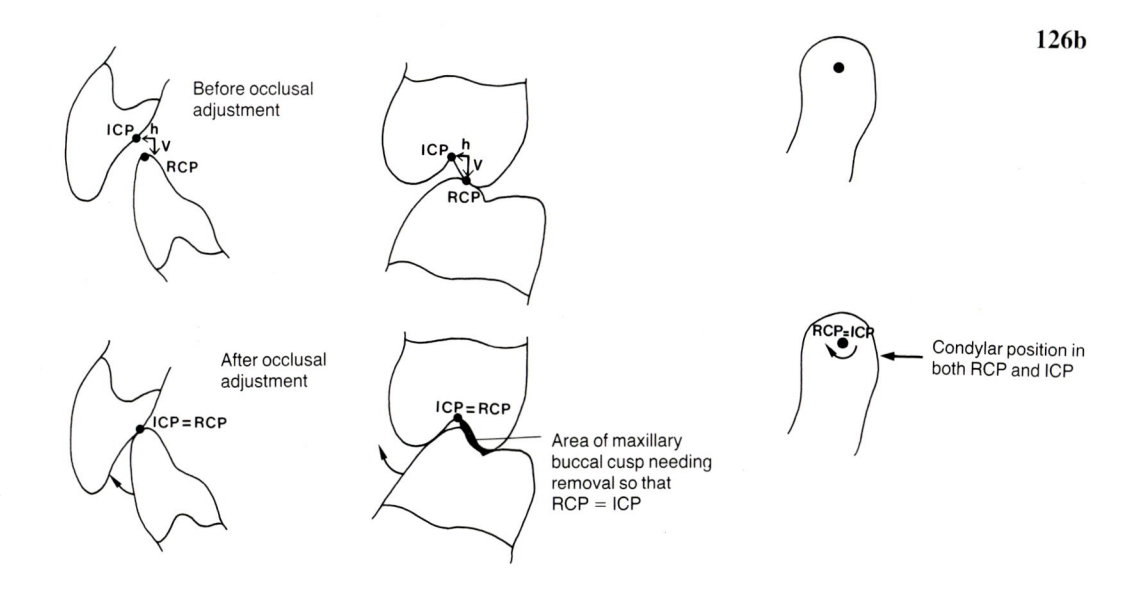

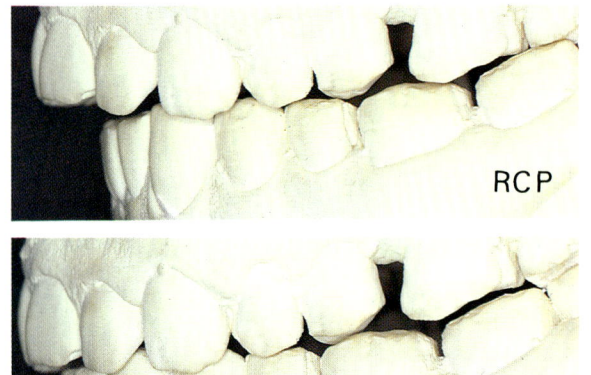

127a, 127b A large horizontal or lateral discrepancy (**127a**) is harder to eliminate and will result in a long or wide centric and no immediate disclusion. During occlusal adjustment the vertical dimension at which the ICP contact occurs is closed on the retruded axis until even, bilateral posterior contact is obtained. This occurs at the same VDO as ICP but posterior to it. The condyles must then translate forwards into ICP to obtain anterior tooth contact (long centric) (**127b**). This makes reorganizing the occlusion more difficult if no anterior restorations are needed which can be built out palatally to provide anterior guidance.

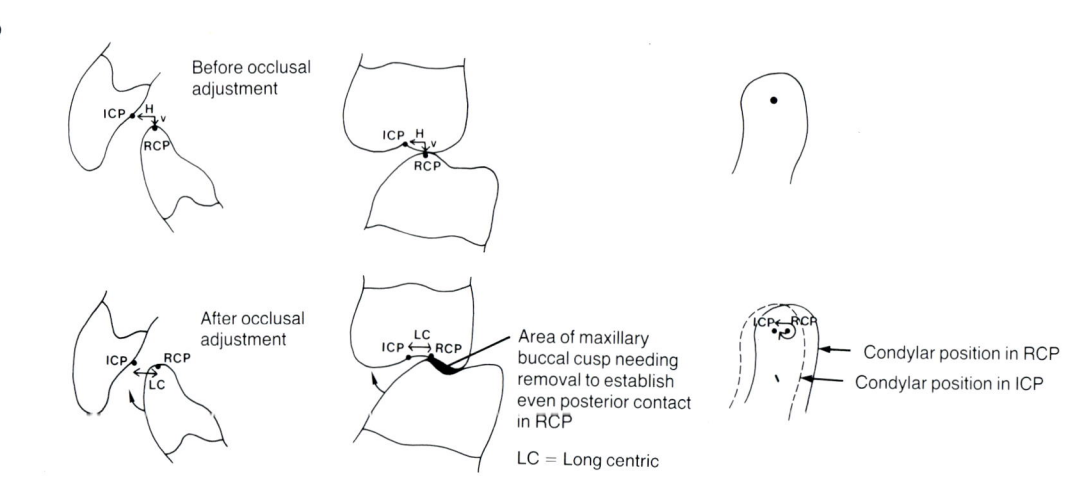

The diagnostic cast analysis for two patients is illustrated. The first had a large vertical, small horizontal discrepancy between RCP and ICP, and the second, a large horizontal, small vertical discrepancy. Further examples are illustrated of patients in whom reorganisation is indicated.

A large vertical, small horizontal (Vh) RCP–ICP discrepancy

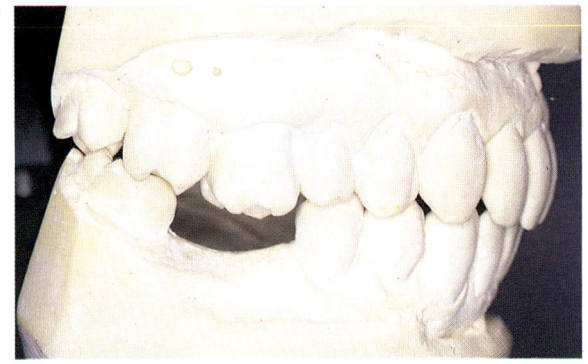

128 This patient needed a bridge to replace a missing mandibular molar and to prevent further over-eruption of the maxillary first molar. It was essential to reduce the height of the over-erupted tooth first, to level the occlusal plane and eliminate lateral or protrusive interferences between 16 and the bridge. This common problem is often dealt with simply by grinding the over-erupted cusps. In this case it was necessary to reduce the occlusal surface of 16 so much that restoration of the tooth with a ¾ crown was needed.

129, 130 Most posterior bridges of this type are made conformatively. The casts revealed that the RCP contact between 18 and 48 would be removed during preparation of the distal abutment. It is possible that by removing this contact and also the ICP contacts when preparing 48,45, posterior stability would be lost. The condyles may then reposition subsequent to tooth preparation, impressions and jaw relations, resulting in a significant occlusal error when the bridge is tried in. The occlusal surfaces of both abutments should be prepared on the casts first and the remaining ICP contacts studied to see if they are stable enough to prevent this. In this case the RCP–ICP discrepancy was small and mainly in a vertical direction.

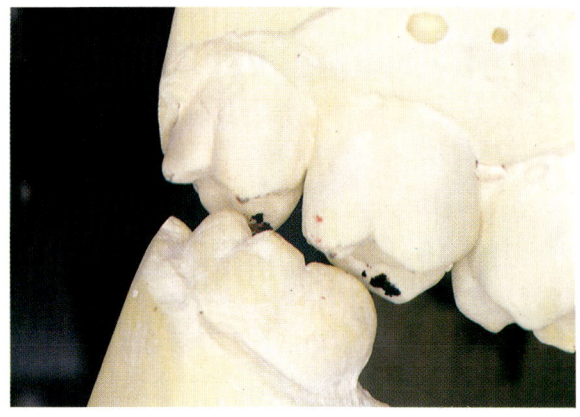

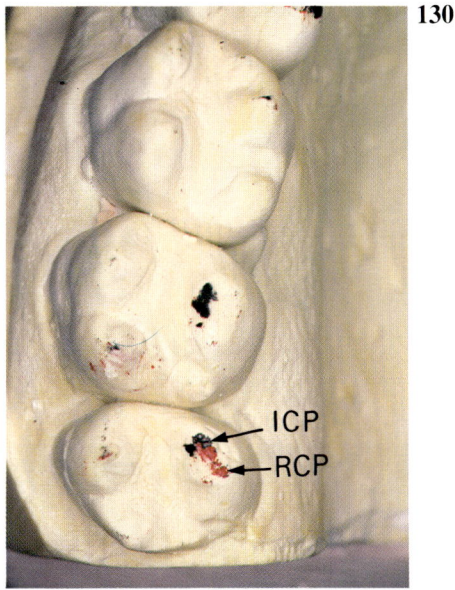

131 A diagnostic occlusal adjustment on the casts showed that this discrepancy could be quickly eliminated, leaving the canine teeth in contact providing adequate anterior guidance for immediate disclusion of the bridge. Consequently, the patient's occlusion was adjusted prior to tooth preparation and the bridge made in a reorganized manner.

If the RCP–ICP discrepancy had a large horizontal component, its elimination would produce a long centric. As this would lose anterior guidance, every effort should then be made to work conformatively. The RCP contact on 48 would be removed and the occlusion observed for stability prior to tooth preparation.

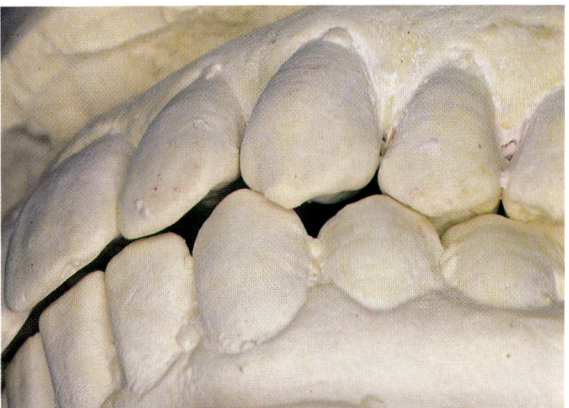

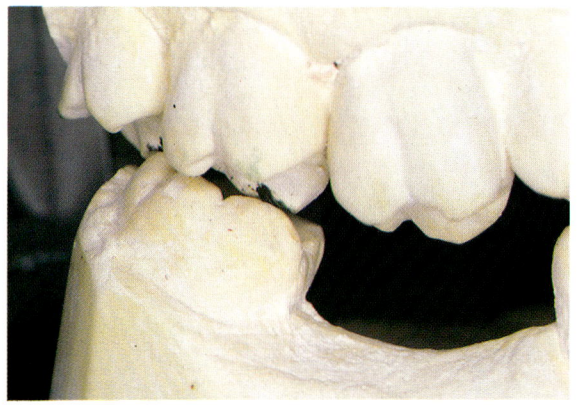

132, 133 A non-working side interference (i) was present between 17 and 48 which was also eliminated prior to tooth preparation. Note that the mesio-palatal cusp of 17 had tilted down and the non-working side interference passed through the ICP contact. It was necessary to reshape this cusp to level the occlusal plane so that stable ICP contacts could be restored without recreating this interference.

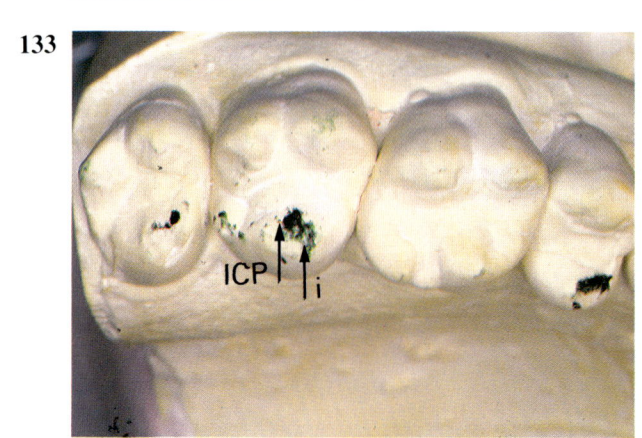

134 The occlusal surface of 16 was reduced and waxed up, the palatal cusp of 17 reshaped, and diagnostic tooth preparation and waxing of the mandibular bridge was carried out.

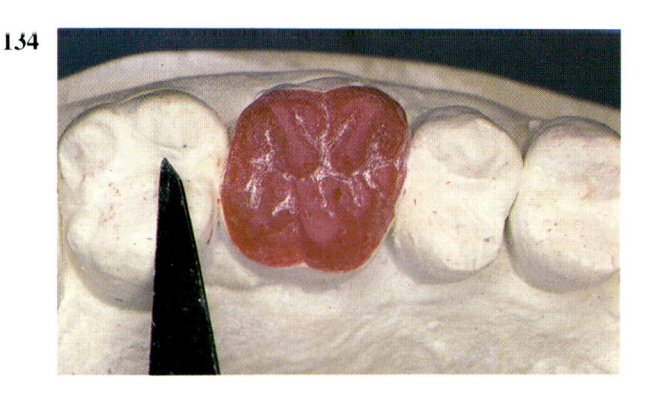

135 The occlusal plane was flattened and a note made to carry out extra occlusal reduction distally on 48 intra-orally.

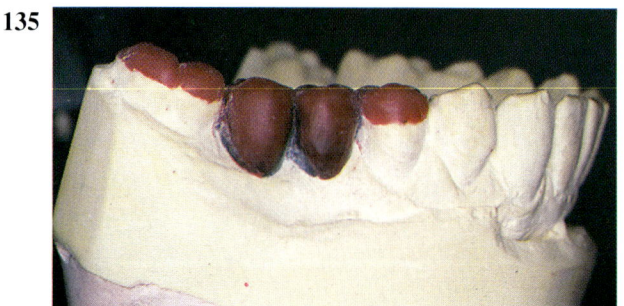

136 Stable ICP contacts were achieved and the non-working side interference eliminated.

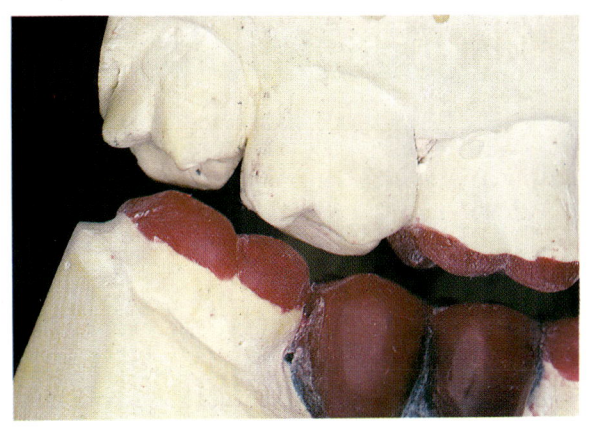

137 Finally the wax-up was duplicated in yellow stone and vacuformed shells made over the casts. These served as matrices for provisional restorations and tooth preparation guides to insure adequate occlusal clearance relative to the intended outline form of the bridge and ¾ crown.

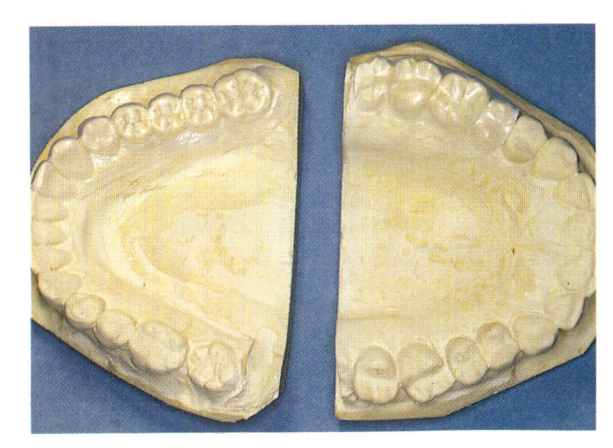

A large horizontal, small vertical (Hv) RCP–ICP discrepancy

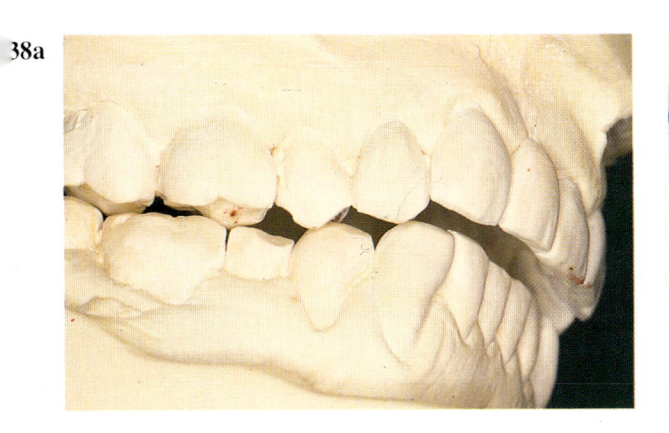

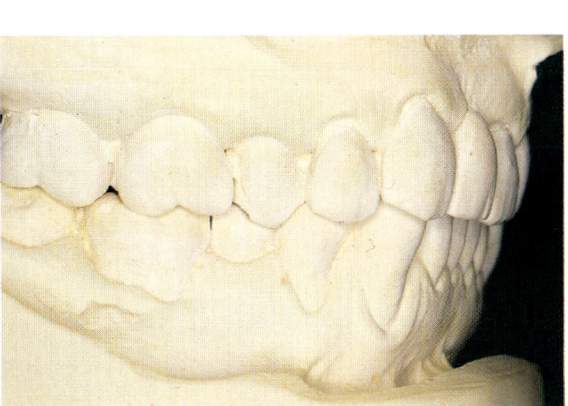

138a, 138b These casts reveal a large horizontal discrepancy between RCP (**138a**) and ICP (**138b**) with only a small vertical component.

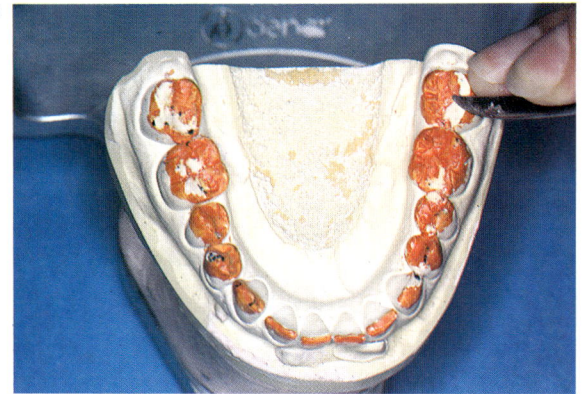

139 Diagnostic casts may be used to practise equilibration to see whether a conservative removal of enamel will produce a satisfactory and stable occlusal relationship. It is essential to be able to envisage the end result before carrying out an irreversible procedure on a patient.

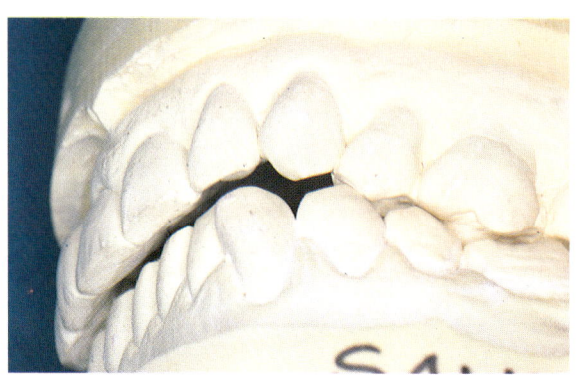

140 Diagnostic cast adjustment has achieved bilateral posterior contact in retruded, but with no anterior contact and consequently compromised anterior guidance.

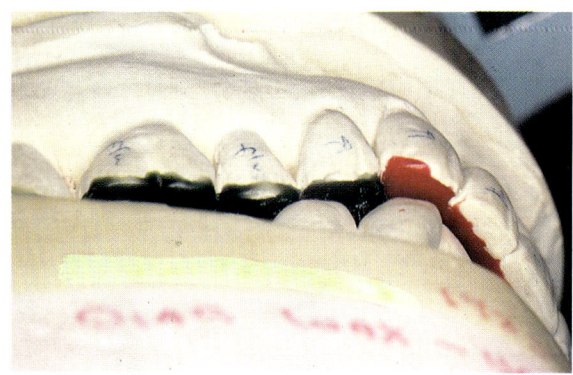

141 The anterior teeth and all maxillary posteriors required restoration and in view of the large number of units involved it was decided to reorganize the occlusion. Building up the cingulum areas of the anterior crowns resulted in contact with the lower incisors and hence immediate disclusion could be achieved. If the anterior teeth had not required restoration, immediate disclusion could have been achieved by reducing the occlusal vertical dimension. If only one quadrant had required restoration, it would have been more sensible to work conformatively.

Reorganizing to create space in the anterior region

142 This patient required restoration of severely worn mandibular anterior teeth with porcelain-fused-to-metal crowns. In ICP there was no space available in which to place the crowns as the anterior teeth were in contact. However, due to a large horizontal discrepancy between RCP and ICP, reorganizing the occlusion created space for longer and more aesthetic restorations. It is helpful to treat patients with anterior wear requiring crowns in this way. If no significant horizontal discrepancy exists, it may be necessary to use an anterior cobalt/chrome biteplane to make room by intruding the lower anterior teeth and allowing the posterior teeth to erupt, as no anterior space will be created by reorganizing the occlusion.

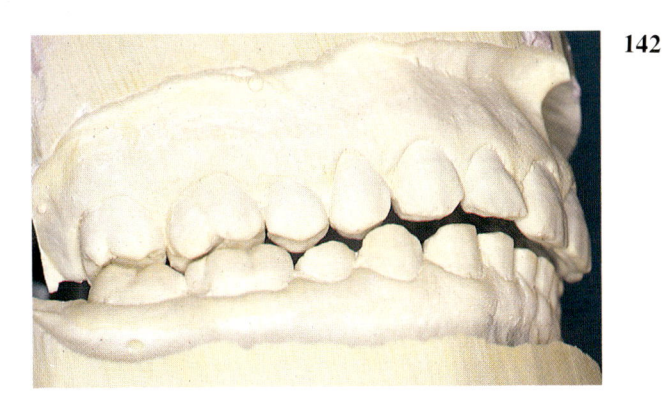

Other indications for reorganizing the occlusion

143 This patient required two mandibular bridges. If there was a large horizontal discrepancy between RCP and ICP, it would be easier to work conformatively to maintain the existing ICP, completing one bridge before starting the other. If the RCP–ICP slide could be easily eliminated, maintaining anterior tooth contact in retruded, it would be more sensible to reorganize the occlusion as the condyles are likely to reposition following tooth preparation.

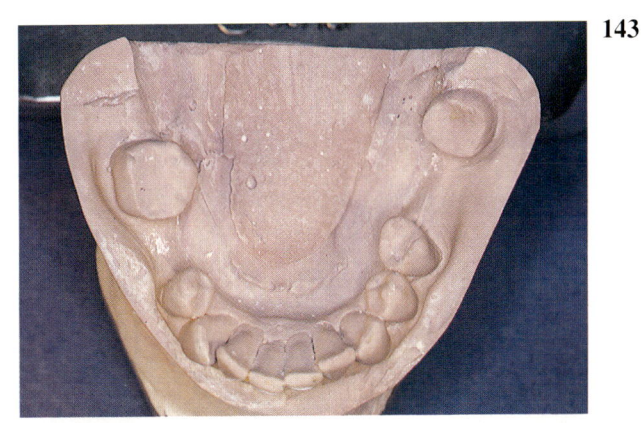

144 As this patient had no stable intercuspal position and required full-mouth restorations, there was no option but to reorganize.

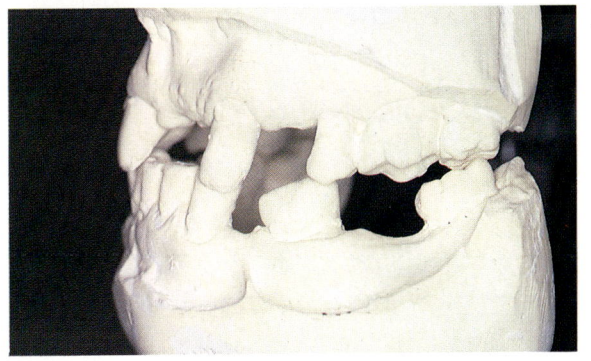

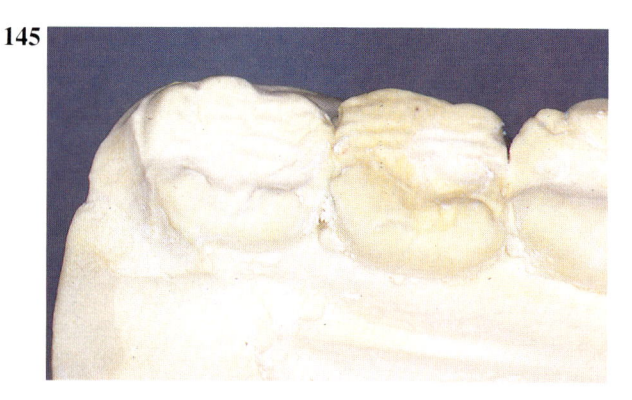

145 This patient presented with acute mandibular dysfunction which occurred after placement of very large and incorrectly shaped fillings. The lack of attention to restoring ICP contacts and the subsequent attempts at 'occlusal adjustment' had caused posterior instability. The dysfunction must be eliminated and the occlusion reorganized before new restorations are made.

The use of diagnostic casts in predicting the outcome of orthodontics and orthognathic surgery

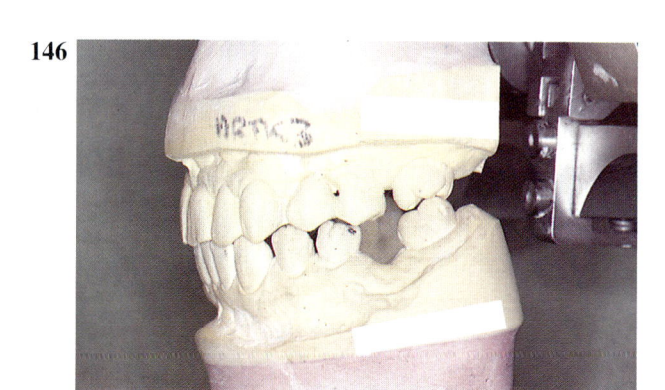

146, 147 Diagnostic casts provide a means of communication between different specialists. A Kessler set-up has been carried out by the restorative dentist, repositioning tilted potential bridge abutments, ideally. The orthodontist will then use this as a guide during tooth movement.

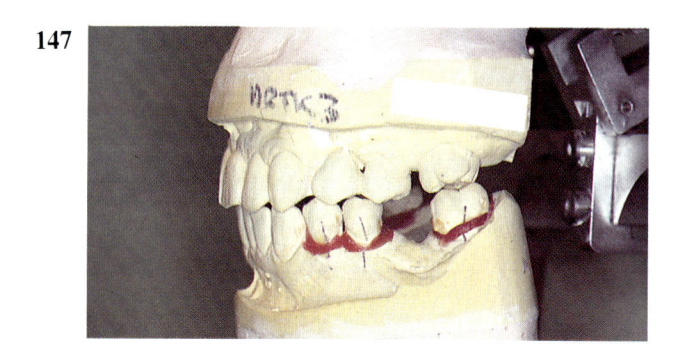

148, 149 Accurately mounted casts should be used prior to orthognathic surgery to enable a satisfactory and predictable functional occlusal relationship to be achieved. The oral surgeon should indicate where the surgical cuts are to be made and the restorative dentist should then section the casts and reposition them so that a surgical splint can be made which will produce the desired occlusion.

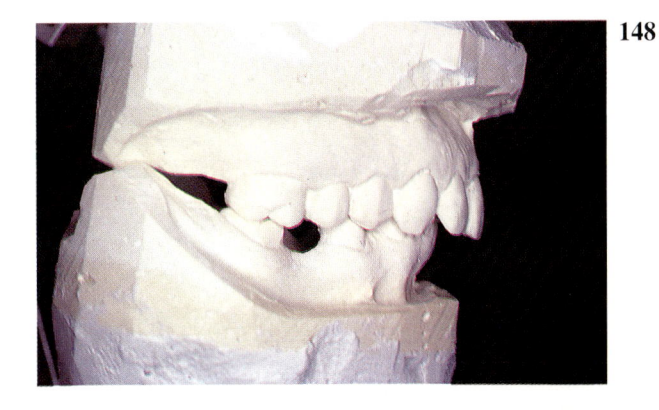

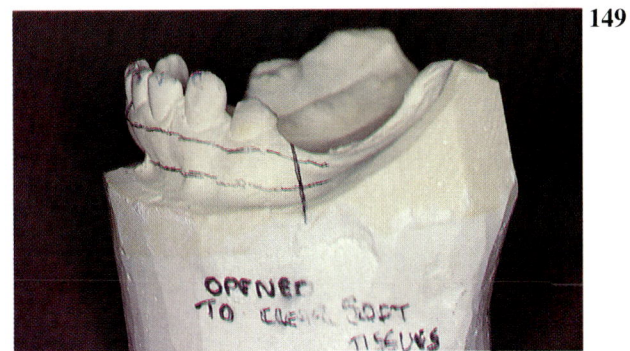

Pantographics

150, 151 Patients with mandibular dysfunction are unable to perform normal, smooth and reproducible mandibular movements. The Denar mechancial and computerized pantographs are able to record the abnormal movements produced by these patients. These recordings may be used to diagnose the presence of dysfunction and subsequently to monitor the changes occurring during treatment such as occlusal splint therapy.

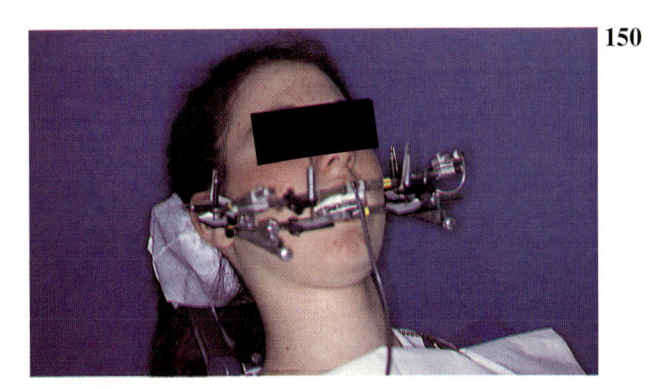

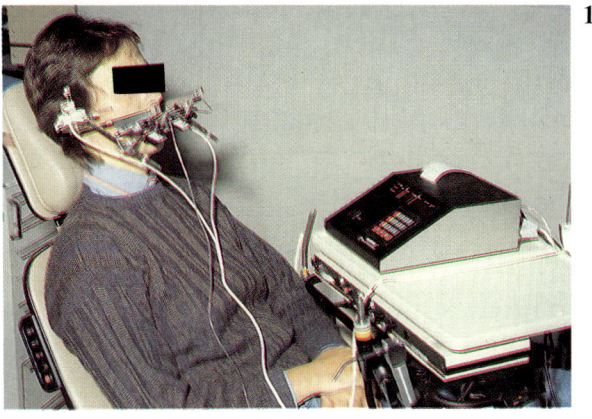

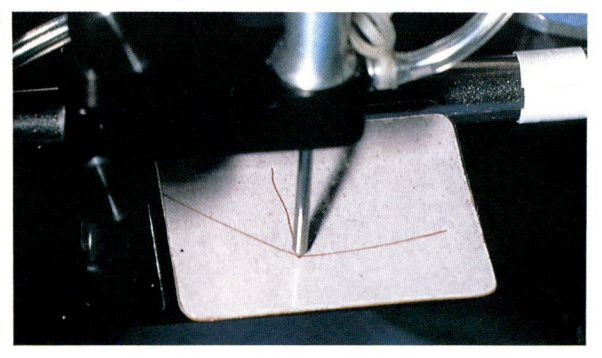

152 This is a tracing representing three successive left and right lateral movements, with the stylus shown at the retruded position. The tracings are exactly superimposed or reproducible, illustrating a lack of dysfunction.

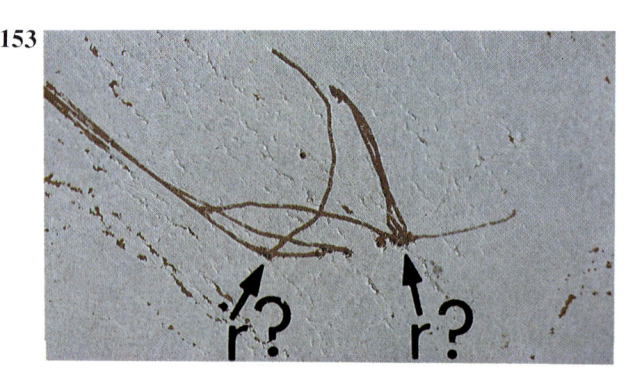

153 A patient with TMJ or muscle dysfunction is often unable to provide a reproducible retruded position. Every time an attempt is made to place the mandible in retruded, different positions are obtained r? and r?. The problems of taking a retruded record for mounting diagnostic or working casts are apparent.

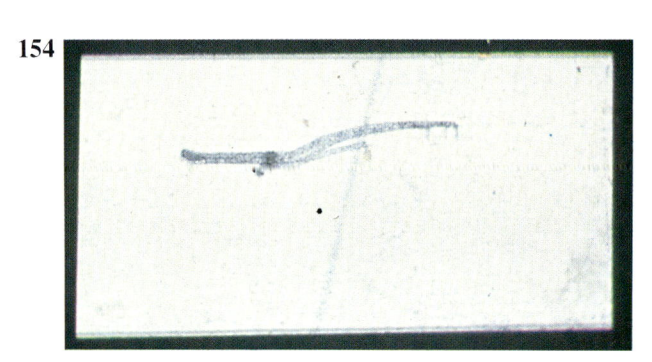

154, 155 These are tracings of condylar movement in a vertical plane before and after occlusal splint therapy, respectively. When the patient was dysfunctional the condylar movements were restricted and non-reproducible and the retruded position was inconsistent (**154**). After wearing an occlusal splint for three months, a normal range of reproducible movement was restored (**155**).

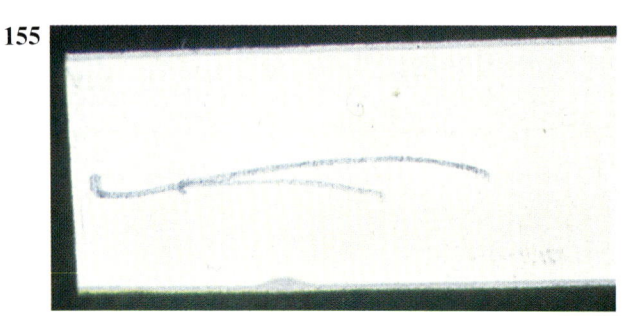

The ability to detect dysfunctional movement is important in restorative dentistry, particularly as it may occur in patients without other obvious signs and symptoms of mandibular dysfunction. The dentist may unknowingly be prevented from recording an accurate jaw relation with the result that occlusal interferences will be incorporated into the new restorations.

Occlusal splint therapy

Many types of occlusal splint have been described, mainly for the treatment of problems associated with the TMJs and muscles of mastication. Restorative dentistry and orthodontics should not be undertaken in patients suffering from these problems as it is impossible to locate the retruded axis for diagnostic and treatment purposes.

A maxillary, full coverage, heat-processed acrylic resin splint may be used as a diagnostic appliance to achieve muscle relaxation and allow condylar respositioning. In this way a correct jaw relationship may subsequently be recorded. For the same reason, this type of splint may also be used prior to extensive restorative dentistry in patients with no obvious signs of joint and muscle problems, particularly if a diagnostic pantographic survey has not been carried out.

Making an occlusal splint

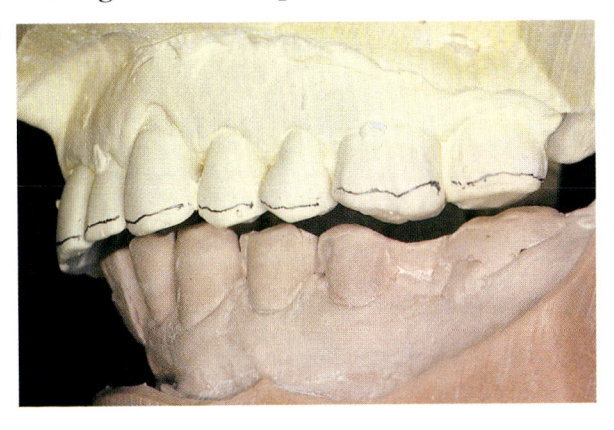

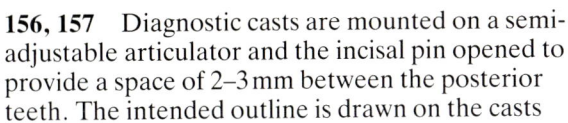

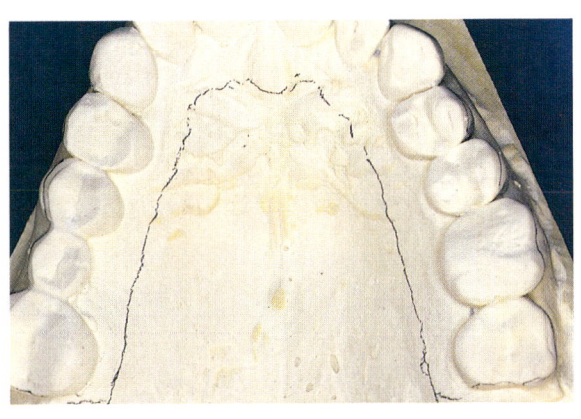

156, 157 Diagnostic casts are mounted on a semi-adjustable articulator and the incisal pin opened to provide a space of 2–3 mm between the posterior teeth. The intended outline is drawn on the casts prior to waxing. The splint is retained by buccal and palatal undercuts and is extended 3–4 mm onto the palate to ensure adequate strength and rigidity.

158 Two thicknesses of baseplate wax are softened in a waterbath, adapted over the maxillary cast and then cut back to the pencilled outline. The articulator is closed until the incisal pin touches the incisal table, the mandibular cusps indenting the softened wax. The indentations are cut back to form a flat occlusal surface against which all mandibular teeth occlude.

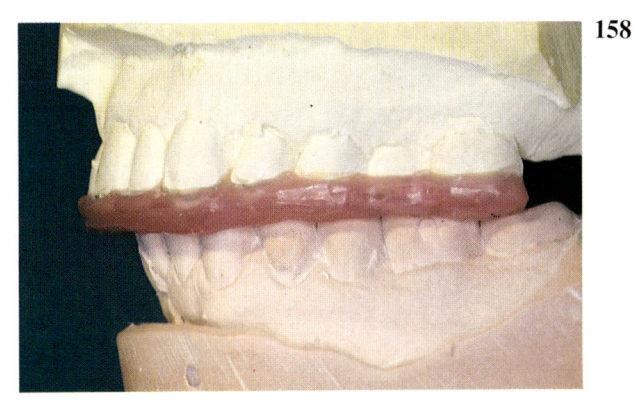

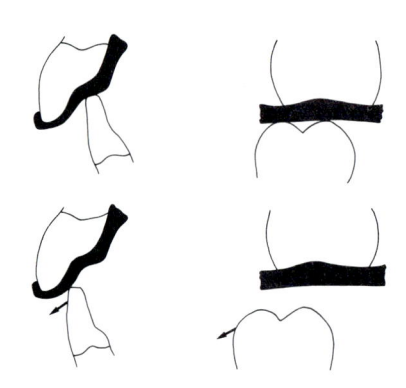

159, 160 Wax is added between the two canines, anterior and lateral to the points of intercuspal contact, to form an anterior guidance surface. This should be smooth, concave and steep enough to disclude the posterior teeth in protrusion.

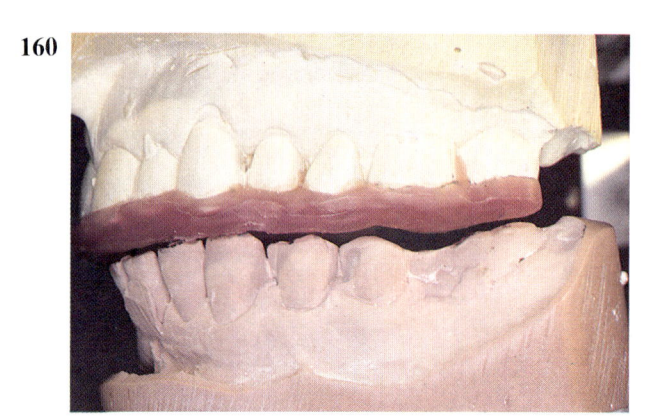

161 Bilateral canine guidance is developed to ensure adequate disclusion of the non-working side.

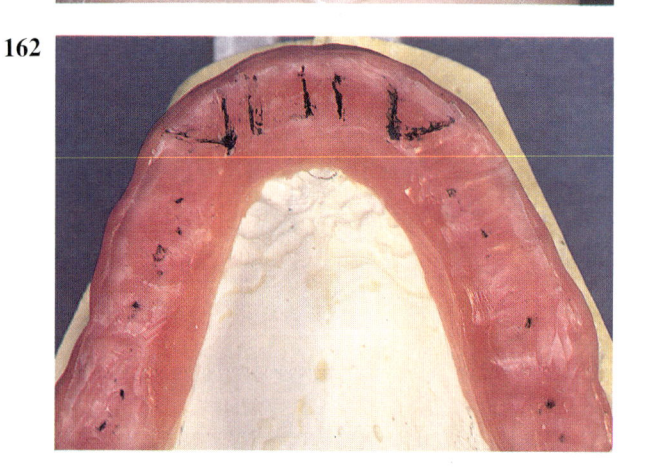

162 The finished wax-up showing centric contacts and the anterior guidance marked with articulating paper. The maxillary cast is then invested in a denture flask, the wax boiled out and the splint processed in clear acrylic resin.

Fitting and adjusting a splint

163 Thin articulating paper held in Miller's forceps, shimstock and a large acrylic trimmer are required for fitting and adjusting the splint.

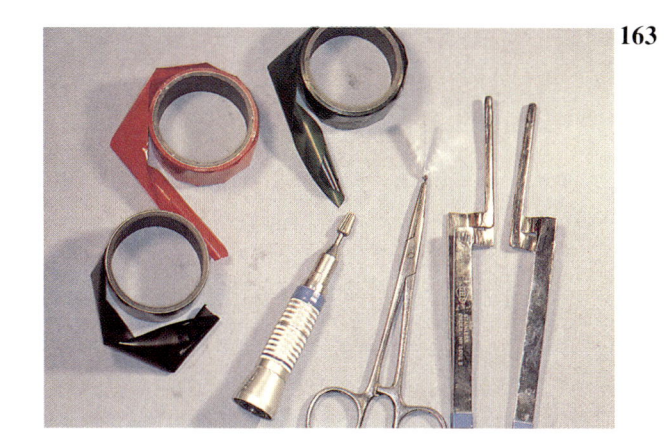

164, 165 The splint is seated and checked for adequate fit and retention. The patient is guided into retruded, and tooth contacts are marked. Initially the splint may occlude with one or two mandibular teeth only. These areas of acrylic are reduced until all mandibular teeth occlude evenly, with the mandible in the retruded position.

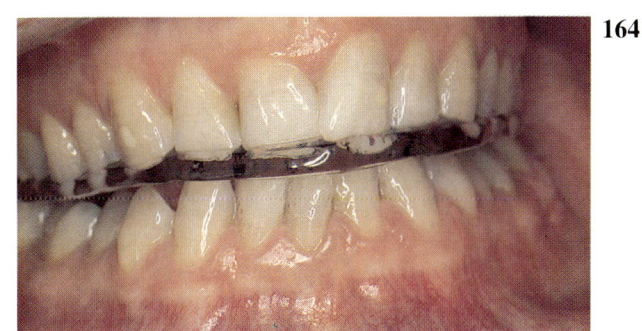

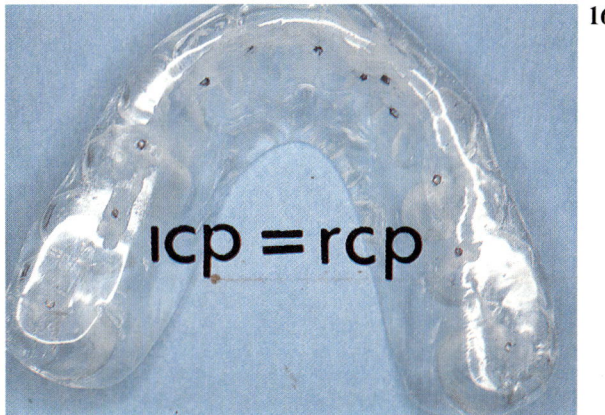

166 The patient is then guided into left and right lateral and protrusive excursions and the splint adjusted to remove all interferences.

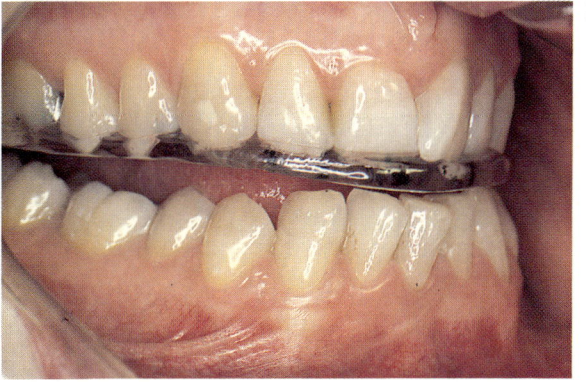

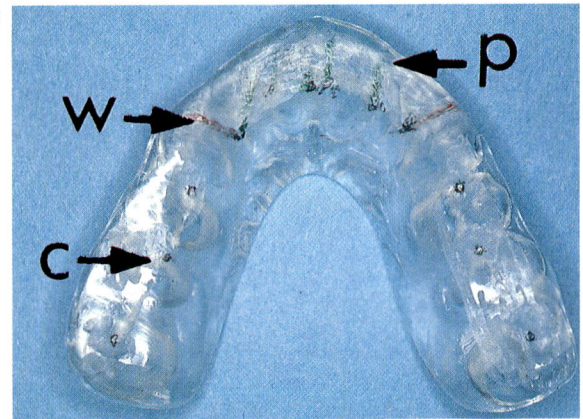

167 c = intercuspal contacts; p = protrusive guidance; w = working side or canine guidance. Note that the guidance lines are straight and continuous, there are no red or green markings in the posterior region which would indicate interferences, and the non-working side has been discluded. A break in the canine guidance line may be due either to a working side or a non-working side interference. Both types of interference should be removed.

The patient is instructed to wear the splint 24 hours a day and to return in 2–3 days and then at weekly intervals for adjustment. As the muscles relax and condyles reposition, the occlusion on the splint will change and require readjustment. The splint is worn until no changes occur between successive appointments whereupon an accurate retruded record can be taken for cast mounting. This may be verified by taking a diagnostic pantograph.

Conclusion

The examination techniques required will depend upon the nature and complexity of the clinical case involved. Extra time spent on examination and diagnosis will save time later on and ensure a better result.

Chapter 5: Orthodontic assessment

Orthodontic assessment of patients has evolved as treatment goals have changed. The narrow traditional approach to diagnosis, based on detecting any deviation from 'normal occlusion', has been replaced by a more rational approach. This involves identifying the causes of dental, skeletal or soft tissue abnormalities, with reference to their effects on functional as well as static occlusion. An overall approach to diagnosis is now recommended where the dental, skeletal and soft tissues are considered together with growth stage, development and facial aesthetics. Growing individuals in early childhood and adolescence constitute the majority of orthodontic patients. However, the adult makes up 20 per cent of orthodontic patients in some countries. In this group, potential growth is of minimal importance whereas mutilated dentitions, periodontal disease and temporomandibular disorders combined with developmental malocclusions are major problems.

The information required to make a diagnosis and treatment plan in orthodontics is collected from the patient's history, the clinical examination and orthodontic records. These records are casts, radiographs and photographs.

History

Present complaint

- Concern about facial and/or dental appearance.
- Facial asymmetry.
- Trauma to protrusive incisors.
- Pain associated with the muscles of mastication and TMJs.
- Gingival/periodontal condition exacerbated by tooth malposition or abnormal frenal attachments.
- In adults, further complaints as in the restorative assessment related to changes in occlusion and breakdown of the dentition.

Dental

- Previous dental treatment.
- Oral health care regimes and diet.
- Dental trauma.
- Orthodontic history in the family.
- Expectations of treatment.
- Dentofacial perception.
- Degree of concern about facial and/or dental appearance.

Medical

- Standardized questionnaire on an interview basis, designed for six-monthly rechecks during treatment.
- Growth and development stage.
- Growth abnormalities.
- Genetic pointers to problems.
- Trauma to head and neck.
- Conditions leading to likely decreased tissue tolerance to treatment techniques.

General

- Suitability for lengthy and complex treatment.
- Family and social history, for example boarding/day school.
- Habits.

73

Examination

An initial appointment for recording the patient's history and to obtain the special orthodontic records is advisable, so that casts, radiographs and photographs are available for the full assessment.

Extra-oral examination

Dentofacial proportions and aesthetics

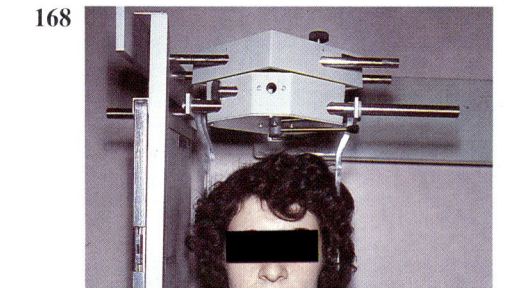

168 **Dentofacial proportions and aesthetics** are considered anteroposteriorly, vertically and transversely. The profile and full face are assessed for underlying bony structures and the soft tissue cover. The patient should be sitting upright and assuming the natural head position by looking into the distance, thus keeping the visual axis level. Natural head position gives the relationship of the head to the true vertical. A lateral skull radiograph taken in the same orientation, with the patient's lips relaxed, is taken routinely.

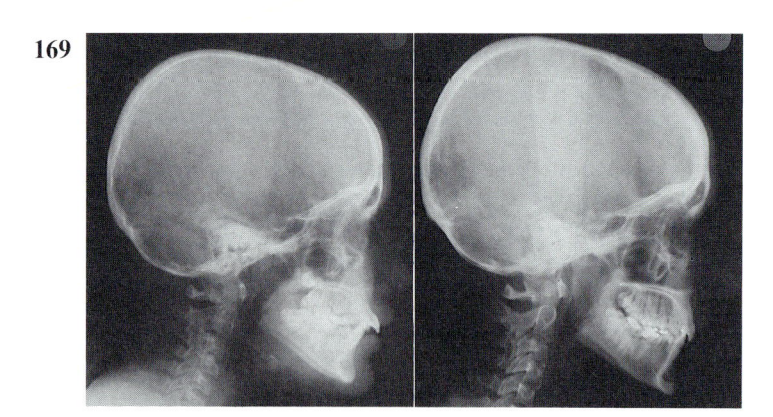

169 Pre- and post-treatment lateral skull radiographs. A postero-anterior cephalometric film is not taken routinely, unless there is evidence of facial asymmetry.

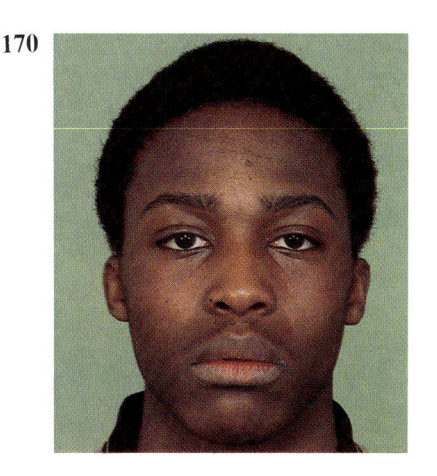

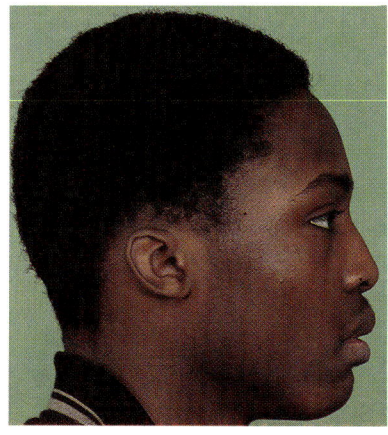

170, 171 Full-face and profile photographs, taken with the teeth in ICP and the lips together, and then repeated with the mandible in rest position and the lips relaxed, are also important pre-treatment records.

172 The presence of any genetic or acquired defects is noted. This nine-year-old patient has a repaired unilateral cleft lip and palate. The lip repair and nasal distortion are clearly evident.

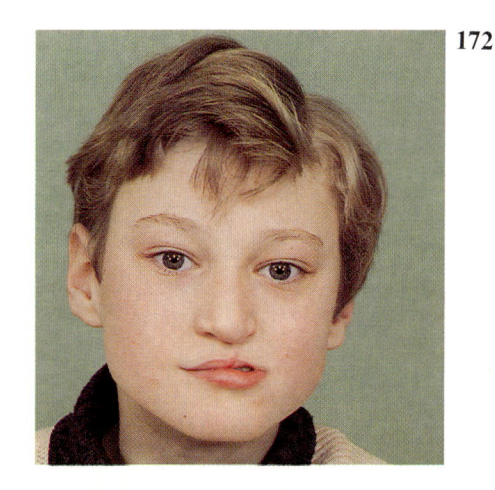

173 The clinical examination of the profile, and the profile diagnostic records are used to establish:

- Prominence in the lips, nose and chin.
- Whether the profile is straight (orthognathic), concave or convex.
- The relative retrusion or prominence of maxilla or mandible and their relation to the cranium.
- The anterior and posterior facial heights and proportions.
- The divergence of the maxilla and mandible.

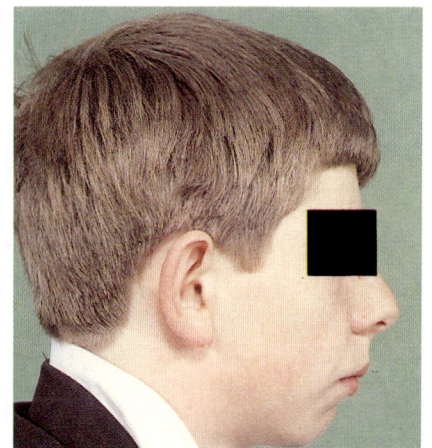

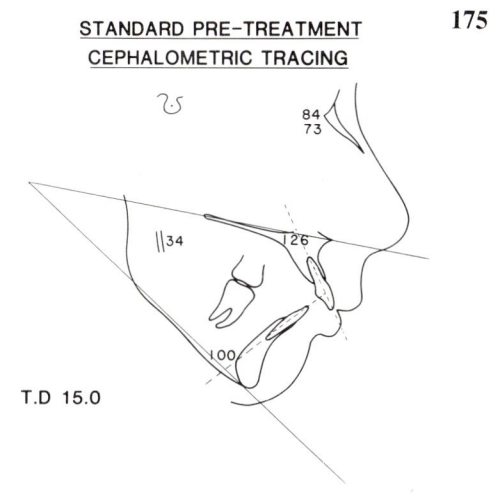

174, 175 This information can be quantified by using cephalometric analyses involving tracing the lateral skull radiograph. This patient has a vertical dysplasia with an increased maxillary to mandibular plane angle of 34° (Mean = 28°), and an anteroposterior discrepancy contributed to by both a protrusive maxilla and a retrusive mandible. Both maxillary and mandibular incisors are proclined.

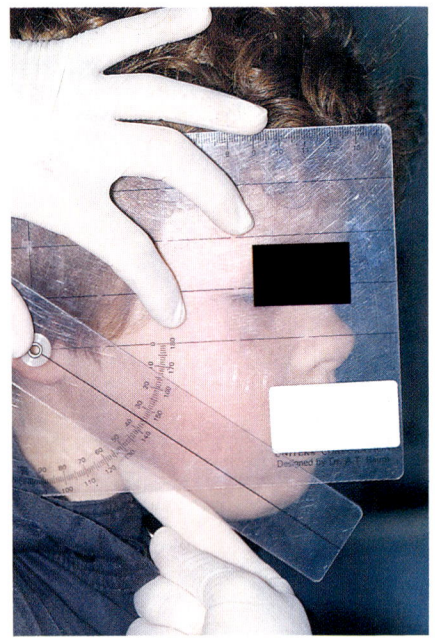

176 When lateral skull radiographs are not routinely available a more extensive clinical examination of the underlying skeletal structures can be obtained. A protractor-ruler device may be used to measure the Frankfort–mandibular plane angle, providing an **estimate of the vertical relationship** of the mandible and maxilla with the teeth in ICP.

177, 178 An **estimate of the anteroposterior skeletal base relationship** in ICP may be obtained by palpating the midline concavities of the maxilla (cephalometric point A) and mandible (cephalometric point B) with and without the lips retracted. The horizontal distance between the fingers indicates the relative protrusion or retrusion of the maxilla and mandible. This method is helpful if there is uncertainty from just viewing the patient.

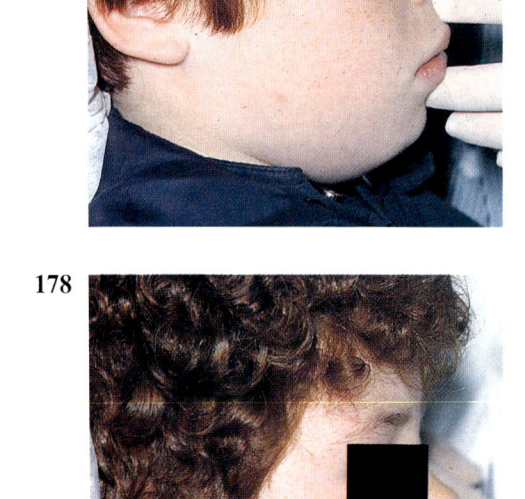

179, 180 **The full face clinical examination and diagnostic records are used to establish:**

- Upper and lower facial proportions.
- Transverse proportions such as inter-canthal width.
- Facial symmetry.
- The relative symmetries of nose, chin and eyes.
- The relative positions of dental, maxillary and mandibular midlines.
- Size and width of the lips and their vertical relationship to the dentition when relaxed and smiling.

This patient has a lower facial asymmetry in which the mandibular centre line is deviated over to the right. There is also a protrusive lower lip and the tongue shows when smiling.

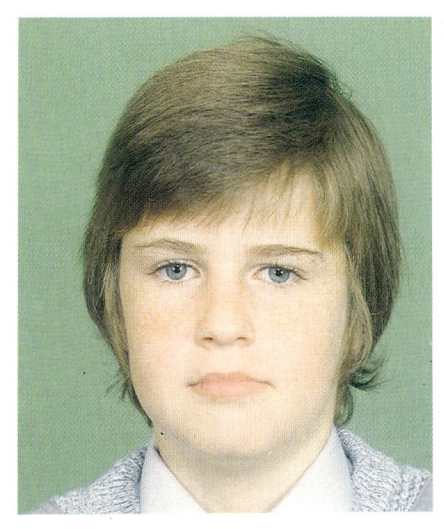

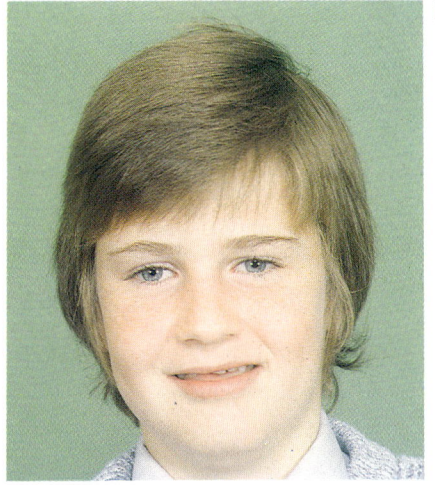

181 The postero-anterior radiograph shows that the asymmetry is only present in the mandible. It also shows the anterior open bite and crossbite.

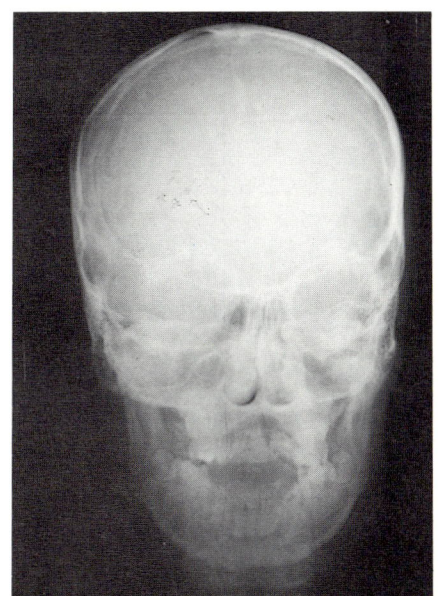

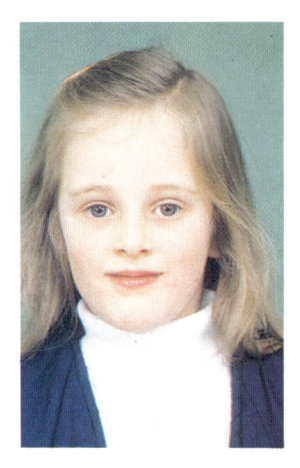

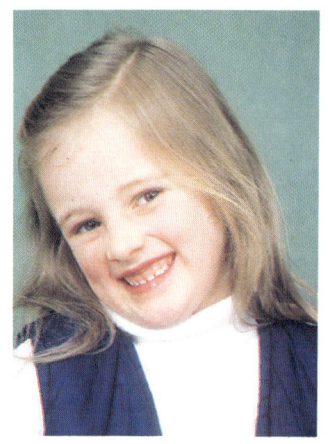

182a, 182b Overall facial proportions may be normal, but the relative sizes of components within one area may be unbalanced. When this patient smiles, a high lip line and alveolar excess are apparent at both the deciduous (**182a**) and mixed dentition stage (**182b**).

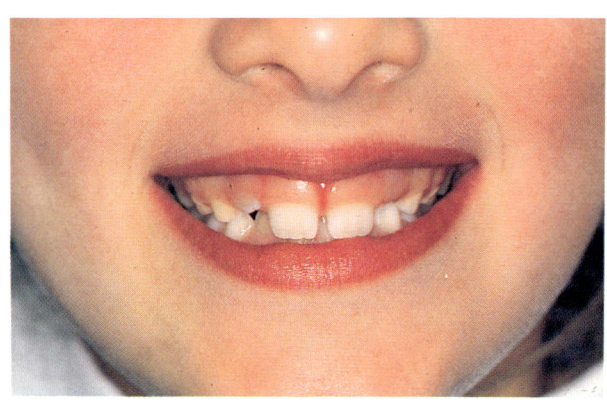

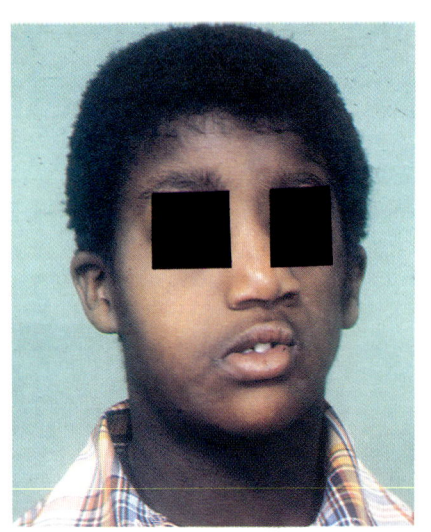

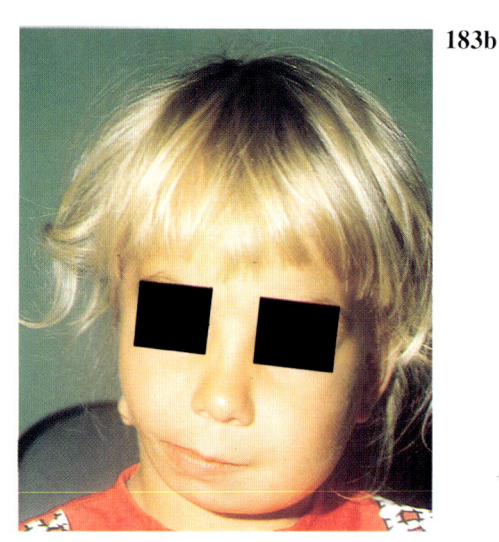

183a, 183b Orofacial muscle balance and function may be abnormal owing to a congenital abnormality affecting development. These patients have plagiocephaly (**183a**), one type of craniosynostosis, and facial microsomia (**183b**) respectively. They both show the distortions which may occur in the hard and soft tissues.
Courtesy of Professor T.D. Foster.

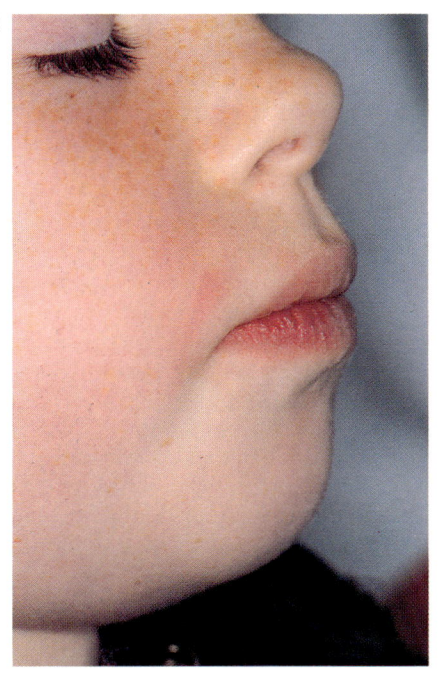

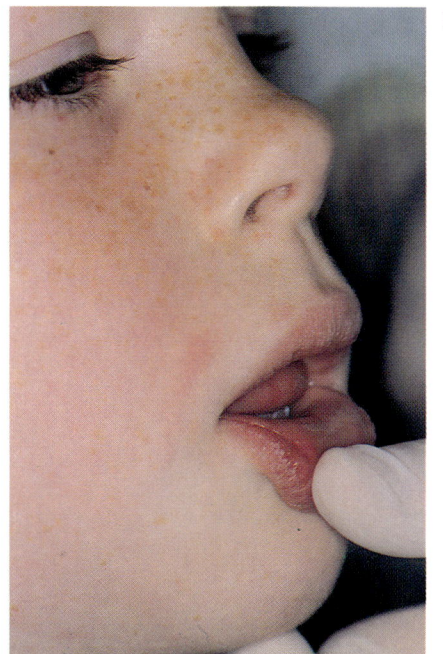

184, 185 The positions of the tongue and lips at rest and in function are noted. The lip positions and action at rest, smiling and during swallowing and speech are examined. The tongue's resting positions, its actions during swallowing and any habits such as tongue thrusting and tongue to lower lip swallowing are noted.

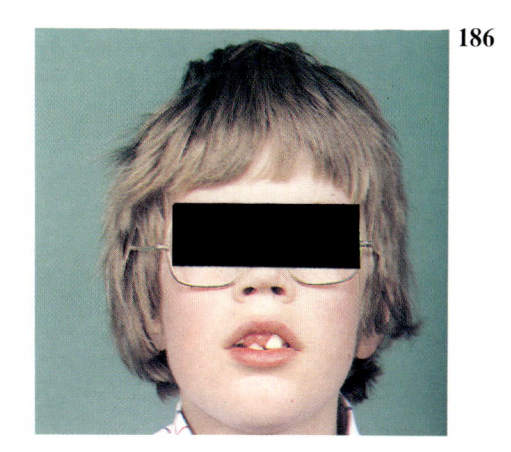

186 Assessment of the potency of the nasal air passages and the positions of the adenoidal and tonsillar tissues on the lateral skull radiograph may be necessary in cases of mouth breathing.

The temporomandibular joints

187 The patient's mandibular movements are checked and any restrictions, deviations, or clicking on opening or in excursions are noted. The presence of any muscle tenderness or evidence of mandibular dysfunction requires further investigation as outlined in Chapters 3 and 4.

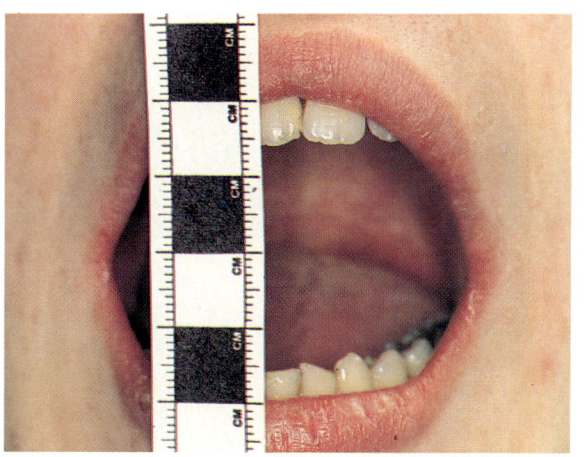

Intra-oral examination

The soft tissues, alveoli, teeth and their supporting structures are assessed. The clinical examination is again complemented by photography, radiography and diagnostic casts.

Orthodontic records

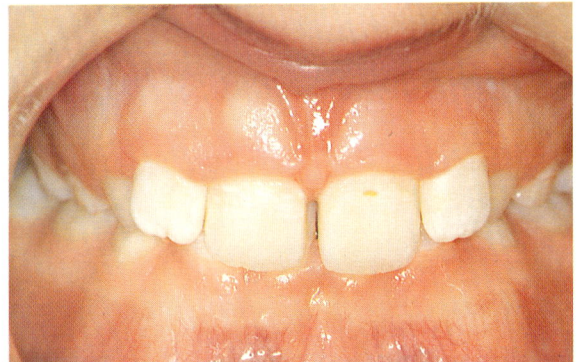

188 Intra-oral photographs showing anterior and side views of the teeth in ICP and occlusal views provide a comprehensive record of the static occlusion. They also show tooth malpositions, caries, restorations and defects of the tooth substance and the soft tissues. This patient has mild enamel hypocalcification. The defects on the incisors here would be recorded, particularly as fixed appliances and poor oral hygiene can create decalcification defects with a similar appearance.

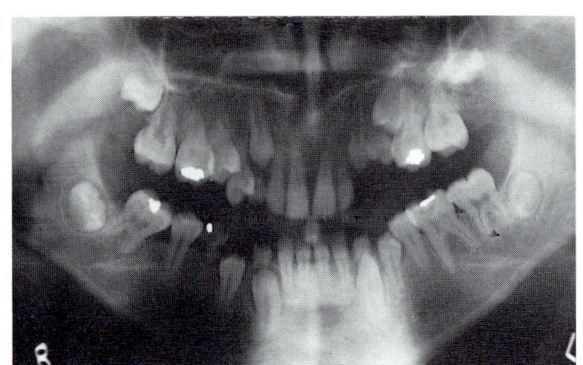

189 A full-mouth screening radiograph such as an orthopantomograph is required for assessing the presence or absence of teeth, their positions and stage of development.

190, 191 Suspected abnormalities on the panoramic radiograph may require more detailed views such as bite-wings for caries, periapicals for shortened or abnormal roots or periodontal conditions, or anterior occlusals for confirming the presence or absence of supernumeraries or the position of unerupted canines.

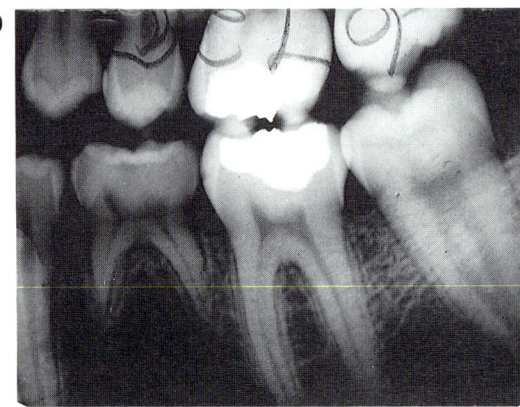

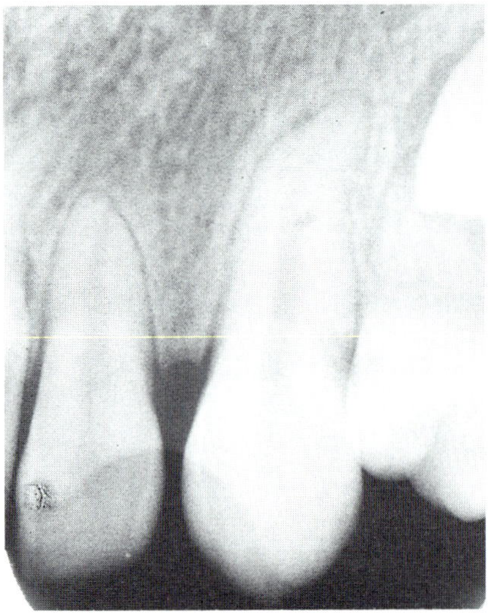

192 Orthodontic study casts show full sulcus depth as well as detailing teeth. The upper and lower casts are related to each other by an ICP occlusal record, usually taken in a wax wafer. The casts are then traditionally trimmed. The use of an ICP occlusal record that prevents full intercuspation of the teeth is inaccurate as some distortion of the way the casts fit together is inevitable. In most cases, a more accurate relationship may be obtained by simply intercuspating the casts in ICP and then checking that the tooth contacts produced correspond with those observed clinically. The wax wafer may prevent damage to the occlusal surfaces while trimming in ICP.

193 Some orthodontists routinely mount study casts on a semi-adjustable articulator as a more complete diagnostic record. These are routinely required in special cases where there is a gross discrepancy between RCP and ICP, or where a skeletal asymmetry is reflected in an abnormally inclined occlusal plane which cannot easily be reproduced in hand-held models. The maxillary cast is mounted using an arbitrary axis facebow record. The mandibular cast is mounted on the retruded axis using an interocclusal record. The casts may be closed together to examine the retruded contact position, intercuspal position and size and direction of the RCP-ICP slide. The tooth contacts in lateral and protrusive movements may also be examined. The procedures for mounting casts on a semi-adjustable articulator have been described in Chapter 2.

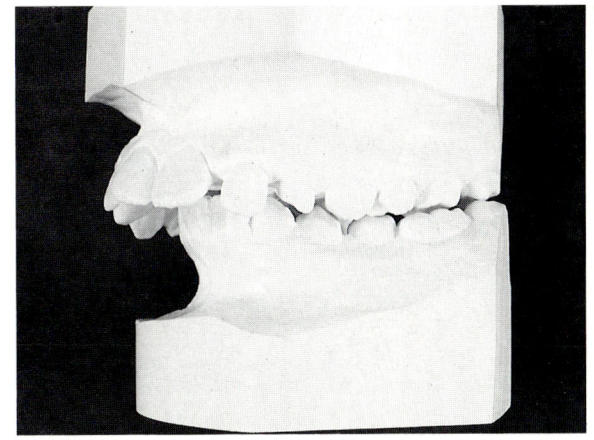

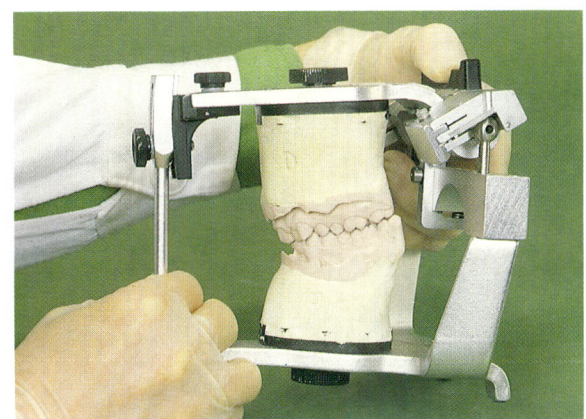

Soft tissue examination

194 The lips, tongue, soft palate, tonsils, cheeks, frena, periodontium and other oral mucosae are examined for any abnormalities in size or form. The general health of the gingivae and periodontium together with the standard of oral hygiene are quantified with the appropriate indices.

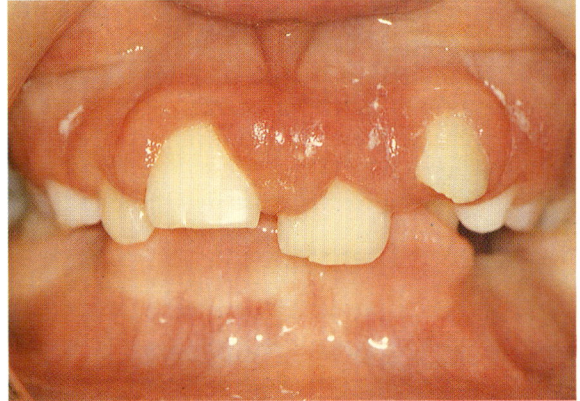

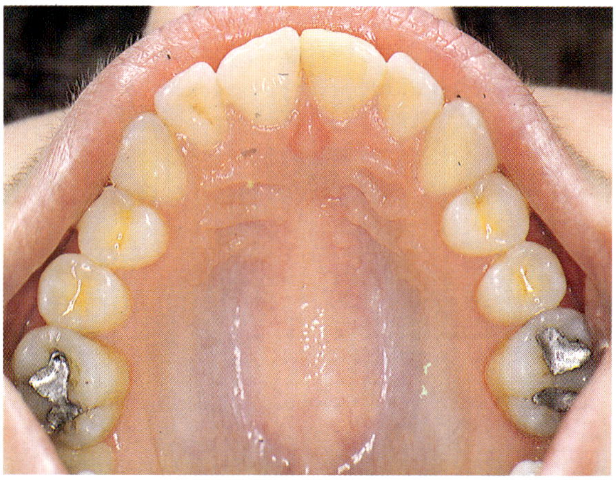

195, 196 Specific anatomical variations, such as high or large frenal attachments, and any secondary effects, such as distortion of marginal gingivae and limitation of mobility of the tongue or diastemas, are noted. The presence of gingival clefts, recession or fibrous hyperplasia needs appropriate treatment prior to orthodontics, or may indicate a lack of underlying bone requiring special care during subsequent tooth movement.

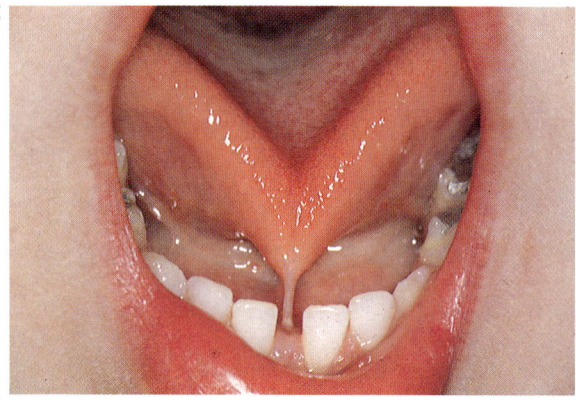

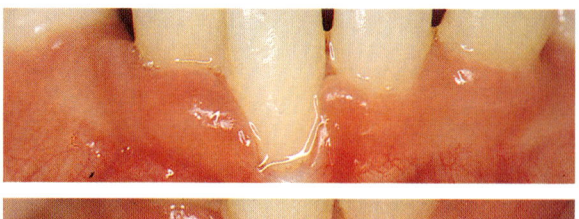

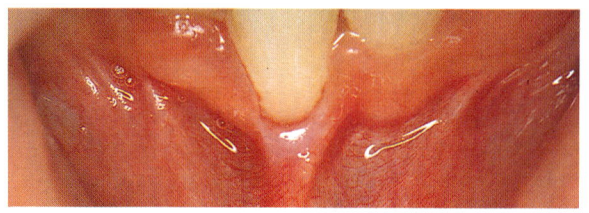

197 During soft tissue examination, abnormalities in the form of the underlying bone may be noted. These may include torus palatinus and mandibularis, which increase in size during the pubertal growth period and can affect appliance comfort.

Examination of the dentitions

The morphological development of the occlusion has been thoroughly documented in a number of texts. If the reader is unfamiliar with the timing of normal tooth development, these texts should be referred to.

The examination of the dentition includes the condition of individual teeth, their position in the arch, and their relationship to teeth in the opposing jaw.

The following features are desirable in both developing and established occlusions:

(i) Maximal and stable occlusal contacts in ICP.
(ii) A normal rest position.
(iii) Coincidence of RCP and ICP.
(iv) Normal mandibular movements.

It is important to identify any conditions which may hinder ideal development.

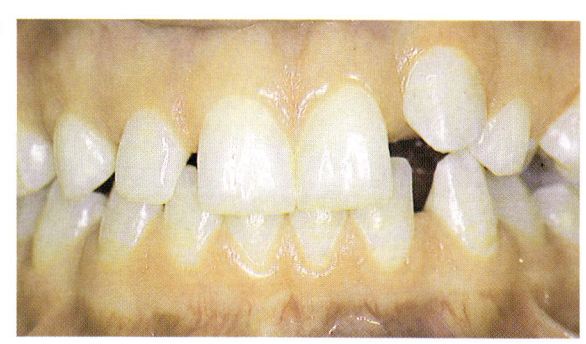

198 The presence or absence of teeth is established by a tooth count clinically and radiographically. In this patient 13 and 22 are not evident clinically. Radiographic examination established 13 to be present and 22 to be congenitally missing.

199 Orthopantomograph showing the absence of 15, 14, 24 and 25 at nine years of age.

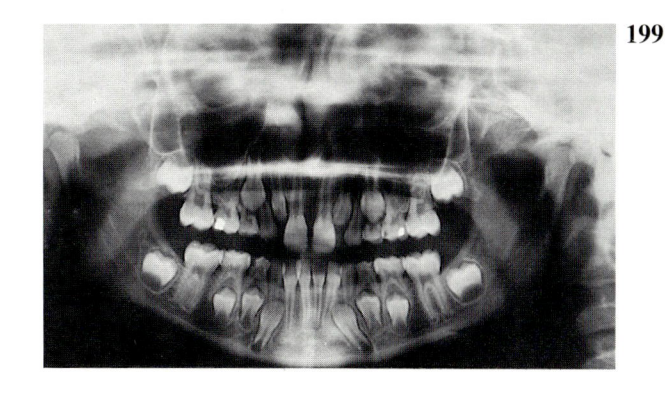

200 Previously traumatized, discoloured or abnormally mobile teeth should be vitality tested and checked radiographically for evidence of periapical changes. 11 exhibited clinical hypermobility. A radiographic examination revealed a middle third root fracture as a result of previous trauma.

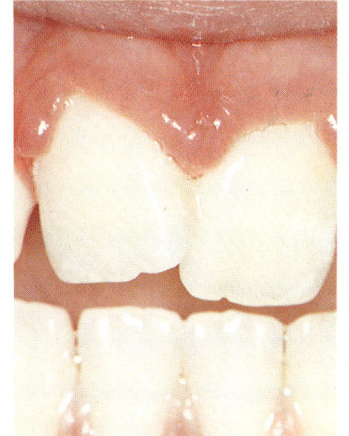

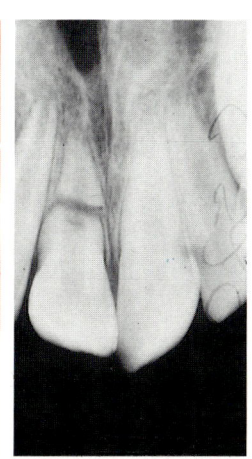

201 The presence of caries, restorations, hypoplasia or hypocalcification, erosion, attrition or abrasion are also noted. Severe wear facets on the maxillary incisors in this patient were associated with a bruxing habit. The tetracycline staining present was confirmed by fluorescence in ultraviolet light. There are **four main groups of parafunctional activity** which should be checked:

- Tooth to tooth contacts.
- Tooth to soft tissue.
- Soft tissue to soft tissue.
- Tooth to foreign objects.

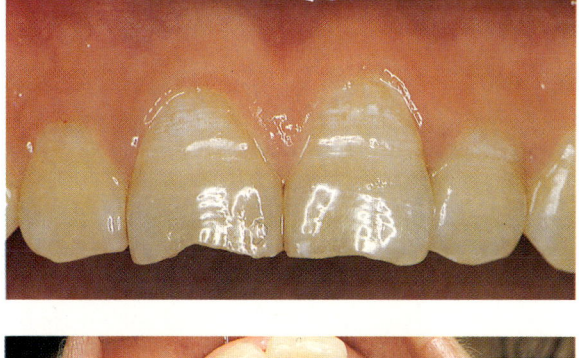

202 Individual tooth size and any discrepancies between the mandibular and maxillary arches are noted. Tooth alignments including axial inclinations and rotations are recorded and the amount of space or crowding present in the arch is estimated.

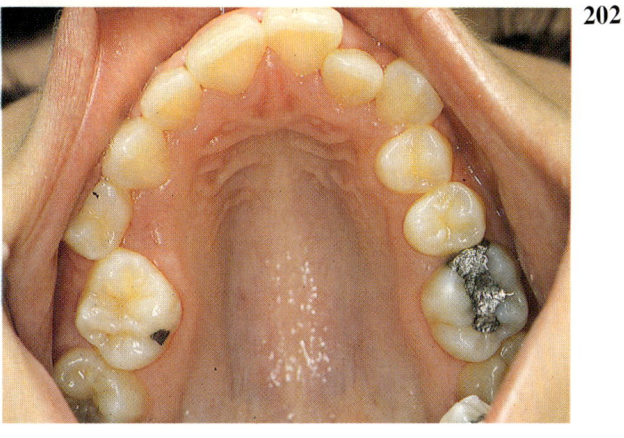

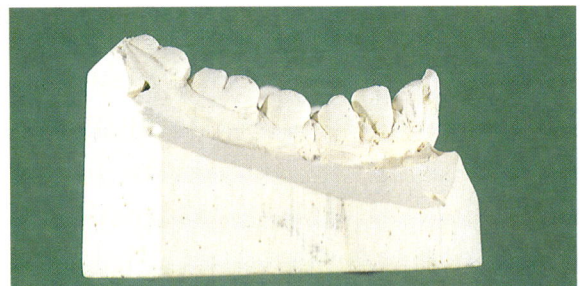

203 The diagnostic casts can be used to quantify the space requirements by direct measurements of the arch dimensions and individual teeth. If there are unerupted teeth, measurements from radiographs are used taking any magnification factor into account. Extractions are often required in orthodontics and the decision is based on the amount of space required, position of crowding, arch form, symmetry and tooth alignment. Levelling the curve of Spee by one millimetre requires the equivalent amount of space within the arch.

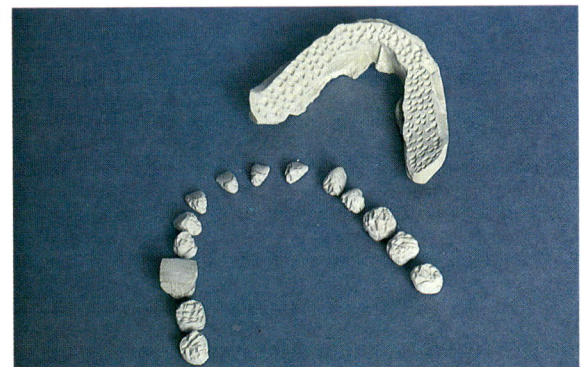

204, 205 In patients in whom the prediction of space required is difficult, a diagnostic set-up using duplicated study casts may be carried out. The teeth are sectioned and repositioned in wax to determine whether, when aligned, they will fit into the space available.

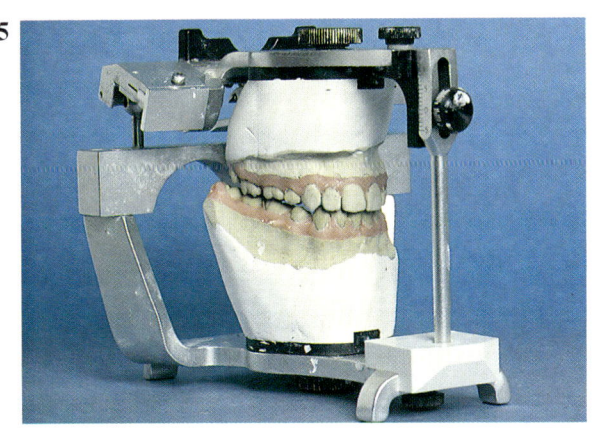

206, 207 The angulations of the incisors can be judged clinically to be proclined, upright or retroclined, in relation to the maxillary or Frankfort plane (for the maxillary incisors), or to the mandibular plane (for the mandibular incisors).

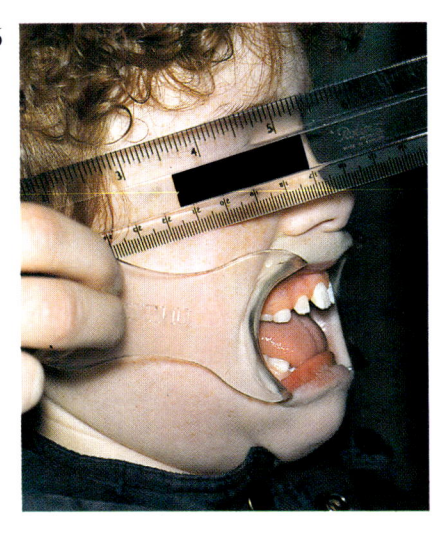

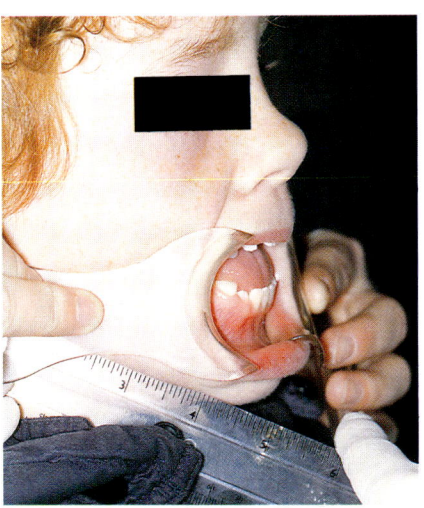

208, 209 Incisal angulations can be assessed more accurately if a profile cephalometric film is available. The angulation of the long axes of the incisors to the maxillary and mandibular planes may be measured directly from tracings of the radiograph. Their position in relation to various facial planes can also be assessed. The results obtained from these measurements may then be compared to average values of the various racial and ethnic groups which serve as baseline measurement.

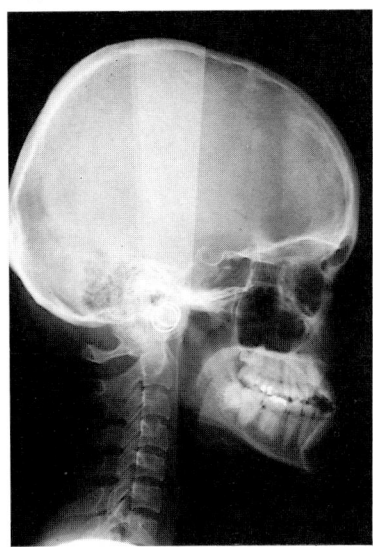

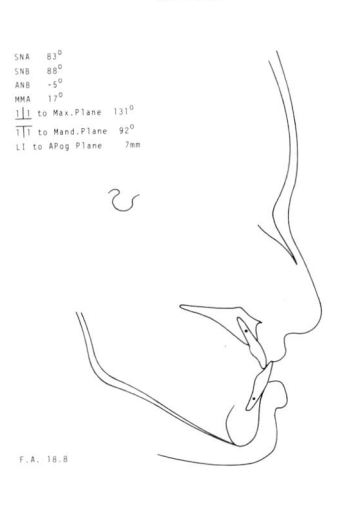

PRE-TREATMENT

SNA 83°
SNB 88°
ANB -5°
MMA 17°
1̄|1 to Max.Plane 131°
1̄|1̄ to Mand.Plane 92°
LI to APog Plane 7mm

F.A. 18.8

(i) Maximal and stable occlusal contacts in ICP

Occlusal contacts are affected by the arch relationship in the anteroposterior, vertical and lateral dimensions. The anterior and posterior parts of the dentition are usually assessed separately.

The deciduous dentition is complete at about three years of age. The change over to the permanent dentition starts at around six to seven and is completed, excluding the third molars, between 11 and 16 years.

(i) Anteroposterior incisal relationship.

The static anteroposterior relationship of the teeth is traditionally classified as Class 1, 2, and 3, based on Angle's original classification.

The incisors and buccal segments have separate criteria. This classification is helpful at the treatment planning stage.

210 Incisor classification is based on the anteroposterior incisor relationship. The following illustrations show deciduous, mixed and permanent dentition examples for each class.

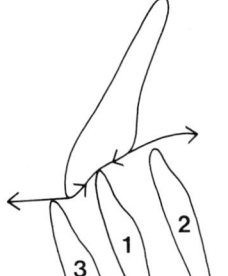

Incisor classification

85

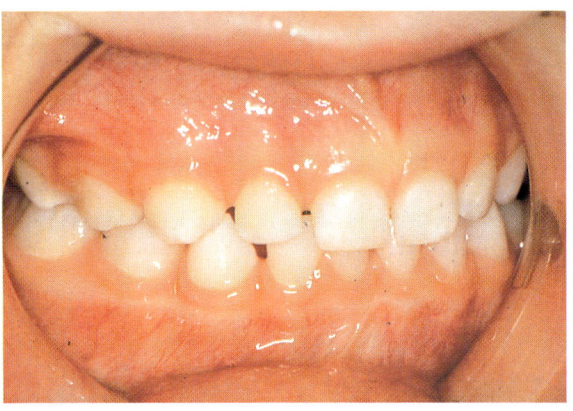

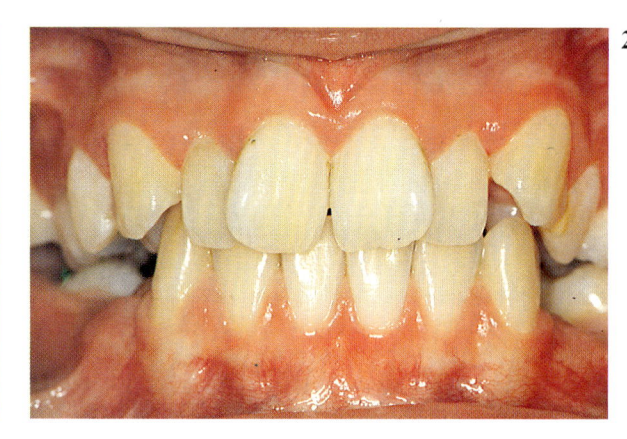

211, 212, 213 Class 1 – The lower incisal edges occlude with or lie immediately below the middle third of the upper central incisors.

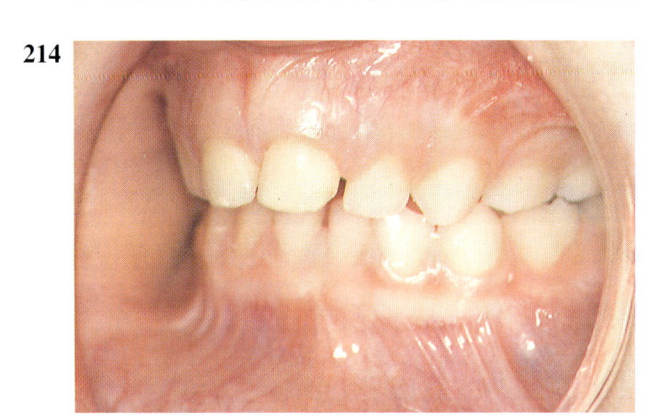

Class 2 – The lower incisal edges lie posterior to the middle third of the upper incisors.
   There are two divisions:

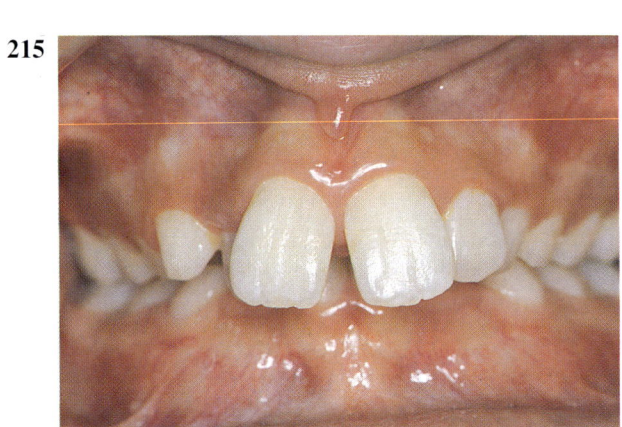

214, 215, 216 Division 1 – There is an increase in overjet and the upper central incisors are usually proclined.

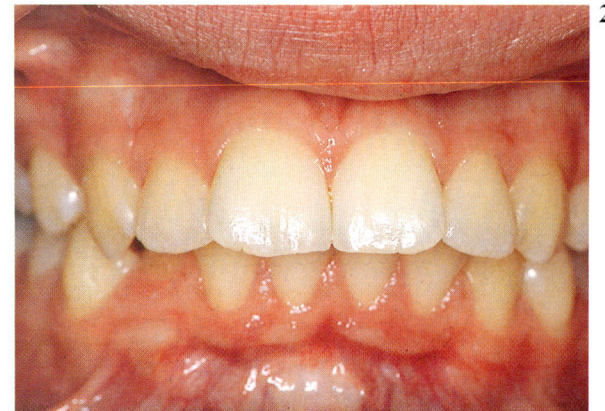

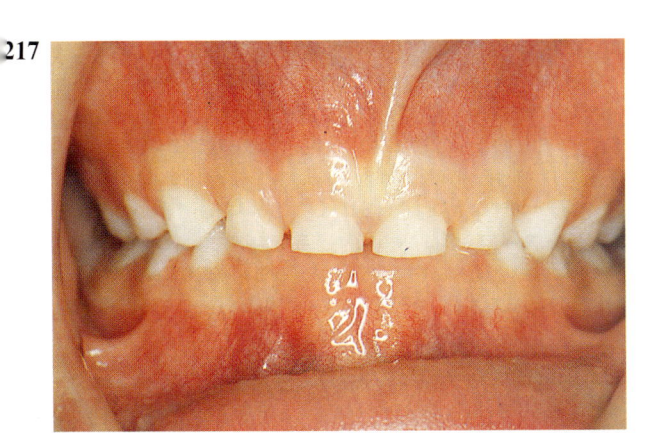

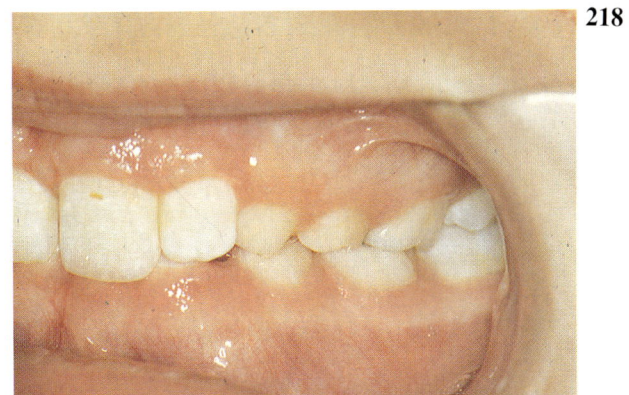

217, 218, 219 Division 2 – The upper central incisors are retroclined. The overjet is usually minimal but may be slightly increased. The overbite is deep and complete.

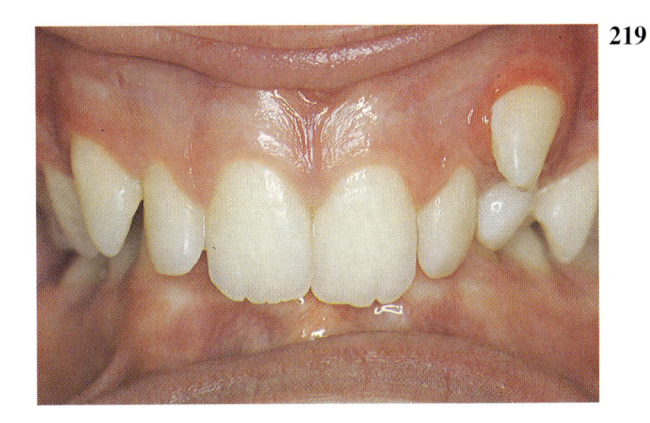

220–223 Class 3 – The lower incisor edges lie anterior to the middle third of the upper incisors. The overjet is reduced or reversed.

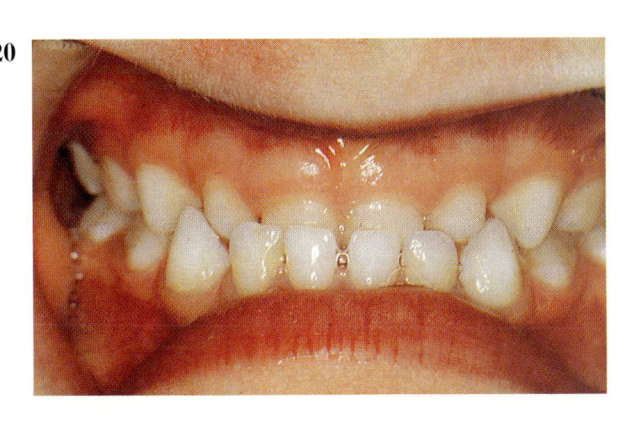

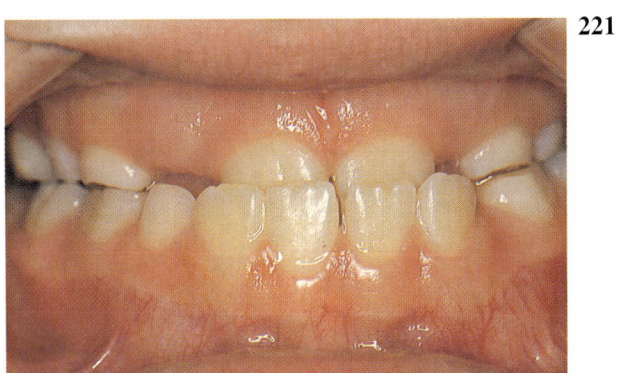

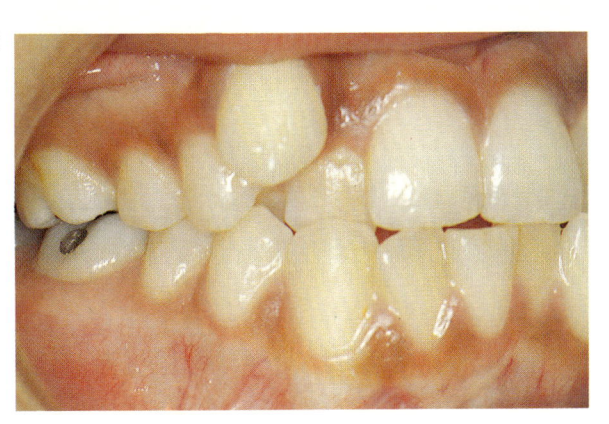

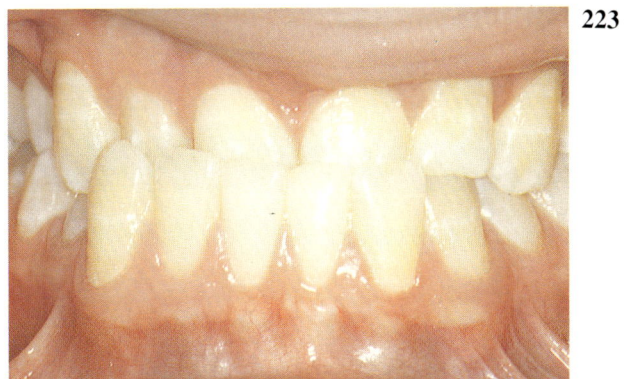

(ii) Vertical incisal relationships.

The vertical incisal relationship is classified as a complete or incomplete overbite. **A complete overbite** is present if the lower incisors contact teeth or soft tissues in the upper arch. The vertical relationship of the teeth is recorded using a millimetre rule, measuring the overlap or opening between the labial segments with the teeth in ICP. A normal complete overbite is 2–4 mm in depth and may be present with a positive or negative overjet. A decreased complete overbite can result in an edge-to-edge incisal relationship. An increased complete overbite can result in soft tissue trauma if the tooth contact is by-passed.

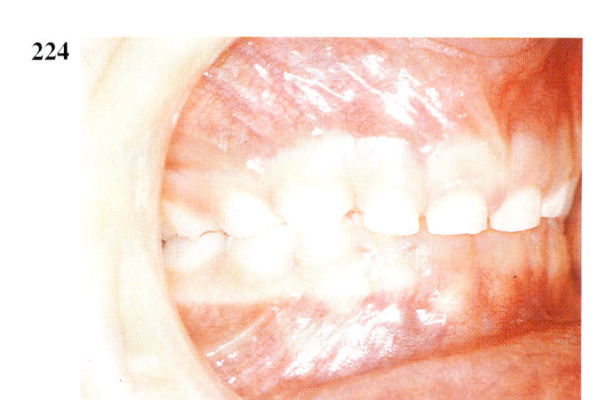

224

224–226 Trauma will be evident either on the lower labial aspect or palatal to the upper incisors. The latter occasionally occurs in Class 2:1 occlusions. Trauma is most commonly associated with Class 2:2.

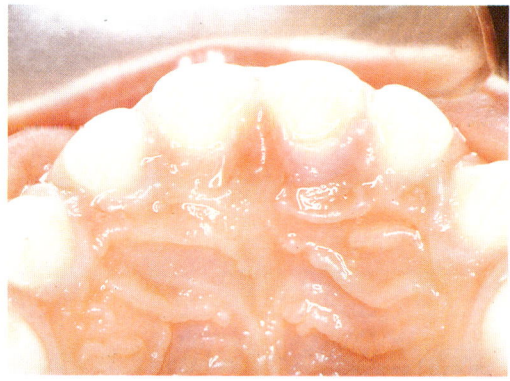

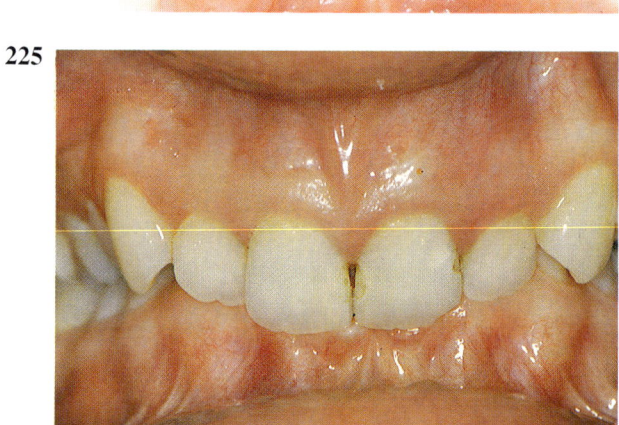

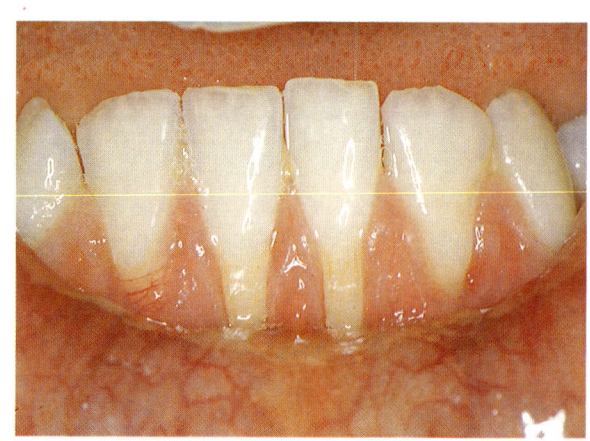

225

226

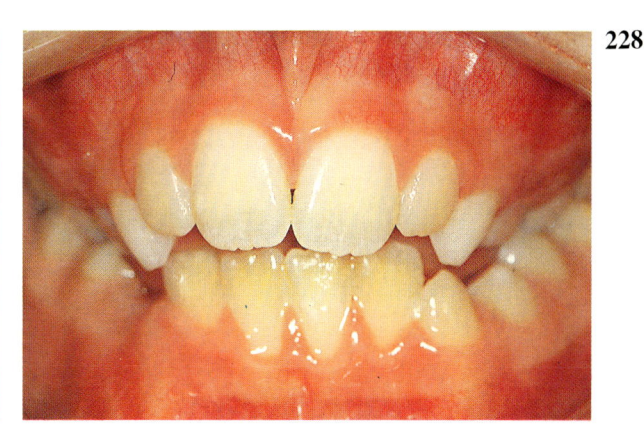

227, 228 An **incomplete overbite** is present if there is a space between the incisors. There may still be a positive overbite.

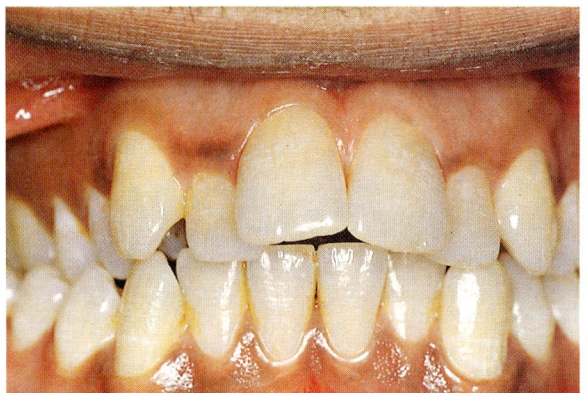

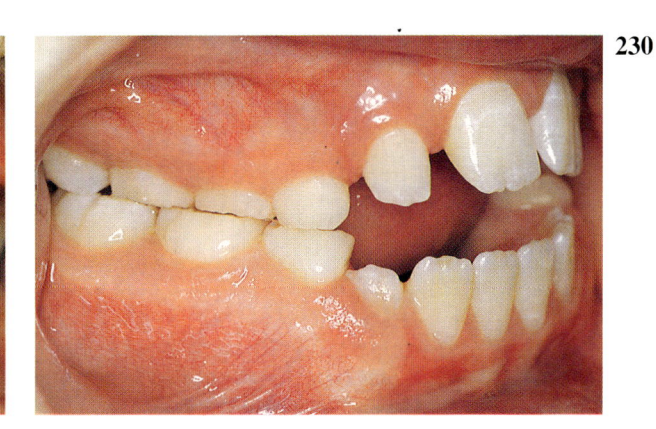

229–231 Alternatively, an **anterior open bite** may be present. Anterior open bites may be of skeletal aetiology. There is increased divergent growth of the maxilla and mandible and increased anterior facial height. In the most severe cases, patients only occlude on the molars. Anterior open bites of dental aetiology are caused by an abnormal vertical position of the teeth due to abnormalities in eruption, or habits such as digit sucking. The patient's history may establish an association with dummy or digit sucking. The habit results in dento-alveolar distortion. The open bite can resolve if the habit stops. However, the proclination of the upper incisors is likely to be retained as the lower lip often comes to rest behind it. The tongue may play a role in the development of the anterior open bite. A tongue thrust maintains the opening as a tongue to lip contact is necessary to produce an anterior oral seal during swallowing. In skeletal open bites, the tongue tends to lie between the teeth. Identification of the aetiology in these patients is often difficult.

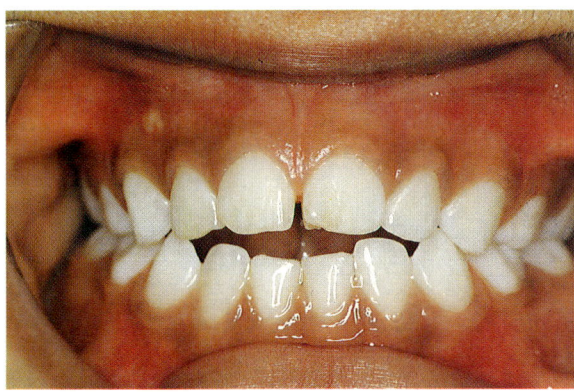

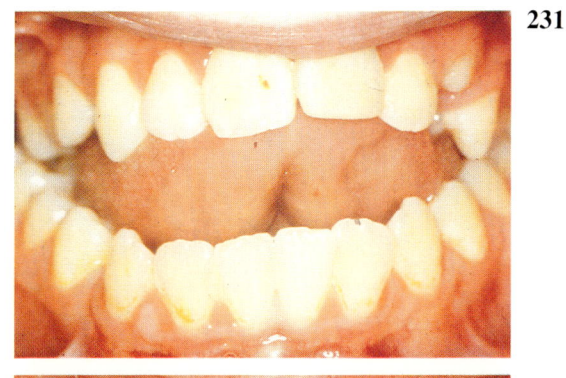

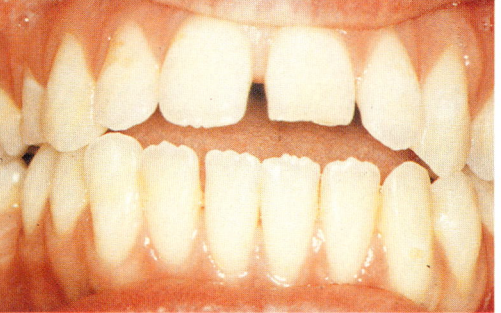

(iii) Lateral incisal relationships.

A lateral discrepancy in the incisor region may present as non-coincidence of upper and lower centre lines. It may be due to malalignment (**212**) or mandibular displacement (**227**).

(iv) Anteroposterior buccal segment relationships.

232a Neutral/Class 1 incisors, canines and molars

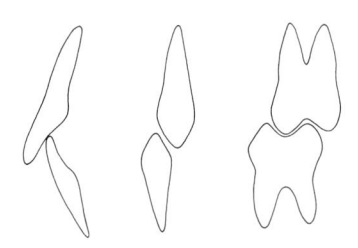

232a–232c Buccal segment classification is based on the anteroposterior relations of the mandibular buccal teeth to the maxillary buccal teeth. (**a**) Class 1 – the mesiolingual cusps of the maxillary first permanent molars rest in the central fossa of the mandibular first molars. (**b**) Class 2 – mandibular teeth are at least one half-cusp width distal to the Class 1 position. (**c**) Class 3 – mandibular teeth are at least one half-cusp width mesial to the Class 1 position. One half-cusp width is also denoted as half a unit, a unit being a pre-molar width or 7 mm.

232b Postnormal/Class 2 canines ½ unit, molars 1 unit

Prenormal/Class 3 canines ½ unit, molars 1 unit **232c**

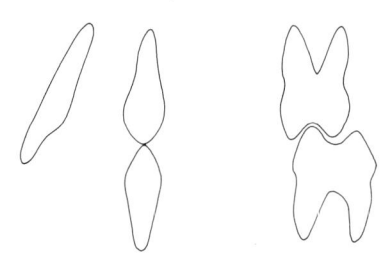

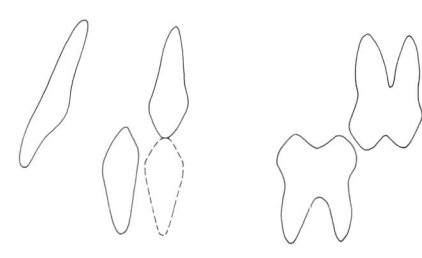

233 Deciduous molars

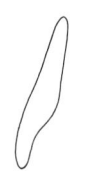

Class 1
Flush
Neutral

Class 2
Distal step
Postnormal

Class 3
Mesial step
Prenormal

233 The classification for the deciduous dentition is the same for incisors and canines. However, the relationship of the molars differs. Flush distal surfaces of the second deciduous molars are designated to Class 1. When the upper molar is mesial to the distal surface of the lower molar, there is a Class 2 relationship. A Class 3 is present if the lower molar is mesial to the distal surface of the lower molar.

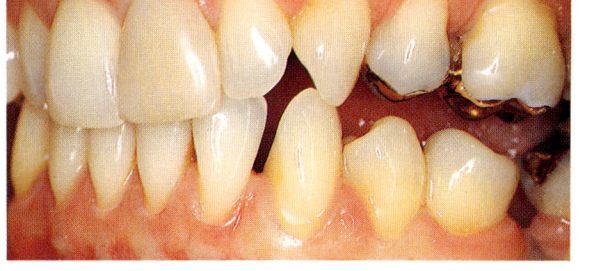

(v) Vertical buccal segment relationships.

234 A vertical space between the posterior teeth is termed a **lateral or posterior open bite**. An anterior open bite may be continuous into the buccal segments with the first contact occurring on the molar. This is of skeletal aetiology.

235a, 235b Posterior open bites are rare, the different types tending to have distinct appearances. They are usually of dental aetiology and may be due to either impaction of individual or groups of teeth (**235a**) or primary failure of eruption (**235b**). Non-eruption due to a particular syndrome, for example cleidocranial dysostosis, is another aetiology.

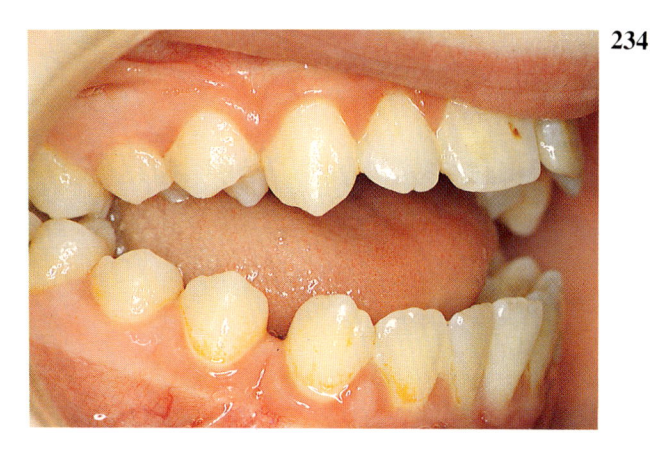

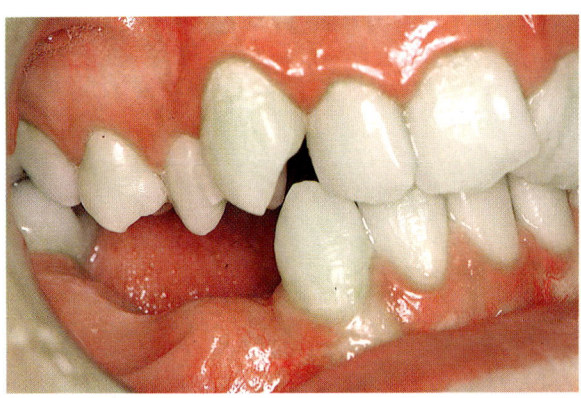

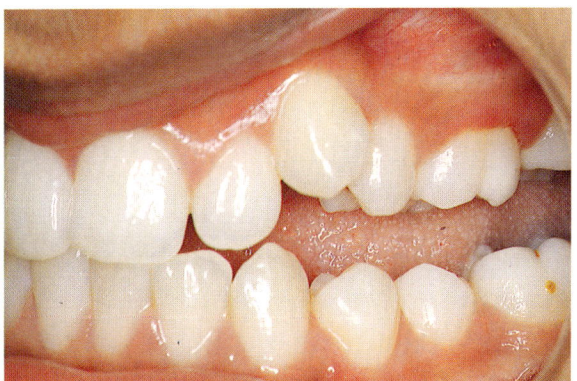

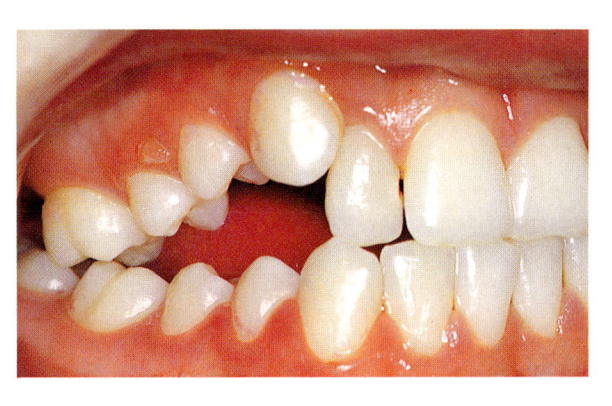

236, 237 Trauma may be the aetiology, as in this patient with a history of an electrical burn.

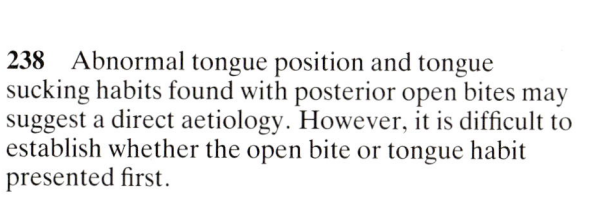

238 Abnormal tongue position and tongue sucking habits found with posterior open bites may suggest a direct aetiology. However, it is difficult to establish whether the open bite or tongue habit presented first.

(vi) Lateral buccal segment relationships.

239 Posterior lateral arch relationships

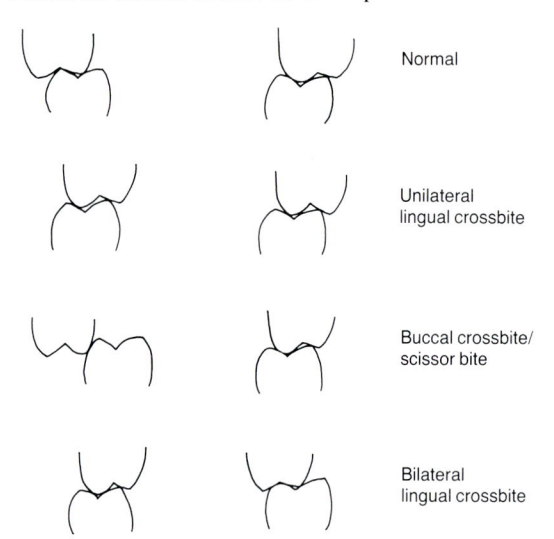

- Normal
- Unilateral lingual crossbite
- Buccal crossbite/scissor bite
- Bilateral lingual crossbite

239 A normal lateral relationship of the dental arches in the buccal segments is present when the lingual cusps of the upper teeth rest in the fossa of the lower teeth. The lateral dimensions of the dental arches may be abnormal. There may be a **lingual crossbite** with all or a few of the maxillary teeth inside the lower arch, or a **buccal crossbite** with some of the upper teeth outside the lower arch (this is termed a **scissor bite** if the whole segment is involved). The lateral discrepancy can be **uni- or bilateral**.

(vii) Variation in maximal and stable occlusal contacts.

240

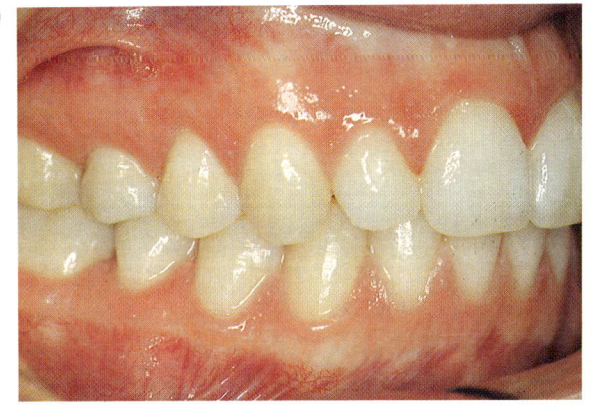

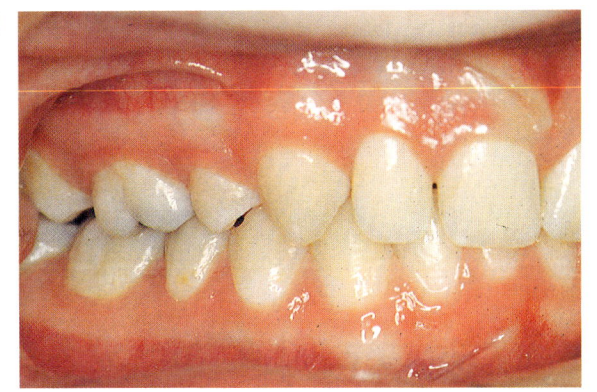

240, 241 Multiple and stable cusp to fossa contacts are present to a greater degree if buccal segments are well aligned in Class 1, or full units of Class 2 or 3.

241

242, 243 When half a unit discrepancies are present cusp to cusp or cusp to ridge, contacts occur on inclined planes which are less stable. Whenever there is an opening in the buccal segments, as in posterior open bites, the number of stable occlusal contacts are correspondingly reduced. In incomplete and anterior open bites, the number of occlusal contacts in ICP is reduced. Occlusal contacts which are stable are also reduced when complete overbites result in tooth-to-soft-tissue instead of tooth-to-tooth contacts. Non-coincidence of centre lines may prevent ideal cusp to fossa relationships, which may reduce the number of stable ICP contacts.

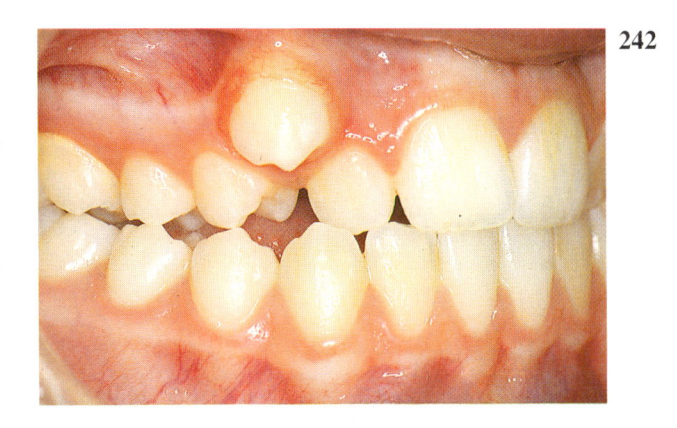

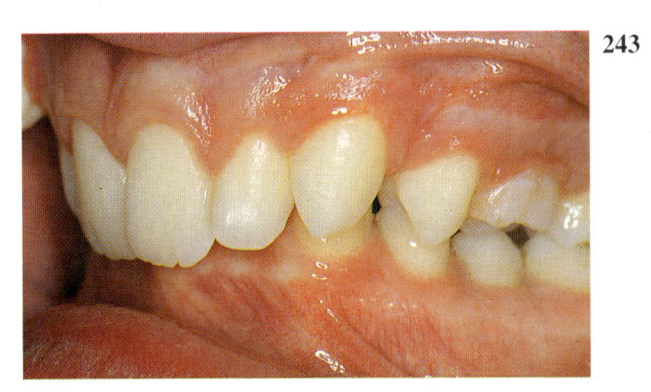

244, 245 The number of occlusal contacts in the intercuspal position with whole segment uni- and bilateral lingual crossbites is not usually reduced.

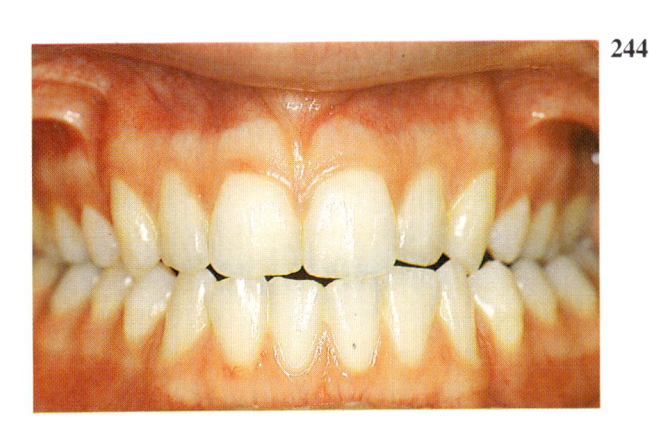

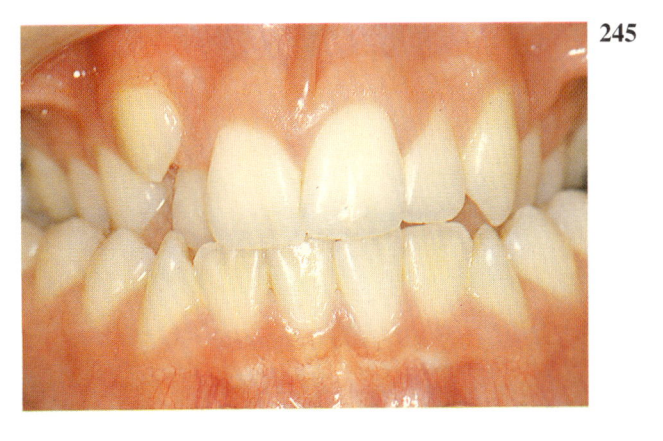

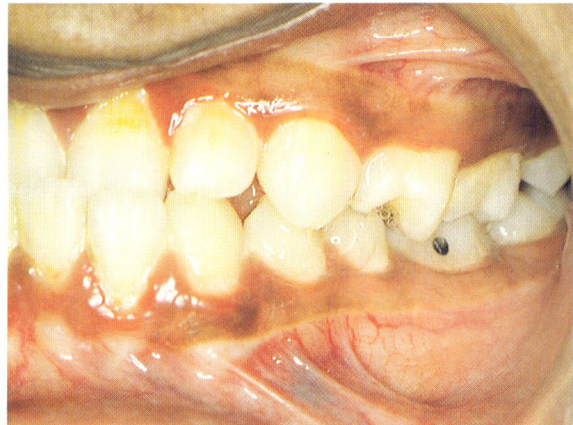

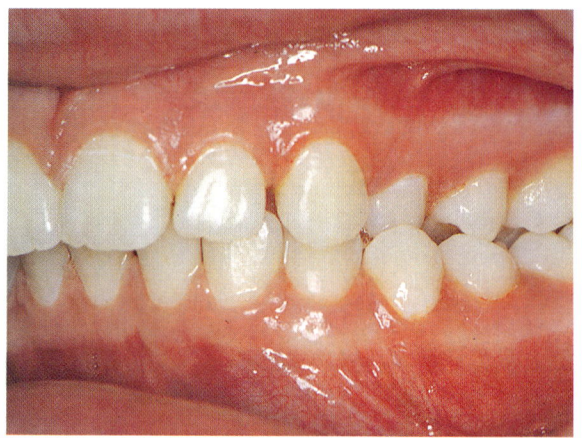

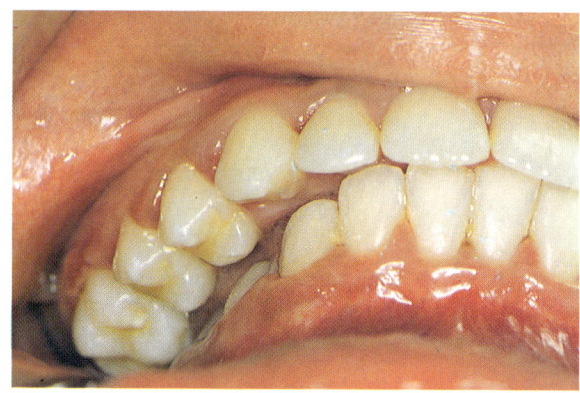

246, 247 Lingual or buccal displacement of single teeth is usually a manifestation of crowding. When only one or two teeth are displaced, the intercuspal occlusal contacts are reduced by the number of teeth involved.

248 In a scissor bite, where there is a buccal occlusion of the whole segment, the multiple stable contacts are substantially reduced as no contacts are present on the involved side.

The occlusal development of the young child and adolescent is characterized by multiple changes occurring, as teeth exfoliate and newly erupted teeth move towards full occlusion with their antagonists. These changes result in a consistently smaller number of multiple and ICP contacts than is usually found in the adult dentition.

(ii) Abnormality in the rest position

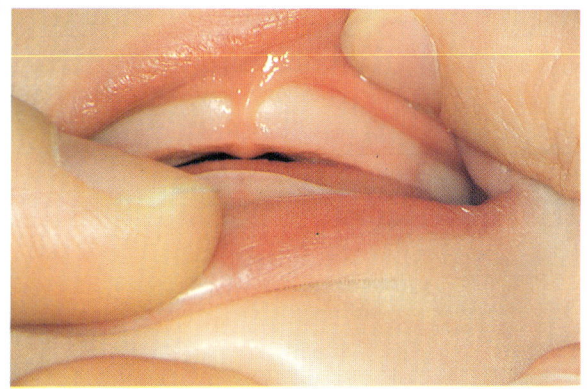

249 The rest position of the mandible is established at birth. Until the teeth erupt the tongue lies at rest between the gum pads in contact with lips and cheeks. Abnormality of the rest position is uncommon.

250 Increases in interocclusal distance occur when the head is tilted back. As head posture is a factor the patient should be in the upright natural head position for assessment. The rest position is considered normal if the interocclusal distance of the first molars is approximately 2–4mm. Deviation is defined as abnormal movement of the mandible in the sagittal plane during closure from a habit rest position posture to intercuspal position.

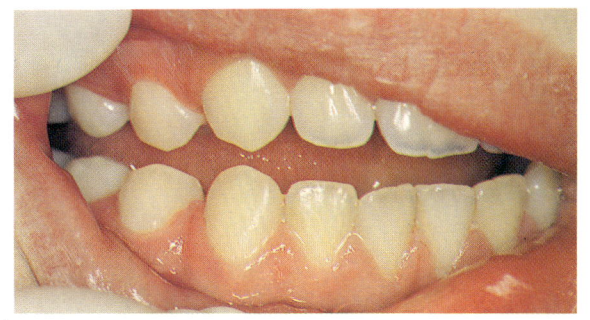

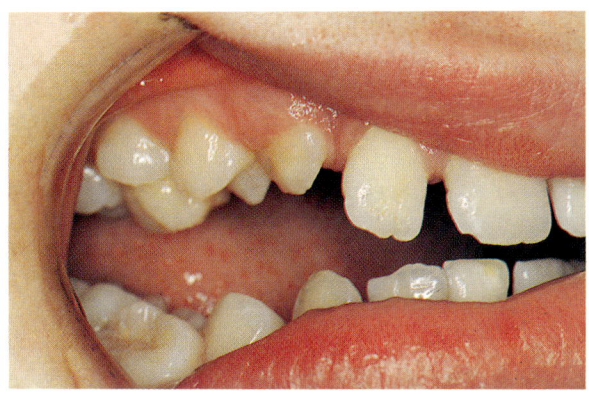

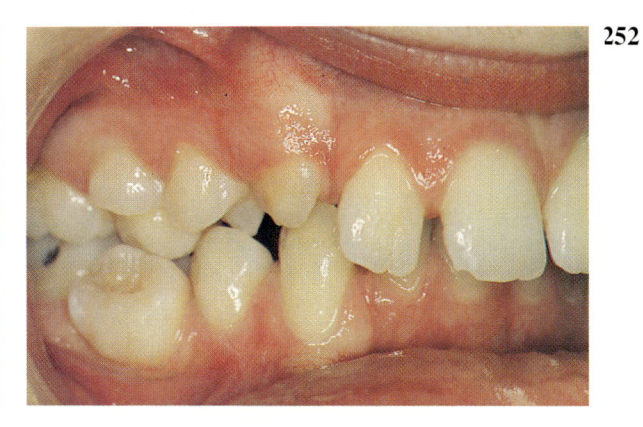

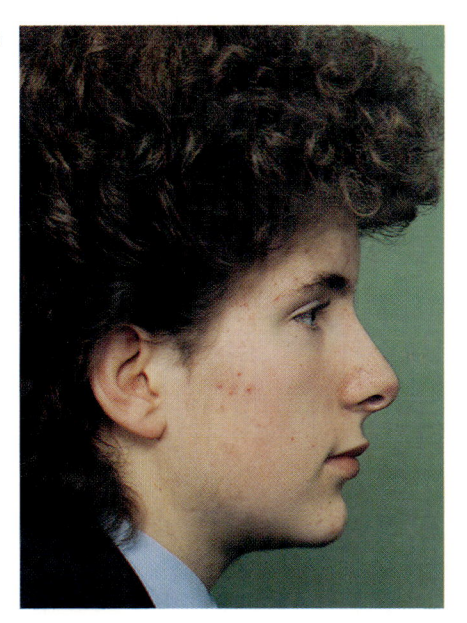

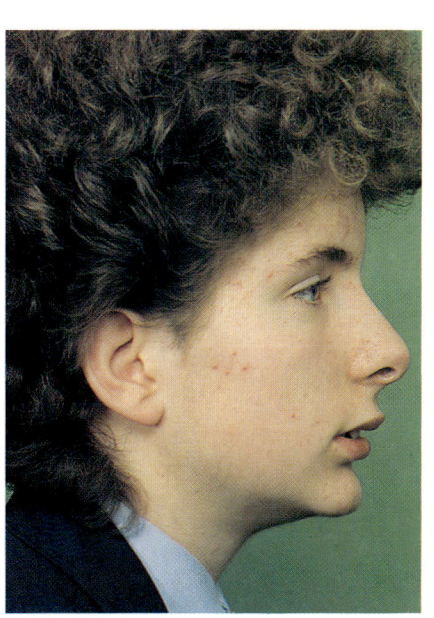

251–254 In Class 2:1 malocclusions, when there is a large anteroposterior discrepancy, to achieve an anterior oral seal the mandible may be held more anteriorly in a more open position (**251, 253**). **Posterior deviation** of the mandible occurs in closing to the intercuspal position (**252, 254**).

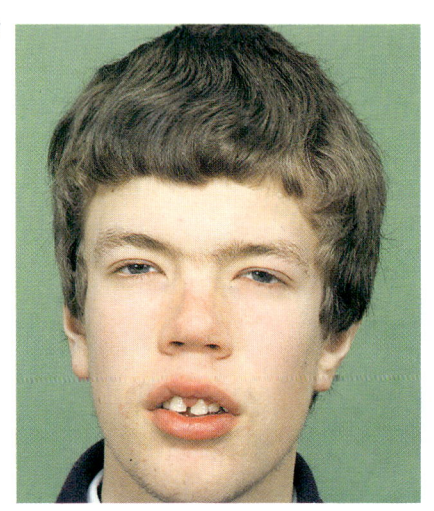

255, 256 In a Class 3 malocclusion, to achieve more pleasing aesthetics, the mandible can be held more posteriorly in a more open position (**255**). **Anterior deviation** of the mandible occurs on closing to the intercuspal position (**256**).

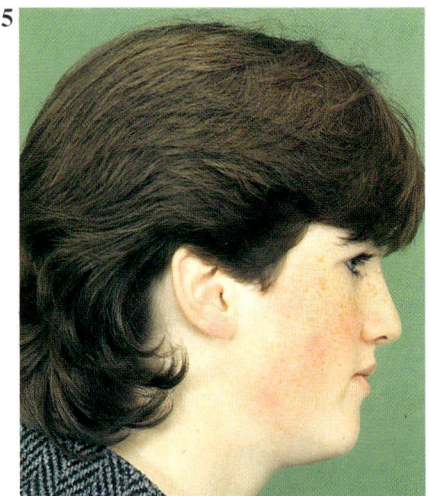

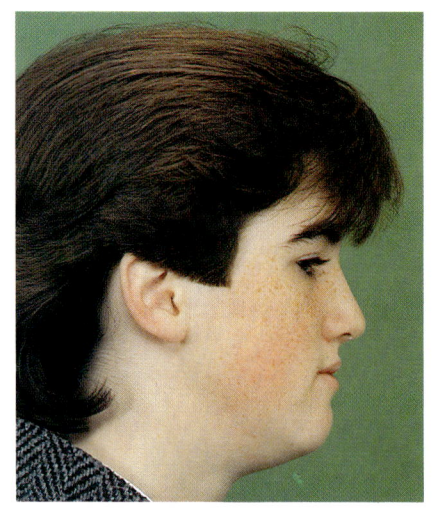

257, 258 **Vertical deviation** occurs when the mandible is held in a more open position to achieve oral respiration when the nasal airway is compromised. Abnormal tongue position due to a large tongue, tonsils encroaching on tongue space, or a tongue between teeth swallow (indicated by facial grimacing) may be instrumental in causing vertical deviations.

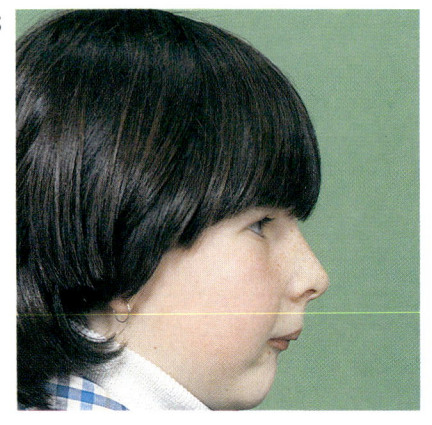

(iii) RCP–ICP discrepancies

The size and direction of any discrepancy between RCP and ICP is noted. Anterior, posterior, lateral and vertical slides between RCP and ICP can occur often in combination, but with the major component in one particular direction. Average non-significant RCP–ICP differences in the deciduous, mixed and permanent dentitions are about 1 mm.

259, 260 During the first few months of life the TMJs and muscles control mandibular movements. The first occlusal contacts are established when the upper deciduous central incisors erupt to contact the lower incisors.

Occlusal contacts assume a role in controlling mandibular movements as soon as the first contact occurs. At this early stage and even before posterior teeth are present, a discrepancy between RCP and ICP may be present, causing a displacement of the condyles on closing. The establishment of the occlusion of the first deciduous molars is also an important stage. The occlusal vertical height is established for the first time with intercuspation between upper and lower molars.

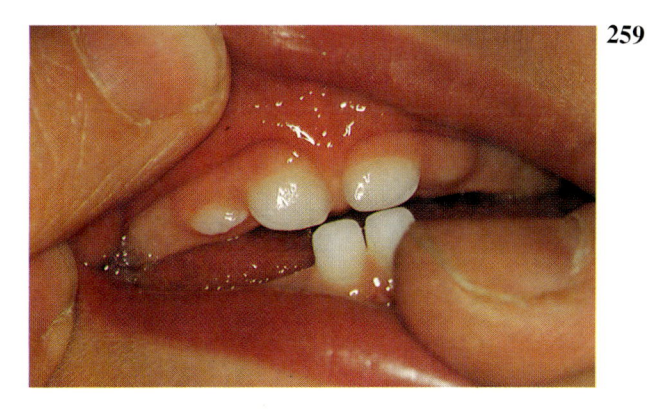

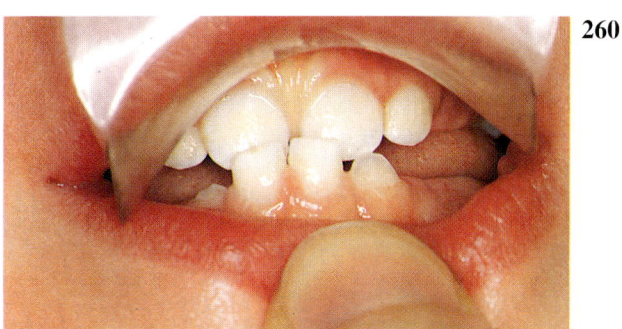

(i) Anterior displacements.

If the anteroposterior relationship of the maxilla and mandible is such that the incisors meet in an edge-to-edge contact on closing in the retruded position, an anterior displacement will occur with further closure. The condyle is pulled downwards and forwards.

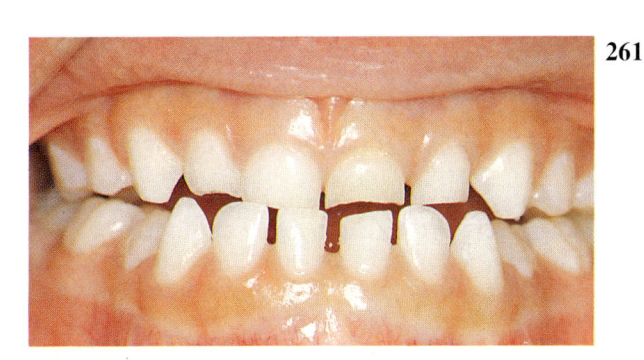

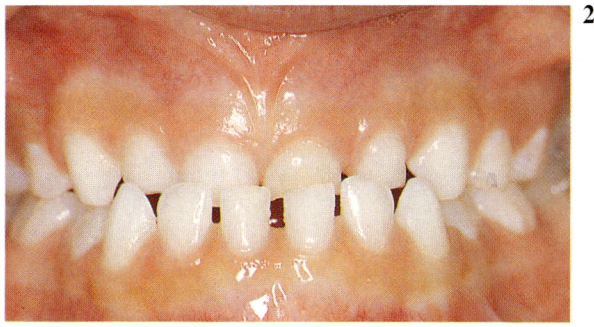

261, 262 Anterior crossbites with displacements are present in the deciduous, mixed, and permanent dentitions. The displacement from the incisal edge-to-edge retruded contact position to the intercuspal position may be composed of anteroposterior, vertical and lateral movements of the mandible. If a more severe anteroposterior jaw discrepancy is present, no displacement occurs as the incisors never meet. Some displacements result in the freeway space looking excessive when the patient is in the rest position, as the displacement may produce a reduced occlusal vertical dimension by interfering with normal vertical dento-alveolar development.

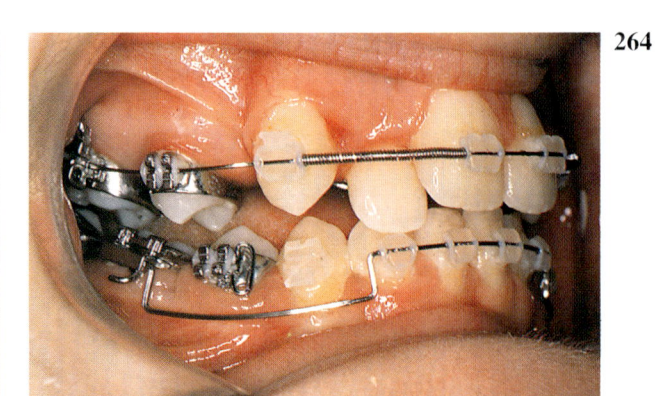

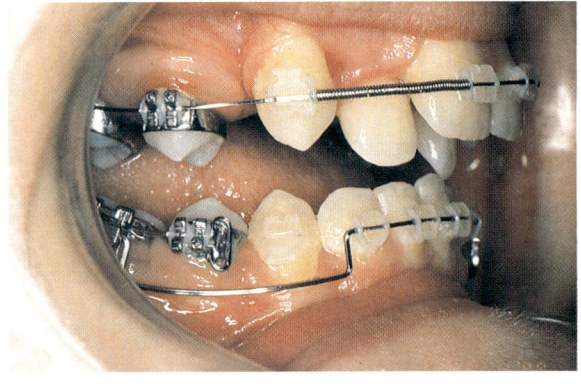

263, 264 Anterior displacements in Class 2:1 malocclusions occur when an instanding upper lateral incisor contacts teeth in the lower labial segment on closing. The mandible is deflected forwards into the intercuspal position, with the lower anterior teeth slotted between the central incisors in front and the lateral incisor(s) behind. The displacement can mask the severity of the anteroposterior arch discrepancy if only the intercuspal relationship is noted. The lateral incisors develop in a more lingual position than the central incisors and their eruption lingually is a manifestation of crowding. Palatally placed lateral incisors also occur in Class 1 and Class 3 malocclusions, but are less often a cause of displacement.
Courtesy of Mr D. Birnie.

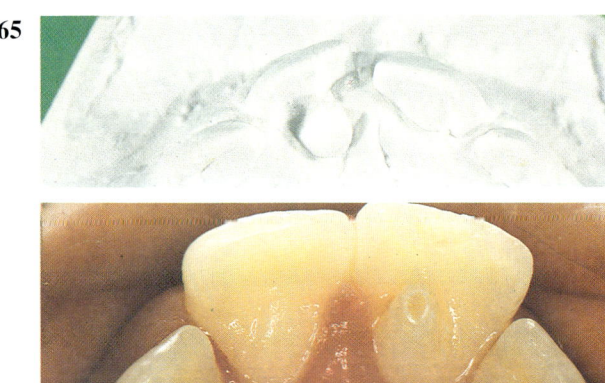

265 Local irregularities may have a similar effect. Talon cusps are additional cusps that project from the lingual surface of anterior teeth. They occur in both deciduous and permanent dentitions, in the upper or lower labial segments. Talon cusps contain enamel, dentine and pulp tissue.

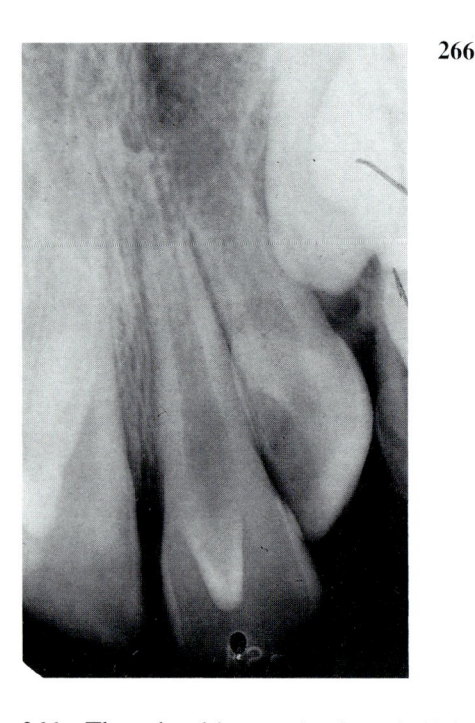

266 They should extend at least half the distance from the cemento-enamel junction to the incisal edge to be classified as talon cusps rather than enlarged cingulae. The talon cusp causes an occlusal interference unless a reduced overbite is present.

(ii) Posterior displacement.

267 Posterior displacement may be present in Class 2:2 malocclusions. Incisal angulations are upright or retroclined. Initial contact occurs in the incisal third; to close into the intercuspal position the mandible must move posteriorly, guided by the steep angulations of the incisors.

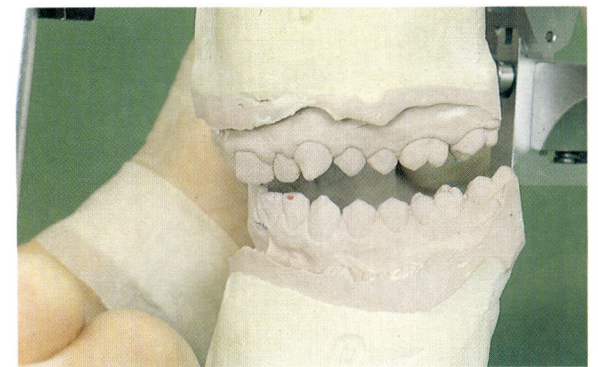

267

(iii) Lateral displacement.

268 Single posterior teeth or whole segments may be involved in lateral displacements related to lingual or buccal crossbites. Seventy-five per cent of unilateral lingual crossbite malocclusions present with a lateral displacement. The displacement in unilateral crossbites occurs because there is an imbalance in dental arch width. As the mandible closes, the lingual cusps of the upper and lower posterior teeth contact. The mandible is moved laterally into the intercuspal position. The side to which the mandible has moved is in crossbite; the opposite side has a normal lateral relationship.

268

269, 270 Although the displacement is mainly lateral (**268, 269** = ICP), anteroposterior and vertical movements may also be present (**270** = RCP). Unilateral crossbites with displacements are present in the deciduous, mixed and permanent dentitions. The imbalance of the lateral dimensions of the arches may be due to mismatch of the skeletal bases. Alternatively, it may be a dento-alveolar type with abnormal inclination of the teeth buccolingually.

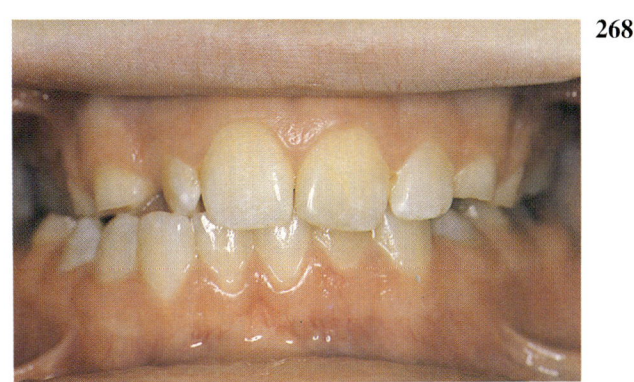

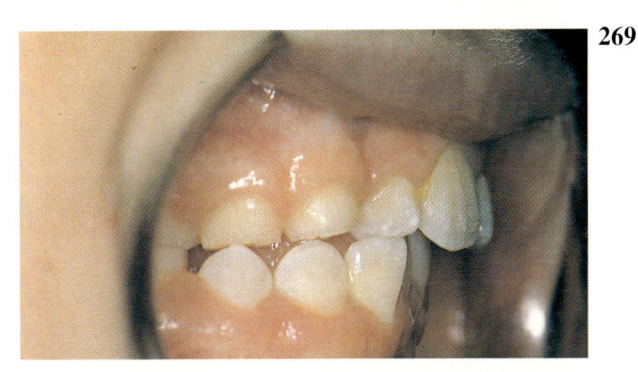

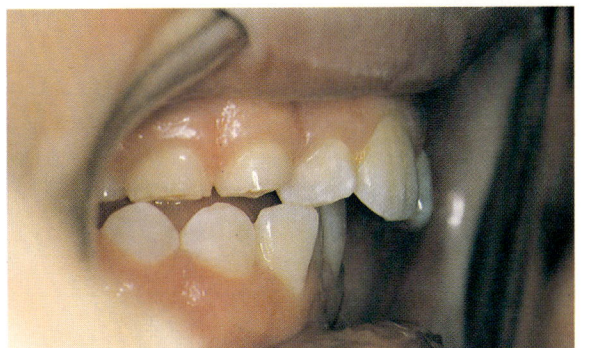

269

270

99

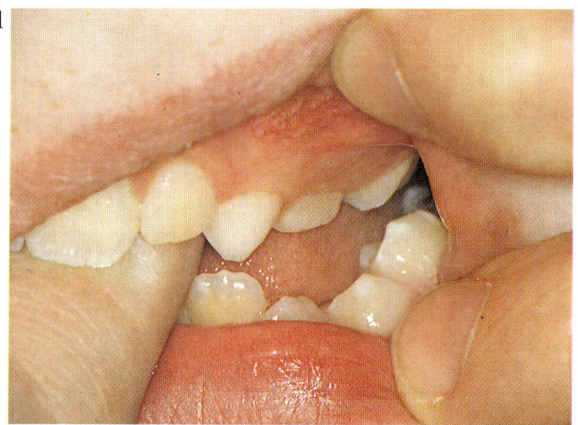

271 Unilateral crossbite may be combined with an increased overjet and reduced overbite as a result of a digit sucking habit. While actively sucking, the teeth are held apart and the intra-oral pressures result in equalization of the mandibular and maxillary arch widths.

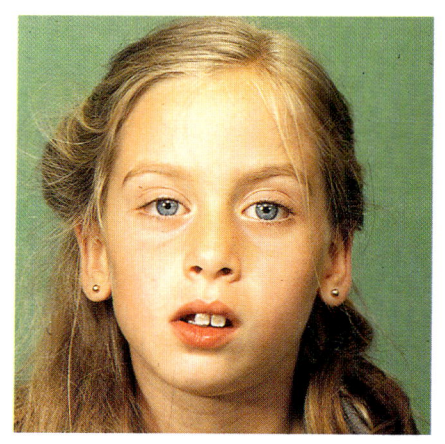

272 Other causes of unilateral crossbite with or without displacement may be related to a specific underlying pathology. Trauma to the condyle at an early age may cause fracture and/or ankylosis. Asymmetric development of the mandible results. Unilateral hyperplasia of the condyle will have a similar effect.

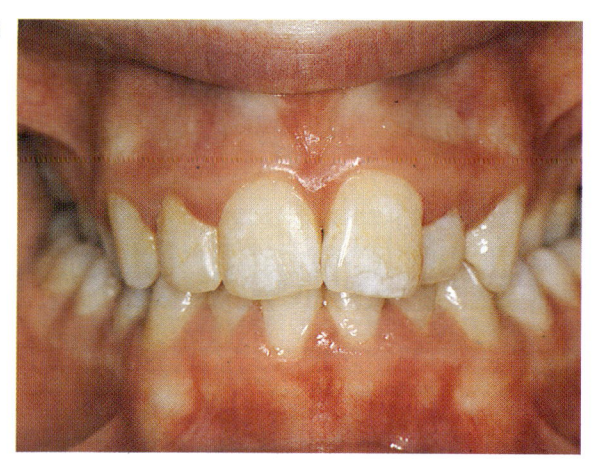

273 If the lateral discrepancy in the jaw or arch size is more severe, a bilateral crossbite occurs. This may occur in Class 1, 2 or 3 malocclusions. It more commonly occurs in Class 3 malocclusions because the posterior, wider part of the lower arch contacts the narrower, more anterior part of the upper arch. Displacement seldom occurs in bilateral crossbite.

274, 275 Unilateral scissor bites may present with displacement. As closure occurs, the buccal cusps of the lower posterior teeth contact the palatal cusps of the upper posterior teeth. To achieve an intercuspal position the mandible displaces to one side. The side to which the mandible has moved has a normal lateral relationship; the opposite side has a scissor bite. In the extremely rare bilateral scissor bite, displacement into the intercuspal position can also occur. If closure occurs on the retruded axis, the lower arch is fully enclosed by the upper arch. To obtain posterior occlusal contacts the mandible is moved to the right or the left on closing.

Scissor bites are caused by an imbalance in the lateral dimensions. A narrow, small mandible may be related to a wide or normal-sized maxilla. Alternatively, a dento-alveolar aetiology may be present if there is abnormal inclination of the teeth.

Scissor bites are more often associated with Class 2 arch relationships. The narrower, anterior part of the lower arch contacts the wider, posterior part of the upper arch.

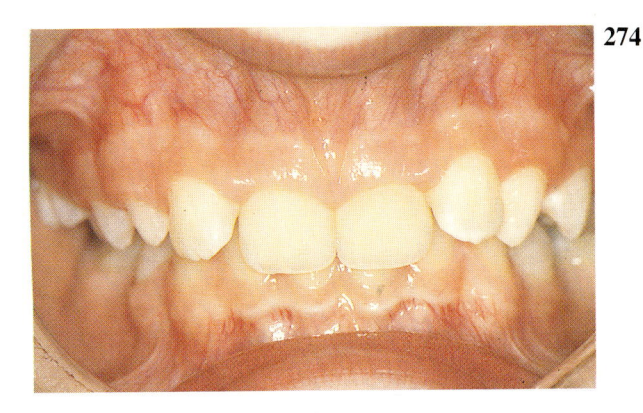

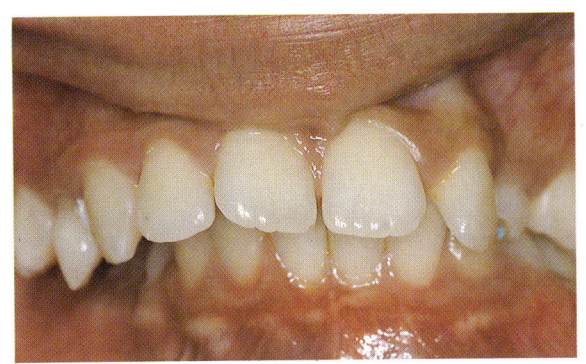

(iv) Vertical displacement.

276, 277 Vertical displacement tends to occur as an integral but smaller part of anteroposterior or lateral displacements. Vertical displacement may occur on its own when pivoting of the mandible occurs around a retruded contact position on a posterior tooth (**276**). To obtain an intercuspal position on the teeth anterior to the pivoting contact, the condyle is moved downwards. At tooth level a substantial increase in the degree of overbite is present with little change anteroposteriorly or laterally (**277**). Individuals with increased divergence of the maxilla and mandible and a tendency to anterior open bite are more likely to present with this type of displacement.

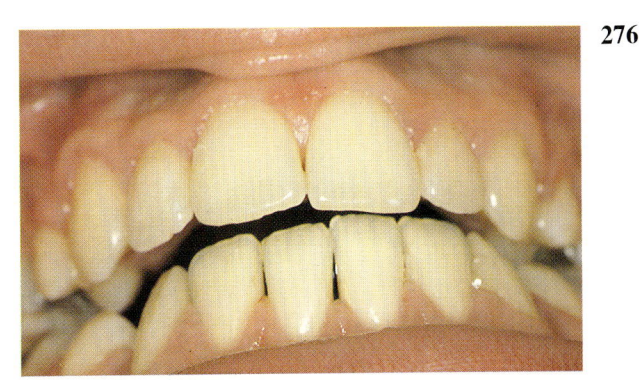

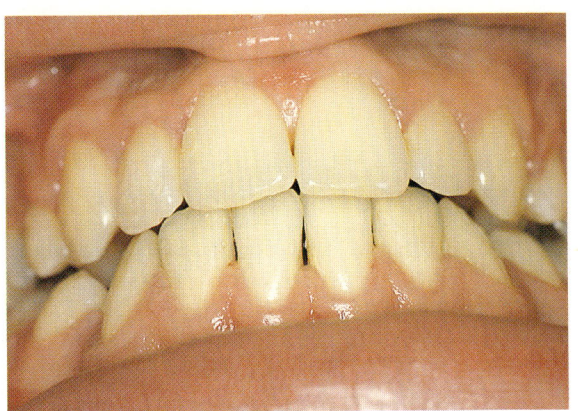

(iv) Mandibular movements

Lateral and protrusive movements start from the intercuspal position. Any significant discrepancy between RCP and ICP must be corrected first before valid judgements can be made about the excursive movements. Anterior guidance in protrusion, canine guidance and group function are all described in Chapter 1.

(i) Excessive occlusal wear.

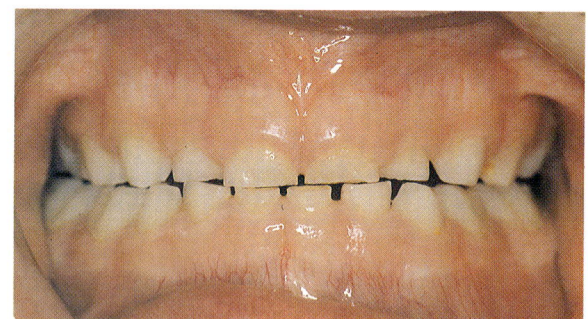

278 Attrition is a common feature in many deciduous dentitions so that disclusion of the teeth seldom occurs in lateral or protrusive movements. The presence of non-working side contacts in lateral excursions and bilateral posterior contacts in protrusion is not harmful, as the contacts do not interfere with the path of mandibular movement. This patient demonstrates this pattern in right lateral movement of the mandible.

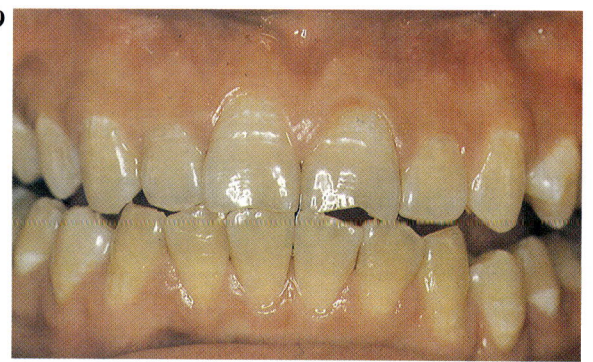

279 Excessive occlusal wear in the mixed or permanent dentition is usually related to parafunctional activity such as clenching, bruxing or a tooth to foreign object habit.

Wear facets may involve all the teeth or just localized areas. The mandibular position producing the abnormal wear should be established and any non-working side interferences checked, as these may exacerbate the bruxing by leading to an increase in muscle activity.

(ii) Protrusive mandibular movements.

280, 281 In the mixed dentition, when a positive overbite is established in Class 1, Class 2 and mild Class 3 (reduced overbite and overjet) malocclusions, protrusion results in disclusion of the posterior teeth (**280**). Crowding resulting in lingual displacement of teeth may prevent smooth movement (**281**).

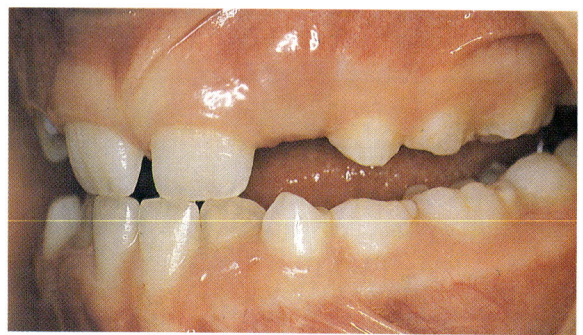

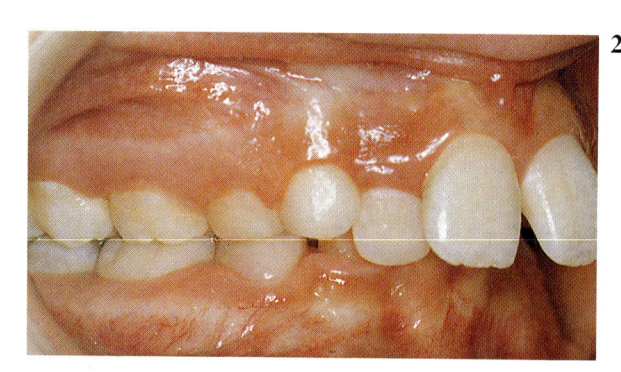

282 Severe Class 2:1 malocclusions with large overjets have no anterior tooth contact in ICP, but there is tooth-to-soft-tissue contact instead. There is therefore no anterior guidance to separate the posterior teeth. Maximum protrusions, as in this patient with a 15mm overjet, may not even achieve an edge-to-edge position.

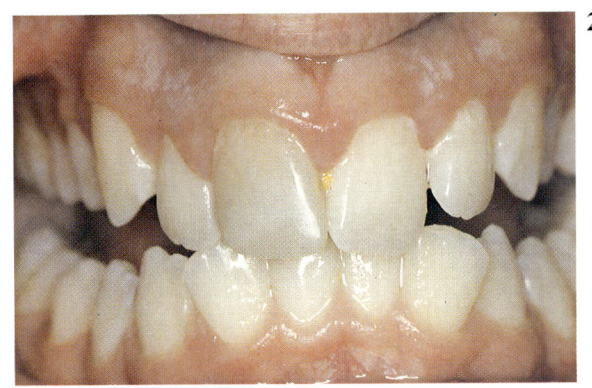

283 Severe Class 2:2 malocclusions may have a protrusive movement resulting in very limited tooth contacts. The proclination of the lateral incisors combined with the retroclination of the central incisors results in only the upper centrals contacting in protrusion.

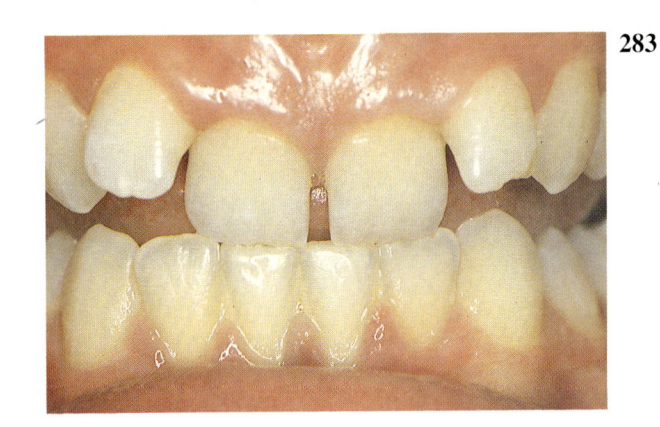

284 In severe Class 3 malocclusions with edge-to-edge and negative overjets, protrusion provides no functional advantage and when it occurs it is guided by contacts on the posterior teeth.

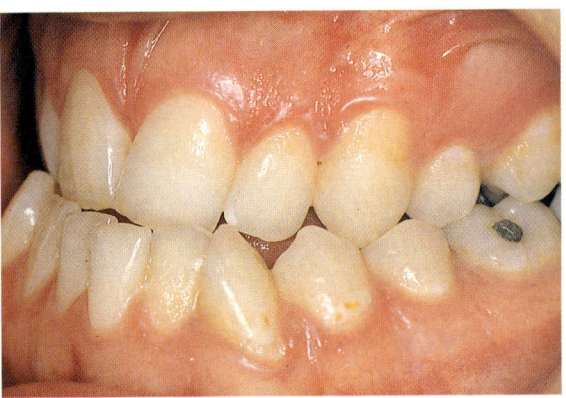

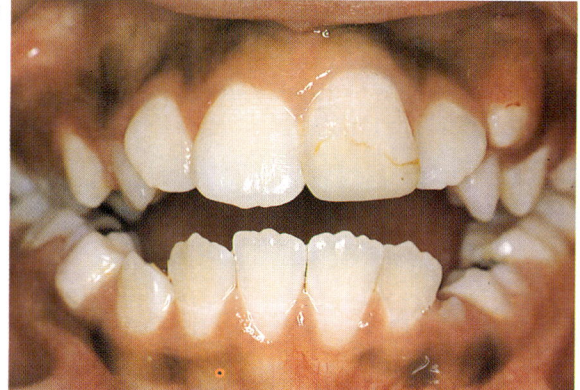

285a, 285b If an incomplete or anterior open bite is present, protrusive movements will be guided by the posterior teeth, whether a positive (**285a**) or negative (**285b**) overjet is present.

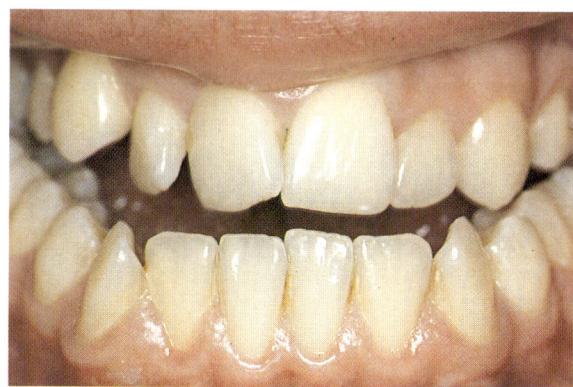

286 Protrusion in individuals with a normal incisal overbite and a posterior open bite will disclude any occluding posterior teeth.

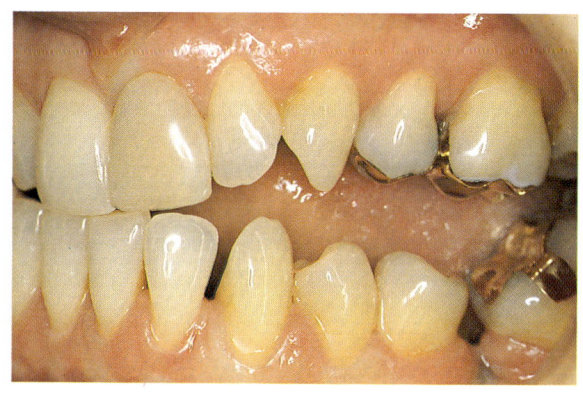

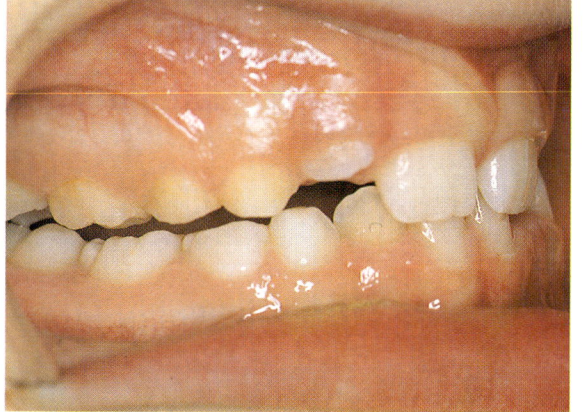

(iii) Lateral mandibular movements.

287 In the mixed dentition, group function is often present in Class 1, 2 and mild Class 3 malocclusions. The more prominent cusps of the first permanent molars are usually involved as well as the deciduous canines. Non-working side interferences are also often present on the first permanent molars and may influence the lateral paths of mandibular movement.

288 Lateral excursions in severe Class 2:1 malocclusions may result in canine to lower incisor contact. The upper and lower canines are too far away from each other to allow canine guidance to occur.

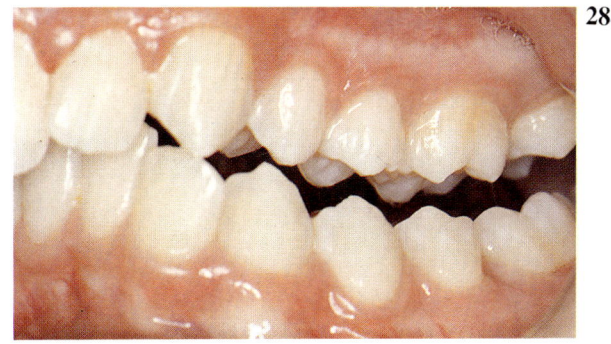

289 Lateral excursion in severe Class 2:2 may be guided by the upper canines and lower incisors or just by the retroclined central incisors.

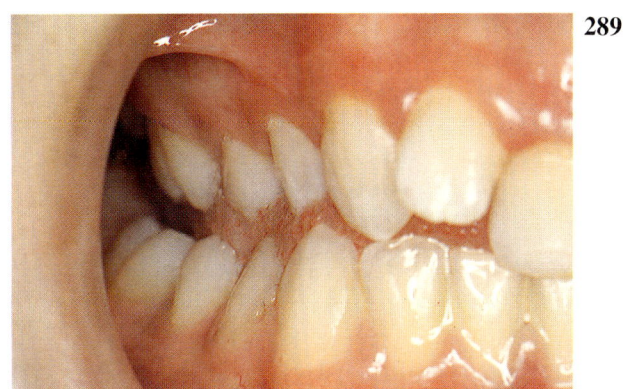

290 In severe Class 3 malocclusions with edge to edge or anterior open bite, guidance from posterior teeth only occurs on lateral movements, and non-working interferences are often present. An association between anterior open bite and non-working side interferences has been established with symptoms of mandibular dysfunction. The presence of signs and symptoms should be checked.

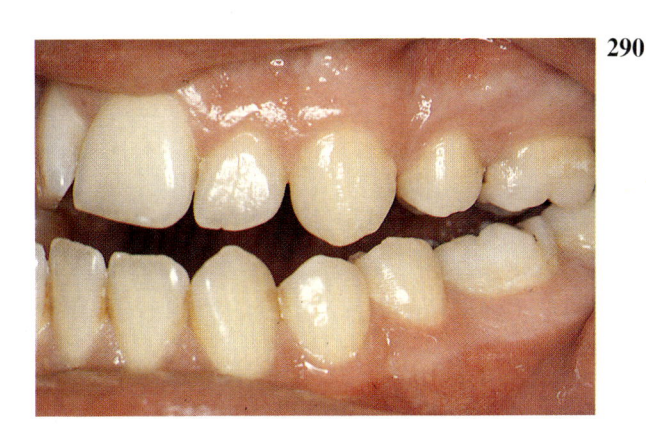

291 Normal or deep overbites associated with reverse overjets may have the canines in a normal lateral relationship giving canine guidance. In the mixed dentition stage, group function may be temporarily established with the first permanent molars contacting until the prominence of the permanent canine comes into function as it erupts. On the non-working side, contacts or interferences may correspondingly occur. This is similar to other occlusal relationships.

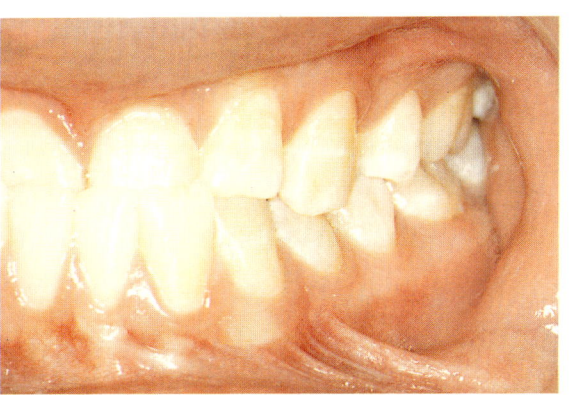

292a Unilateral left side lingual crossbite

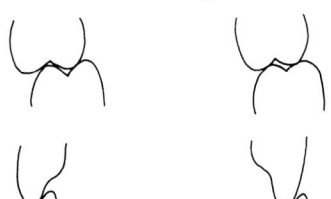

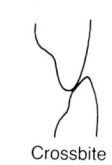

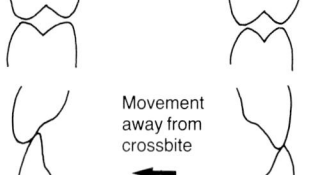

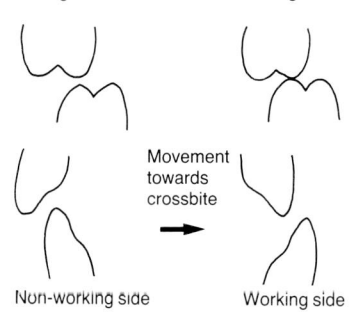

292a–292c Unilateral lingual crossbite occurs without RCP–ICP discrepancies in 25 per cent of cases.

292a A unilateral left side lingual crossbite is represented for canines and molars.

292b Lateral guidance is provided by the working side canines when moving away from the crossbite. Non-working side contacts may occur between the teeth in crossbite.

292c Movement towards the crossbite is usually guided by the posterior teeth, not the canines.

293a Bilateral lingual crossbite

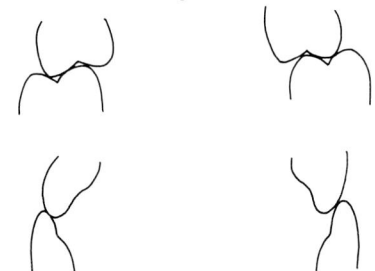

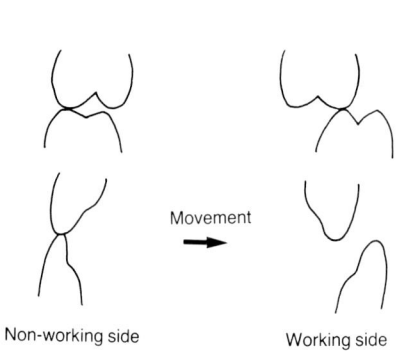

293a, 293b Bilateral lingual crossbite is seldom associated with an RCP–ICP displacement.

293a A bilateral crossbite is represented for canines and molars.

293b Movement to either the right or the left will be guided by the posterior teeth, with or without non-working side contacts from either the canines or posterior teeth.

294 Unilateral scissor bite

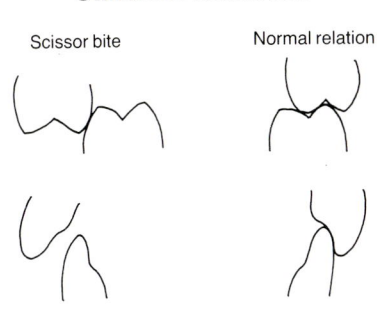

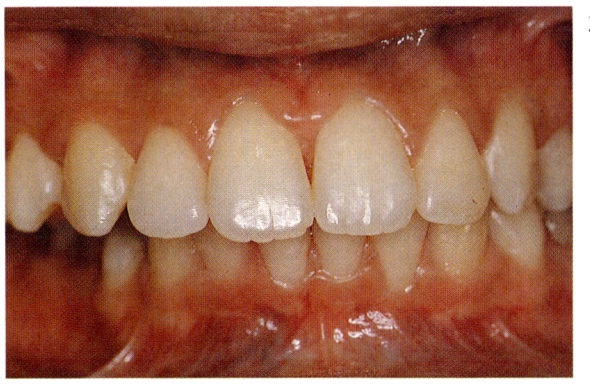

294, 295 A scissor bite more commonly occurs in Class 2 relationships because of the post-normal relationship of the arches. It very rarely occurs bilaterally. A scissor bite on the right side, involving the whole buccal segment, is illustrated.

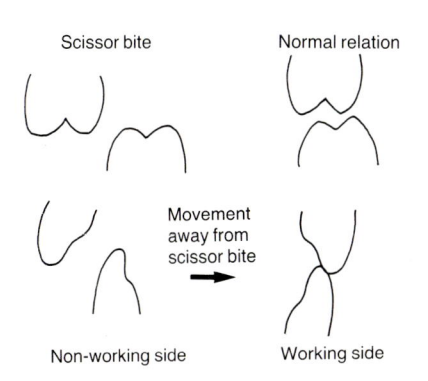

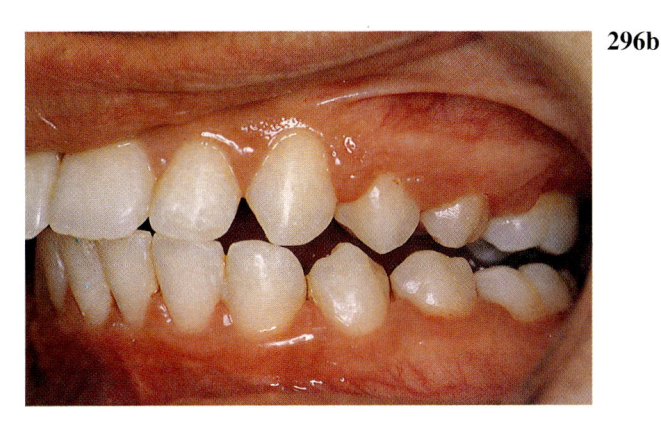

296a, 296b On the normal side, lateral guidance generally occurs from the working side canines.

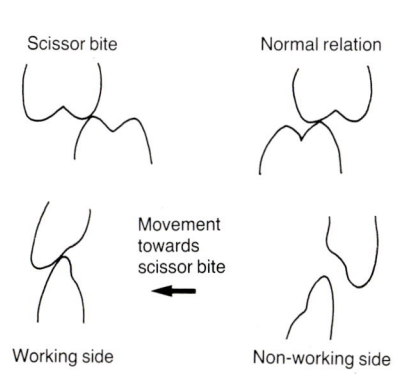

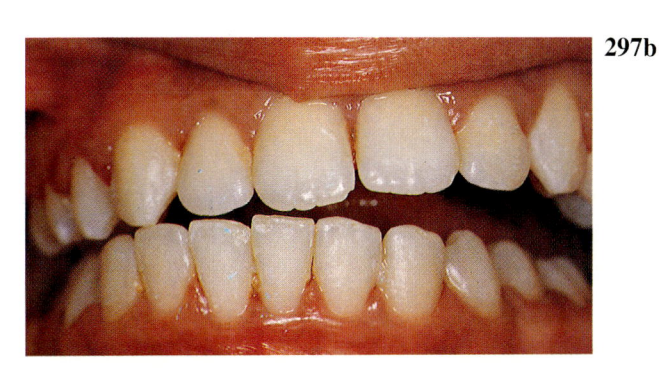

297a, 297b When the mandible moves towards the scissor bite side, the severity of the condition will determine whether the working side teeth contact at all. In the case illustrated, guidance was from the non-working side molars. Contact between the working side canine and a lower tooth required gross lateral movement. In less severe cases, the palatal aspects of the teeth on the working scissor bite side may give some guidance.

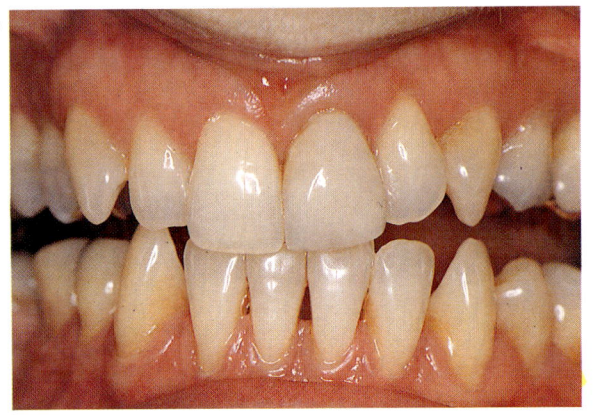

298 In posterior open bites, lateral movements towards the open bite side may be guided by the canines if the position of the upper canine permits contact with the lower canine. However, the guidance may be insufficient to disclude the posterior teeth on the non-working side. If canine contact does not occur on the working open bite side, the guidance will be totally from the non-working side.

The examination of static and functional relations of the dentitions is complete when mandibular movements have been assessed. The many changes occurring during the occlusal development of the young child and adolescent may result in: variations in the number and stability of occlusal contacts in ICP; abnormal rest positions; large variations and abnormalities in mandibular movements. Non-coincidence of RCP and ICP may result in mandibular displacements on closing, in all directions.

Conclusion

The extra-oral and intra-oral clinical examinations need to provide information on dento-facial aesthetics, TMJ function, soft tissues and the dentitions. Combination of the clinical assessment with additional information from study casts, radiographs and cephalometric measurements produces a comprehensive diagnosis for the patient requiring orthodontic treatment. The aetiology of each individual's variation is sought so that fully informed decisions can be made in treatment planning.

Chapter 6: Orthodontic special investigations

In some situations, further investigations are required to formulate a diagnosis and treatment plan; these include, where appropriate:
- General growth and development.
- Occlusal splint therapy (see Chapter 4).
- Instrumental analysis of diagnostic casts.
- ICP–RCP conversion on lateral skull radiographs.

General growth and development

General growth and development influence orthodontic treatment prognosis. The timing of the pubertal growth spurt is important in planning orthodontic treatment. In younger patients it is often necessary to make a prediction of the likely skeletal and dental relationships after growth has ceased.

Numerous methods have been used to predict the onset of the pubertal growth spurt. Ossification of the adductor sesamoid bone in the hand sometimes coincides with the onset. Radiograph examination to show this is often advocated but seldom used.

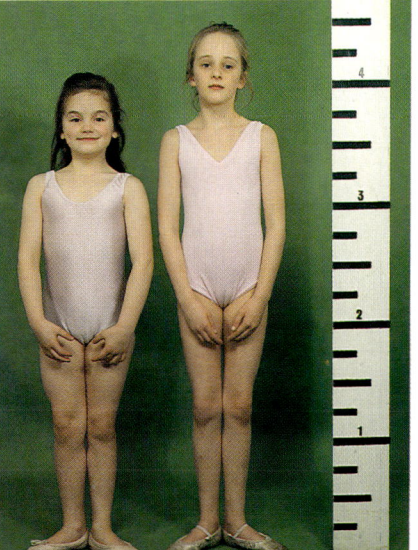

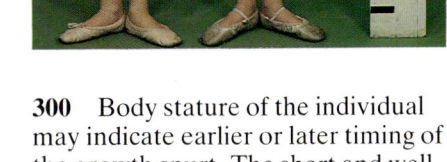

299 Comparison with standard height growth charts is often used and is a useful indicator as facial growth follows the body height growth curve.
Reproduced with permission, Castlemead Publications ©. Chart prepared by J.M. Tanner and R.H. Whitehouse. Published in Archives of Disease in Childhood, *1966, Volume 41. Chart ref: 11A.*

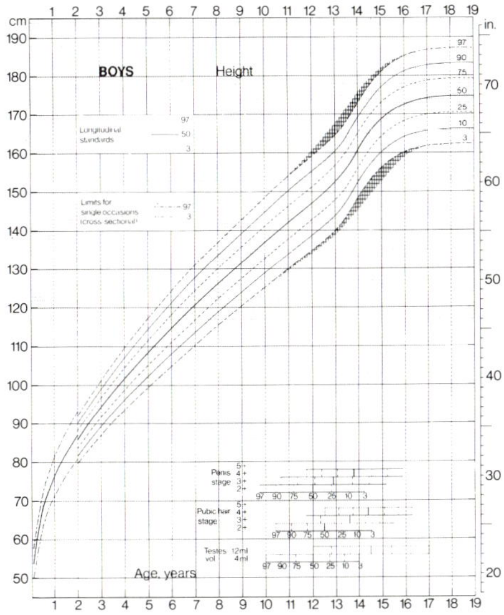

300 Body stature of the individual may indicate earlier or later timing of the growth spurt. The short and well covered endomorphic type grows faster and reaches the pubertal growth spurt earlier than the tall and lean ectomorphic or average mesomorphic individual. These eight-year-olds with birthdays three weeks apart demonstrate typical endomorphic and ectomorphic types.

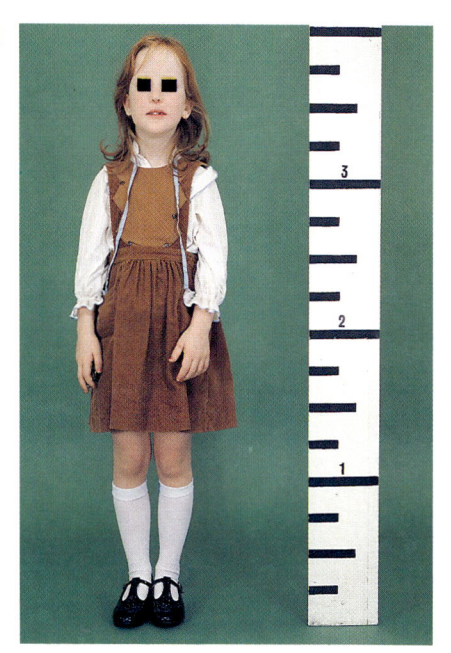

301 Problems associated with general growth abnormalities, neuromuscular development and coordination often require a team approach with other specialists. This patient has a history of hydrocephalus causing a disproportion of head to body size and poor coordination.

302 Superimposed tracings on De Coster's line

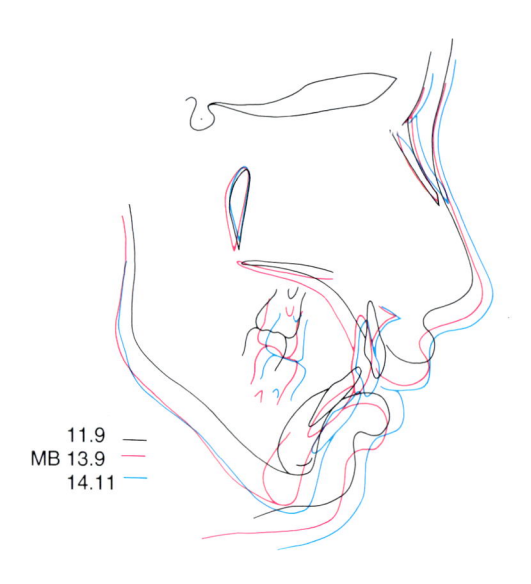

Superimposed tracings on maxillary outline **303**

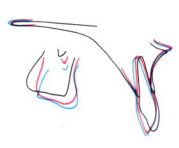

Superimposed tracings on Bjork's landmarks

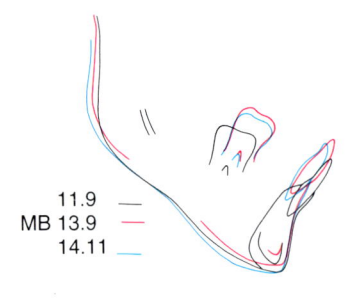

11.9
MB 13.9
14.11

11.9
MB 13.9
14.11

302, 303 Serial cephalometric films will establish directions of growth and type of growth rotation. The ability to produce changes in craniofacial relationships by orthognathic surgery and orthopaedic functional orthodontic appliances has been established in the last fifteen years. The more recent cephalometric analyses that have arisen have therefore been designed to be more sensitive to predicting and measuring these changes. Computerized data banks and programmes are available for analysis against standard norms, treatment planning and growth prediction. For moderate skeletal discrepancies, timing of treatment can be related to the growth spurt. For severe skeletal discrepancies, an early start to treatment gives a longer period over which the facial development can be influenced. The adolescent growth spurt is also used, but in the later stages of treatment.

Instrumental analysis of diagnostic casts

Study casts mounted in a semi-adjustable articulator provide the opportunity for:

- Occlusal analysis.
- Presentation and explanation of the orthodontic treatment plan to the patient.
- The construction of an occlusal splint.
- Diagnostic occlusal adjustment, usually performed with a duplicate set of casts.

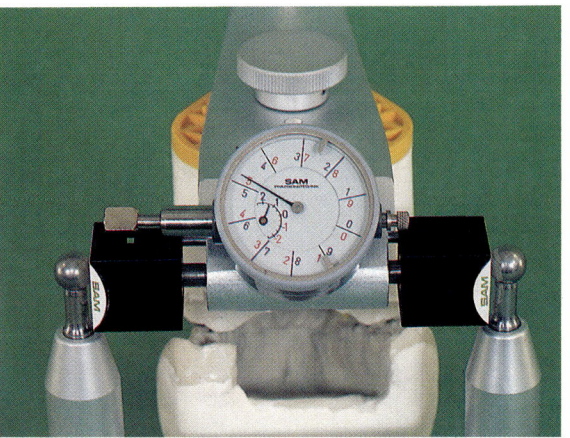

304, 305 The Denar MK11 and the Sam 2 systems can both be extended to provide a graphical analysis of the ICP–RCP difference. The extra instrumentation is called an MPI (Mandibular Position Indicator) in the Sam system, and a CMP (Cranio Mandibular Positioner) in the Denar system. The MPI and CMP are alternative upper members of the articulator. They differ from the standard upper member by having no condylar housing. The housings are replaced by laterally sliding blocks that can contact the condylar heads of the lower member. Coordinates are measured on adhesive graph papers which are added to the patient's diagnostic records.

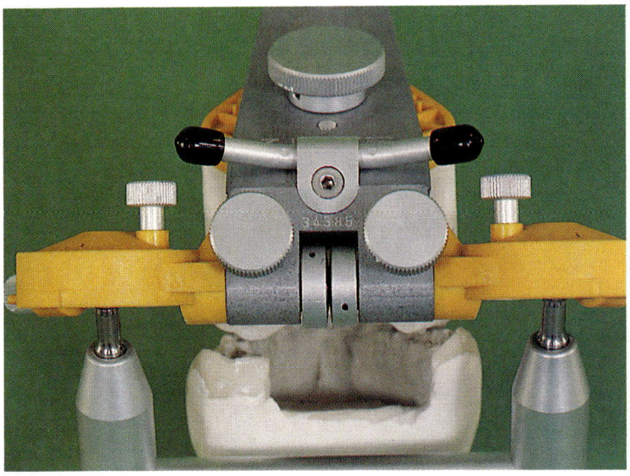

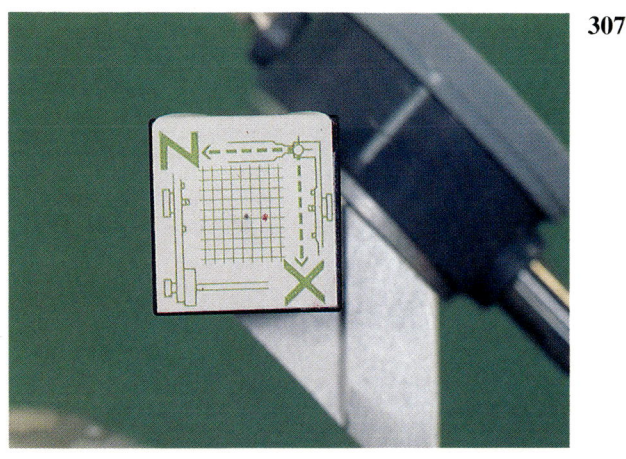

306, 307 The coordinates for ICP–RCP differences at condylar level are given by the dial gauge readings for the transverse dimension. The anteroposterior and vertical dimension differences are read from the ICP point recordings, marked by articulating paper, and the pin-perforation points made by the RCP 'hinge axis' needles through the graph papers attached to the MPI/CMP sliding blocks. The size and directions of the ICP–RCP differences help to establish more clearly in which direction tooth movements must be made to achieve ICP–RCP coincidence.

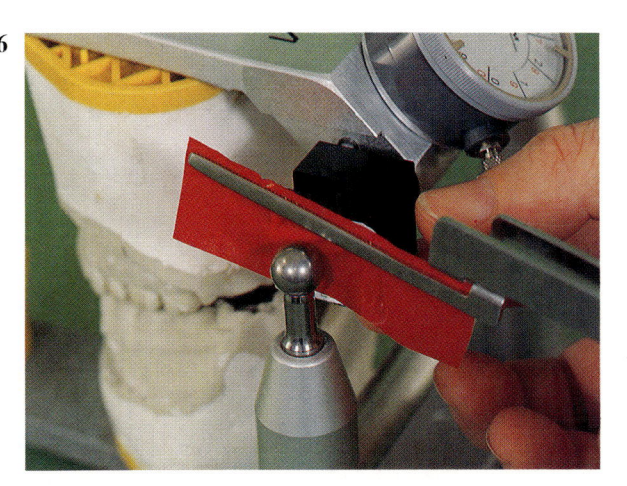

ICP–RCP conversion on lateral cephalometric radiograph

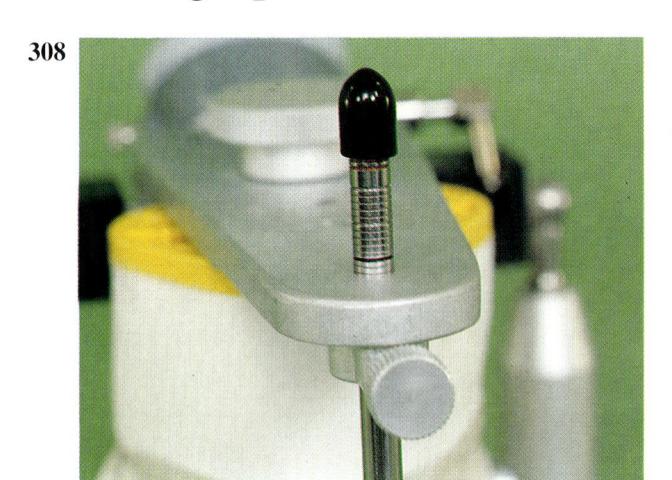

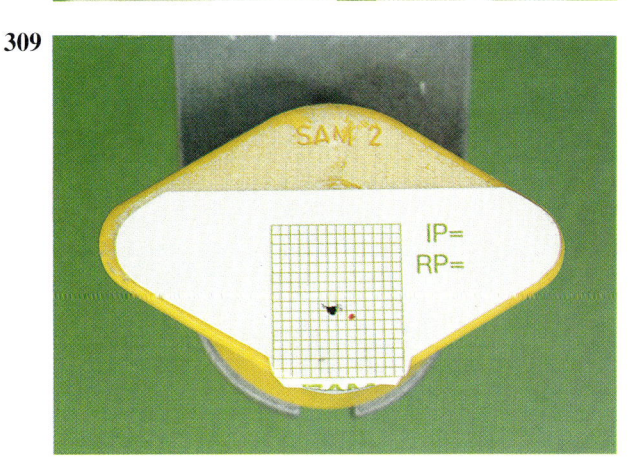

308

309

308, 309 This procedure requires a lateral skull radiograph taken of the patient after radio-opaque markers have been attached to the skin, locating the hinge axis and orbitale level, and MPI/CMP readings. The markers on the radiograph allow the cephalometric tracing to be directly related to the patient in the hinge axis-orbitale plane. The vertical incisal pin difference measured off the incisal ring scale, and the anteroposterior horizontal incisal pin differences measured off the incisal table graph are the measurements used for adjusting the incisal positions on lateral skull cephalometric tracings for ICP–RCP conversions. The first set of measurements is made with the models on the articulator mounted in RCP, and the second set, which gives the difference, is made with the models held in ICP, after the upper member of the articulator has been replaced by the MPI/CMP instrument. A tracing of the mandible and mandibular teeth can be moved from ICP to RCP after use of mathematical conversion charts. Diagnostic information in both positions can then be compared. Computerized programmes are also available for this type of conversion.

Conclusion

Five major aspects of a patient's occlusion should be examined: facial aesthetics, the degree of alignment and symmetry of the dental arches, and the lateral (transverse), anteroposterior (sagittal) and vertical relationship.

An orthodontic assessment should provide sufficient information to identify problems as well as their severity. It should also reveal the aetiological factors responsible for the malocclusion and the problems of facial aesthetics.

Chapter 7: Complete denture assessment

The goals in the restoration of the edentulous mouth are no different from those in restoring dentate patients, namely the restoration of appearance and function while limiting harmful effects to the remaining tissues. However, differences between artificial and natural teeth make it necessary to consider complete dentures as a special problem with different requirements.

Complete dentures differ from the natural dentition in that they lack the innervation and support of the periodontal ligament. Proprioception from the periodontal receptors assists the neuromuscular control of mandibular movements and allows the natural dentition to function around a stable intercuspal position. Without periodontal proprioceptive feedback, the edentulous patient cannot control mandibular movements or avoid deflective occlusal contact in the same way as the dentate patient. While a malocclusion in the natural dentition may be accommodated without many problems, errors in complete denture occlusion evoke an immediate response. Unequal occlusal contact causes movement in the denture base, resulting in pressure and irritation to underlying supporting tissues.

Aside from the patient's medical and dental history, assessment includes the examination of the health of supporting tissues and factors that influence retention and stability of the dentures. Satisfactory complete denture occlusion requires well-supported, retentive and stable bases during record making and in function.

Existing dentures are evaluated for base extension and adaptation, the occlusal contact and the artificial tooth selection and placement. Many complete dentures are unsuccessful because patients experience discomfort, difficulty in chewing and speaking or are dissatisfied with their appearance. Errors in jaw relationships and tooth placement are some of the main reasons for the failure of complete dentures.

History

Present complaint

- Looseness of dentures.
- Pain and ulceration associated with the dentures.
- Unable to chew effectively.
- Artificial tooth arrangement or facial appearance unaesthetic.
- Gagging.

Dental

- Previous denture experiences.
- Length of time edentulous.
- Reason for tooth loss.

Medical

- Oral infections.
- Nutritional deficiencies.
- Bone disease.
- Skin disorders.
- Hormonal disturbances.
- Malignant disease.
- Neuromuscular disorders.
- Medication.
- A full medical questionnaire should be taken.

General

- Occupation.
- Age.
- Social circumstances.
- Personality and mental attitude towards dental care, dentists, dentures.
- Expectations of treatment.

Examination

Extra-oral examination

This involves observation of the facial profile and appearance, as well as an examination of the temporomandibular joints at rest and in function.

The facial profile and appearance

310

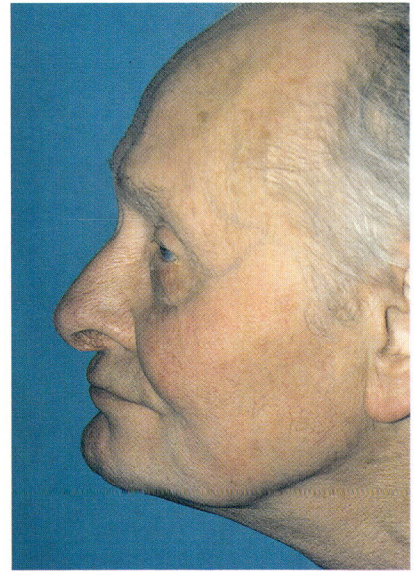

The face and neck are observed and palpated for abnormalities in size and symmetry.

310 Facial profile is affected by alterations in vertical jaw relation and by the relative jaw size. An increase or decrease in occlusal vertical relation with existing dentures not only affects appearance, but may also have a detrimental effect on speech, mastication and denture comfort.
Variation in lip form should be noted because of its influence on the anterior arrangement of teeth. Ulceration and fissuring at the corners of the mouth (angular chelitis) may be an indication of infection, reduced occlusal vertical relation and inadequate nutrition, especially Vitamin B deficiency.

311

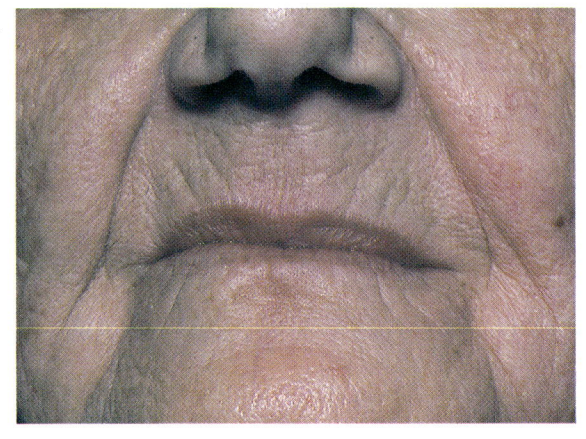

311 Wrinkles around the mouth are usually caused by loss of tissue elasticity and are part of the natural ageing process. These skin changes are seldom corrected by prosthodontic techniques.

The temporomandibular joints

The temporomandibular joints are checked for tenderness, crepitus and clicking on opening and closing of the mandible. Painful or limited opening and difficulty in performing eccentric movements are assessed because they affect the ability to record accurate jaw relationships.

Intra-oral examination

A thorough intra-oral examination includes an evaluation of the supporting tissues, factors that influence retention and stability of the denture bases and the design of existing dentures.

The supporting tissues

312 Mucosa and submucosa vary in their ability to tolerate pressure, depending on their thickness and resiliency, which varies in different parts of the denture bearing area. The soft tissues may be able to adapt to errors in base adaptation and occlusion by displacing viscoelastically.

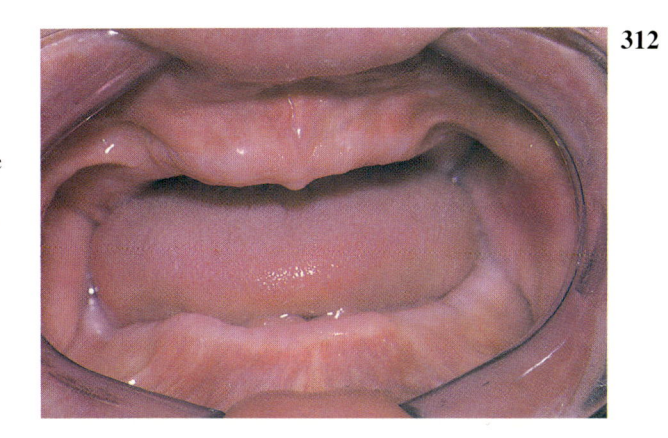

313, 314 If however, the soft tissue tolerance level is exceeded, inflammation and/or ulceration will often occur.

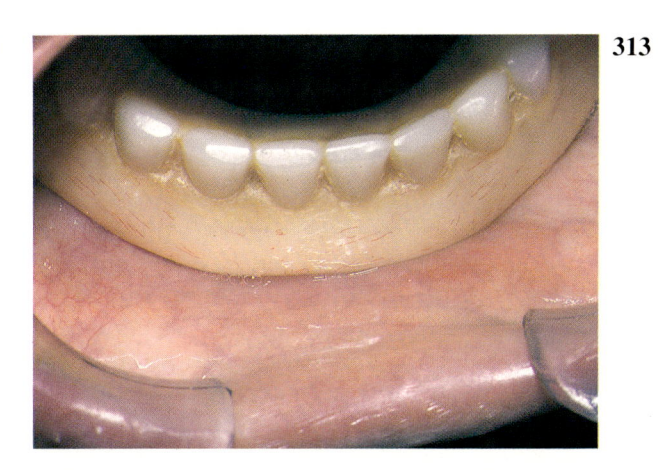

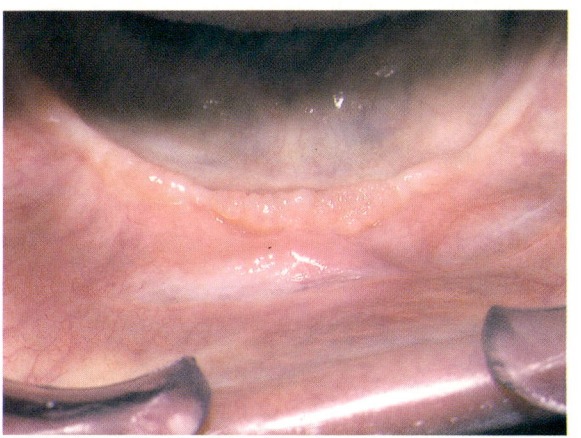

315

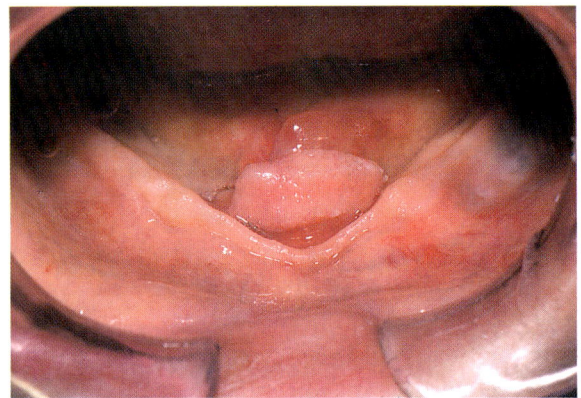

316

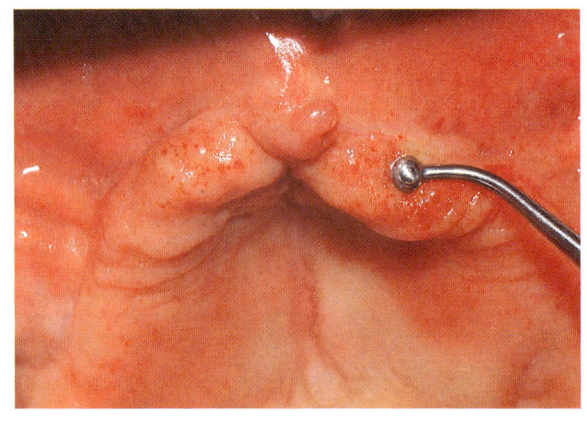

315, 316 Trauma of longer duration may lead to a hyperplastic response of the soft tissues, fibrotic change, or an acceleration in the rate of bone resorption, all of which leave an unstable base.

It is essential that these soft tissues are healthy before impression making takes place. Inflammation, ulceration and excessive amounts of hyperplastic or fibrous tissue must be eliminated, or at least reduced, because distorted or movable soft tissues do not provide the foundation on which to record accurate jaw relations or stabilize the denture bases in function.

The residual bony ridges provide the primary support for the denture bases. Their size (extent of bone resorption) and shape (presence of exostoses, palatal vault form, tuberosities and sharp bony prominences) indicate the quality and quantity of bone support for the dentures.

317

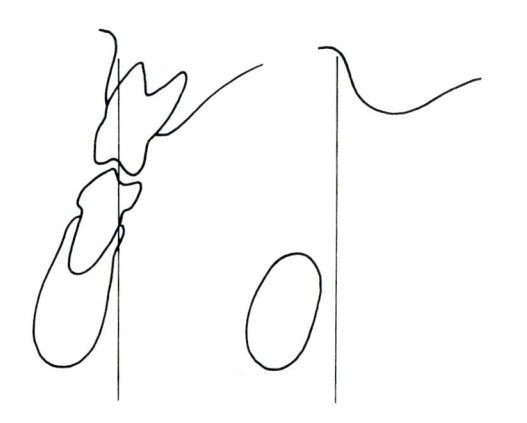

317 Following the loss of natural teeth, bone resorption patterns create a disparity in relative jaw size. The maxilla becomes smaller, resorbing upwards and inwards, while the mandibular bone appears static or widens posteriorly. Pressure from a denture will accelerate bone resorption, particularly if it is excessive and uneven. One of the factors in controlling the pressure to the bone is the denture occlusion.

Factors influencing retention and stability of dentures

318 Tongue size, position and activity relative to the oral cavity should be noted. Although impression making is made more difficult, a thick broad tongue helps maintain lingual border seal for the mandibular denture, while its relation to the polished surfaces assists in denture stability. In most patients, the tongue fills the floor of the mouth with its lateral borders just above the lower posterior teeth and its tip resting on the incisal edges of the lower anterior teeth.

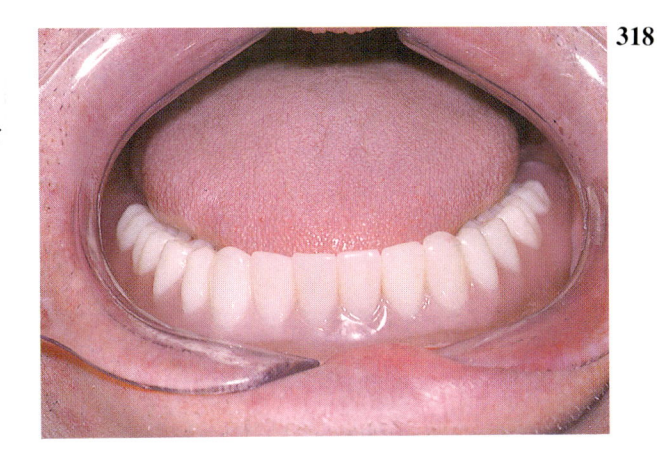

319 In approximately 25 per cent of patients, however, its position is retracted and does not contribute effectively to the retention and stability of the dentures, particularly the mandibular prosthesis. Tongue posture is observed without the dentures in place, and the mouth opened wide enough to accept food.

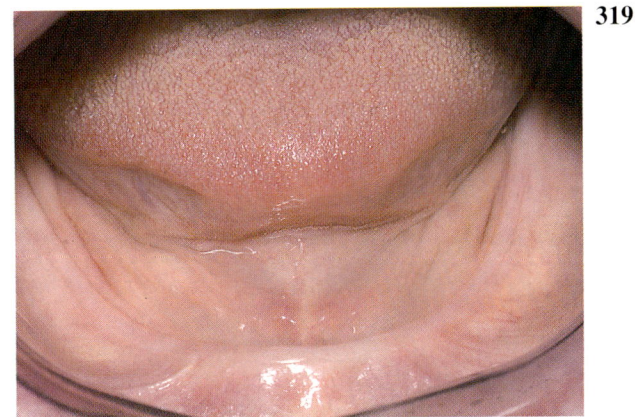

320 The relationship of soft tissue attachments to residual ridges is assessed because of its effect on the degree of denture base extension. The form and activity of the lingual sulcus, and especially the retromylohyoid region, are best evaluated with digital palpation to give an indication of the extension into the sulcus before impression making. The position and extent of the posterior palatal area (vibrating line) develop the retentive seal of the maxillary denture. Posterior extension is placed at the junction of the fixed and movable soft palate, determined clinically as the patient says 'AH'.

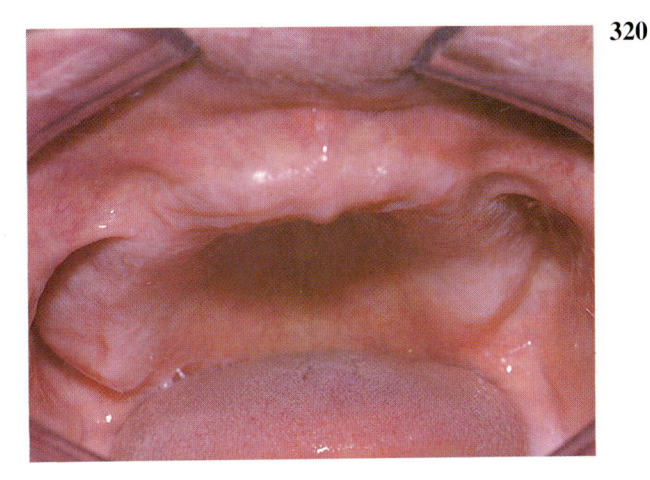

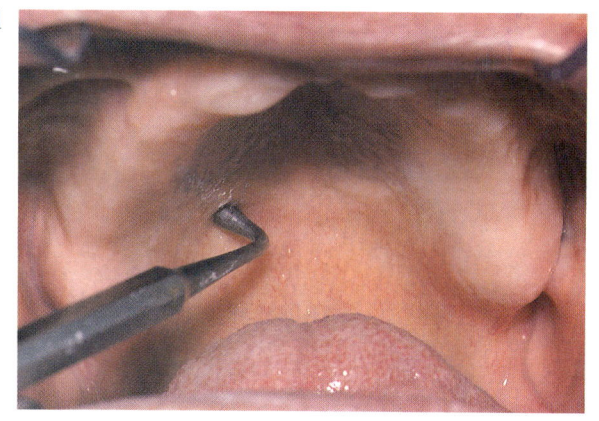

321 The consistency and displaceability of the tissues in this region are assessed with a ball-ended burnisher. The information provides an indication of the depth to which the cast is adjusted to form an arbitrary palatal seal area or, if clinically determined, the quantity of displacing impression material needed to secure effective retention.

The width of palatal tissue to be displaced by the denture base is decided by the degree of vertical movement of the soft palate. The greater the vertical movement, the shorter the width.

The amount and viscosity of the saliva influence the retention of dentures. If the saliva is too mucous, or excessive in quantity, the salivary film thickness will limit the adaptation of the denture reducing retention. When there is insufficient salivary flow, lack of lubrication causes the dentures to irritate the oral tissues.

Existing dentures

If the patient has complete dentures, these are examined intra-orally for:

- Base extension and adaptation.
- Occlusal contact of the artificial teeth.
- Artificial tooth selection and placement.

Denture base retention is improved if the borders are extended to the maximum support area and the base is in intimate contact with the tissues. Displaceability of the soft tissues at the denture base periphery creates a retentive border seal. Overextension or underextension of the bases disrupts the seal with a subsequent loss of denture retention.

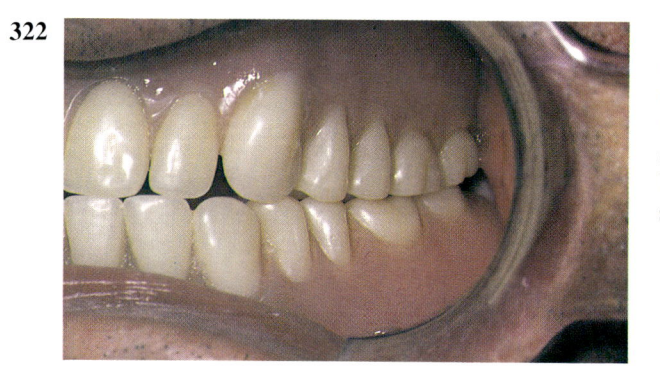

322 Occlusal contact of the artificial teeth at the retruded position should coincide with the intercuspal position. Uneven contact results in unstable denture bases and irritation to the supporting tissues. Initial contact of the teeth may be observed while ensuring that the bases remain seated on the supporting tissues.

If a more accurate assessment of the occlusion is required or occlusal adjustment is anticipated, the dentures are mounted in a suitable articulator with facebow transfer, and an interocclusal record is made on the retruded axis. Occlusal contacts may then be examined with indicator paper outside the patient's mouth on the firm foundation of stone casts. Indicator paper used intra-orally is inaccurate because errors in occlusion will be hidden by denture base displacement. Interocclusal distance (freeway space) may be assessed by comparing vertical dimension of rest (VDR) and vertical dimension of occlusion (VDO). Measurements are made with dividers, a ruler or a Willis gauge between two arbitrary points above and below the lips, firstly with the jaws at rest (VDR), and then with the teeth together (VDO). A distance of 2–4 mm between VDR and VDO is considered acceptable in most patients. The degree of visibility of the teeth, the facial profile and sibilant speech sounds are also used to help evaluate adequate interocclusal distance.

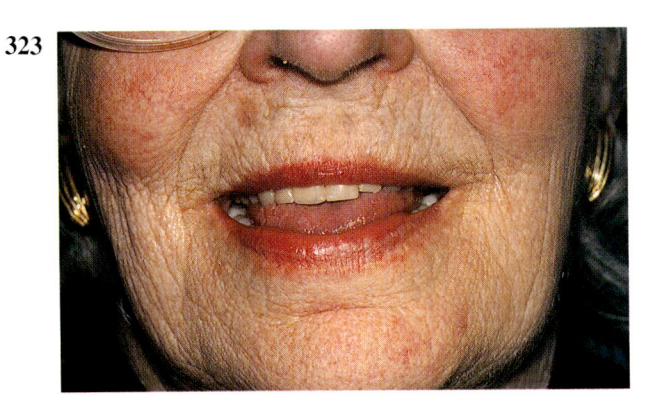

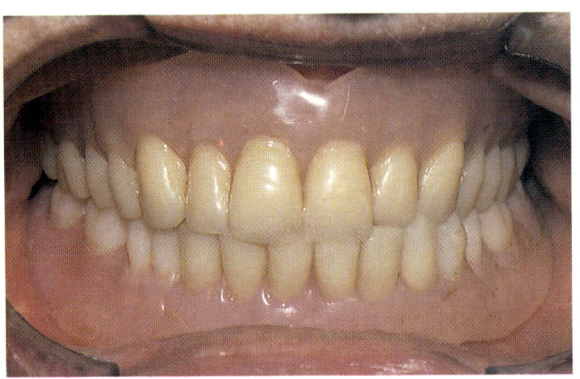

323, 324 Tooth selection and arrangement is assessed by its influence on the appearance and function of the dentures. In this patient, the size and position of anterior teeth created a poor appearance and influenced the stability of the dentures.

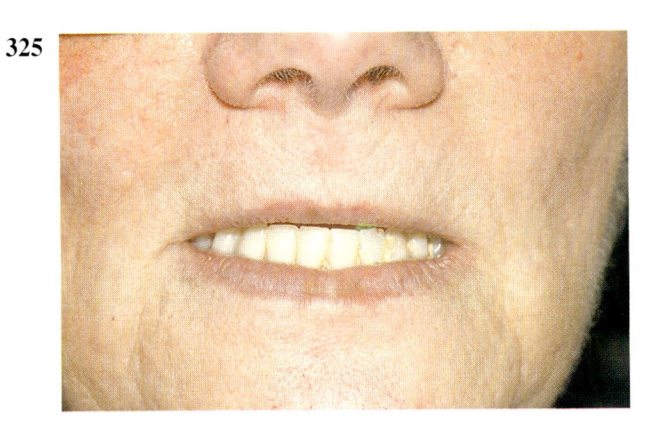

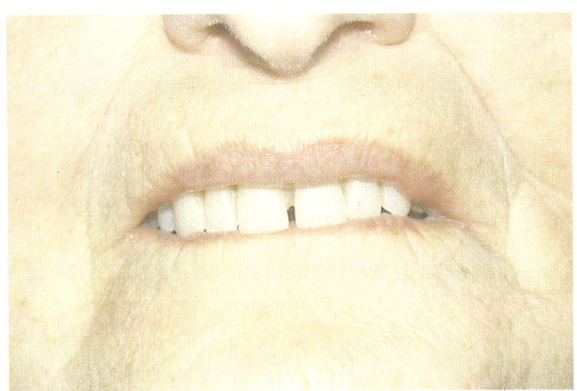

325, 326 In these patients, errors in height of the occlusal plane affected the appearance and stability of the dentures.

327 If the dentures are immediate replacements, artificial tooth shape, shade and position are carefully noted. This valuable information may be considered when selecting and positioning teeth in subsequent dentures.

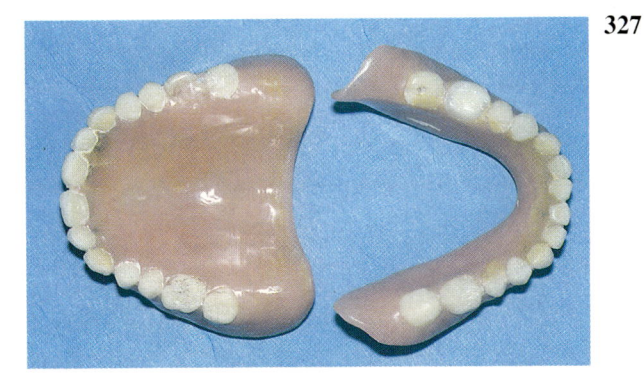

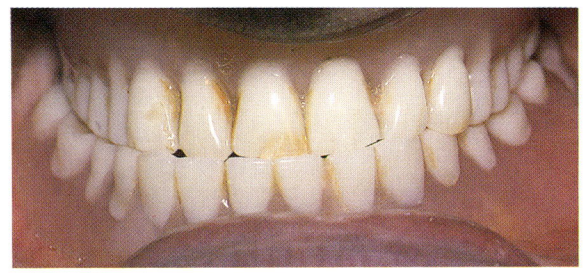

328, 329 Occlusal form, size and position of the posterior teeth and the materials used may provide a helpful guide when planning the occlusal scheme in new dentures. Occlusal wear is often seen in acrylic resin denture teeth.

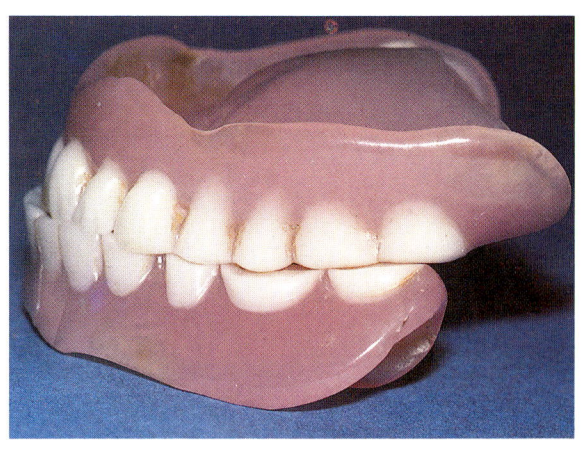

Special investigations

Radiographs

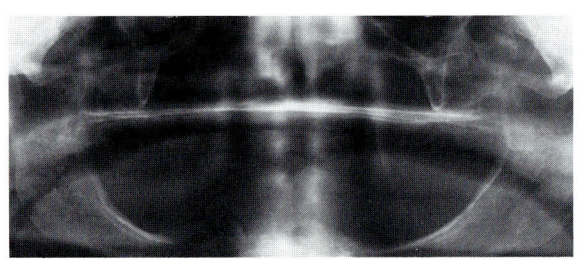

330 Radiographic survey of the mouth is usually with a screening radiograph such as an orthopantomogram. Unerupted teeth, retained roots and changes in bone structure may be seen and require further investigation prior to making new dentures. Further radiographs may be indicated if more detail is needed, and choice of radiographic techniques will depend on the location of the suspected pathological lesion. Unerupted teeth and root remnants need not always be removed, but the patient should at least be informed of their presence.

Mounted diagnostic casts

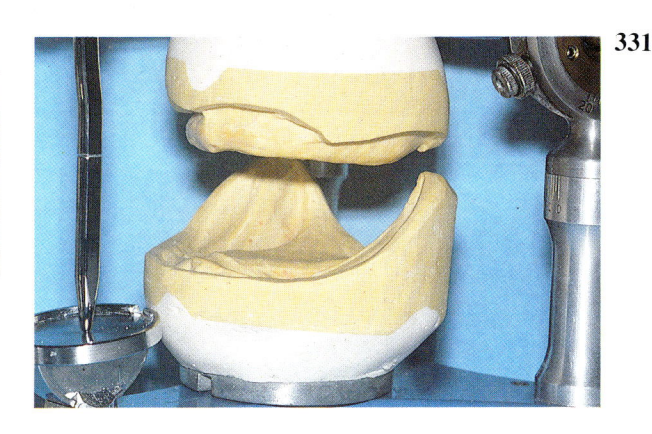

331 Maxillary and mandibular casts of the edentulous ridges help assess the size and form of the bony structures and palatal vault. The only effective way to evaluate the amount of interarch space and ridge relationship is by mounting the casts in an articulator at the established vertical dimension of occlusion in the retruded position.

Conclusion

An assessment of the edentulous patient provides essential diagnostic information when considering complete denture treatment. The biomechanics for successful denture occlusion are evaluated by careful examination of the denture base supporting tissues, factors that influence their retention and stability and the existing dentures.

Part III   Optimizing the occlusion

This section illustrates the restorative, orthodontic and complete denture techniques which may be used for conformative or reorganized treatment for optimizing the occlusion.

Chapter 8:   The conformative–reorganized equation

One of the aims of occlusal assessment is to decide whether or not the patient's existing ICP is stable and treatment can be conformative, or whether the occlusion needs reorganizing.

A summary of the criteria on which this decision is based for the orthodontic, restorative and complete denture patient is listed in the table overleaf.

Criteria for conforming or reorganizing

	Indications for conforming	**Indications for reorganizing**
Orthodontic	1 Tooth movement in a growing individual when RCP=ICP. 2 Tooth movement in an adult when there is no indication to eliminate an RCP–ICP slide, or there is no slide present. 3 Tooth movement combined with orthognathic surgery in non-growing individuals, in which there is no pre-treatment RCP–ICP discrepancy.	1 Presence of RCP–ICP slide in a growing individual. 2 Presence of RCP–ICP slide in patients with occlusal pathology. 3 Adults requiring full-mouth orthodontics in whom there is an RCP–ICP slide. 4 Severe skeletal base discrepancies, in a growing individual, needing functional appliance therapy. 5 Severe skeletal base discrepancies needing orthognathic surgery with a pre-treatment slide between RCP–ICP.
Restorative	1 Stable posterior occlusion. 2 Small number of units to be restored. 3 Large horizontal, small vertical RCP–ICP slide. 4 No need to create space anteriorly. 5 No mandibular dysfunction.	1 Unstable posterior occlusion. 2 Large number of units to be restored. 3 Large vertical, small horizontal RCP–ICP slide. 4 Need to create space anteriorly. 5 Presence of mandibular dysfunction.
Complete Dentures	1 Ill-fitting existing dentures with correct jaw relations.	1 Old dentures with incorrect jaw relations.

▼ *Treat to existing ICP*

▼ *Need to establish RCP=ICP*
Achieved by:
1 Occlusal splint therapy where there is evidence of dysfunction or difficulty in recording a correct retruded position.
2 Re-assessment of diagnostic casts to plan the desirability and ways of eliminating the RCP–ICP discrepancy.

Most restorative treatment is carried out conformatively, as relatively few patients exhibit the signs and symptoms of occlusal pathology indicative of the need to reorganize. Much orthodontic treatment is also carried out conformatively, as the majority of patients have malocclusions falling into the simpler categories and do not present with occlusal pathology. Theoretically, the fabrication of new complete dentures should also conform to the existing retruded jaw relationship. However, this is rarely the case, as ridge resorption, occlusal wear and inaccuracies in the jaw relations of old complete dentures often necessitate the establishment of a new anteroposterior jaw relation and, consequently, the use of a reorganized approach.

The treatment techniques for achieving these objectives are illustrated in the following chapters.

Chapter 9: Introduction to restoration of the occlusion

Following assessment of the occlusion, restorative treatment may proceed along the following routes:

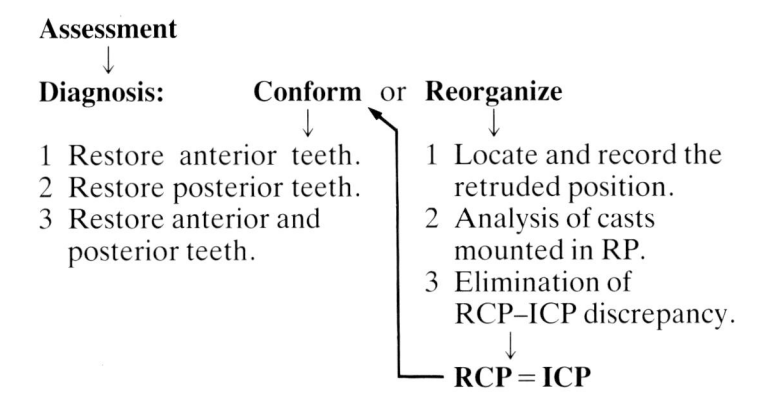

Assessment
↓
Diagnosis: **Conform** or **Reorganize**
↓   ↓

1. Restore anterior teeth.
2. Restore posterior teeth.
3. Restore anterior and posterior teeth.

1. Locate and record the retruded position.
2. Analysis of casts mounted in RP.
3. Elimination of RCP–ICP discrepancy.
↓
RCP = ICP

To avoid unnecessary repetition of both text and illustrations, this first chapter illustrates the treatment stages required to locate the retruded position, and then to eliminate the RCP–ICP discrepancy prior to making restorations, in cases requiring a reorganized approach. Once this has been achieved and the new jaw relationship established, all subsequent restorative dentistry becomes conformative.

It should be emphasized that only the relatively small number of patients who present with the signs and symptoms of loss of posterior occlusal stability require this approach, most restorative dentistry being carried out conformatively.

Once the decision has been made to reorganize, treatment should be undertaken to place the condyles in the retruded position, analyse the resultant occlusal relationships, and finally to eliminate the RCP–ICP discrepancy prior to the provision of definitive restorations. This may involve the following stages of treatment:

- Occlusal splint therapy to place the condyles in RP.
- Analysis of diagnostic casts mounted in RP.
- Eliminating the RCP–ICP discrepancy prior to provision of the final restorations. This may be achieved by the following treatment modalities:

(i) Occlusal equilibration.
(ii) The use of provisional restorations to establish anterior guidance and posterior stability at the retruded position.
(iii) Reorganized orthodontics.
(iv) Orthognathic surgery.
(v) Additions to existing dentures.

When these measures have been carried out, and the anteroposterior jaw relation established, final restorations are made, conforming to the new intercuspal position.

Occlusal splint therapy

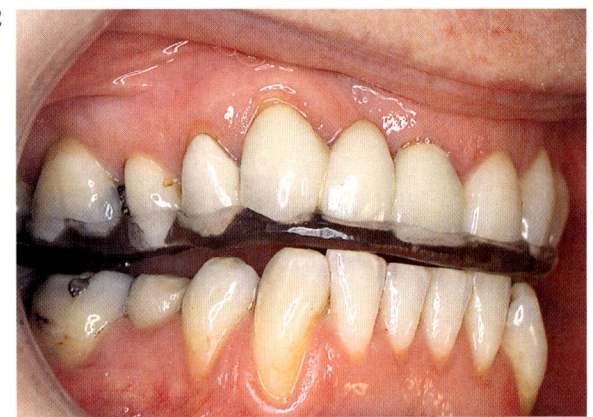

332 The fabrication, fitting and adjustment of occlusal splints has been described in the section on 'Special Investigations' prior to restorative dentistry. The use of occlusal splints prior to reorganized restorative dentistry and orthodontics is indicated when:

- Difficulty is experienced in recording RP.
- The patient exhibits signs and symptoms of mandibular dysfunction.
- As a routine prior to full mouth restoration.
- When a patient cannot produce reproducible pantographic tracings.

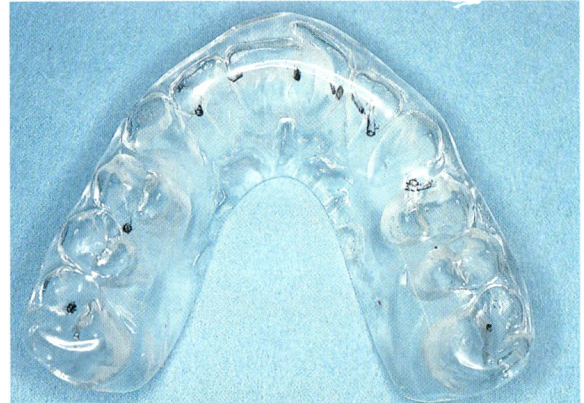

333a, 333b Splint therapy is continued until:

- All signs and symptoms of mandibular dysfunction have gone.
- The occlusal contacts on the splint remain stable between appointments (**333a**).
- The patient can provide reproducible pantographic tracings (**333b**).

For clinicians unfamiliar with the pantograph, the first two criteria are sufficient.

Analysis of diagnostic casts mounted in RP

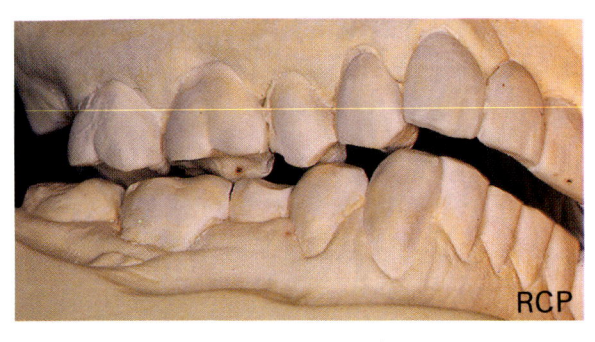

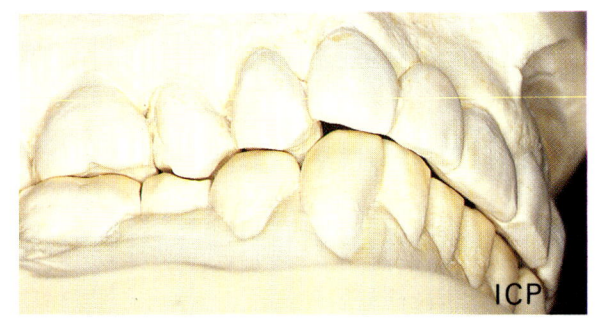

334a, 334b Once a stable and reproducible retruded position has been achieved, a new set of diagnostic casts are mounted and the occlusal relationship analysed to decide upon the appropriate means of eliminating the discrepancy between RCP (**334a**) and ICP (**334b**).

Eliminating the RCP–ICP discrepancy

(i) Occlusal equilibration

335 In many cases where the discrepancy is not too great, occlusal equilibration is sufficient to remove the RCP–ICP slide. In order to learn the mechanics of carrying out an equilibration, readers are referred to more detailed texts on the subject and encouraged to practise on mounted casts. For clinical cases, trial adjustment on mounted casts is advised for two reasons: firstly as a learning process, and secondly to ascertain whether a satisfactory result can be achieved by the conservative removal of tooth structure.

If the teeth are designated for restoration, occlusal adjustment can be more radical and is easier to perform. If not, the amount of enamel which can be safely removed is more limited and a trial adjustment must demonstrate that a stable result can be achieved before the procedure is carried out on the patient. Occlusal equilibration should always be preceded by the successful use of an occlusal splint in patients suffering from mandibular dysfunction. This demonstrates that occlusal therapy will benefit the patient and that a stable jaw relation has been achieved before commencing the adjustment on the patient's teeth. Trial adjustment will also indicate whether the resultant jaw and tooth relations will help or hinder subsequent restorative dentistry.

336 Once it has been ascertained that occlusal equilibration is both possible and also helpful, it may be carried out on the patient's teeth. It is probably one of the more difficult dental procedures and should not be undertaken by inexperienced operators, as it has the capacity to cause great damage both to individual teeth and to the occlusion as a whole.

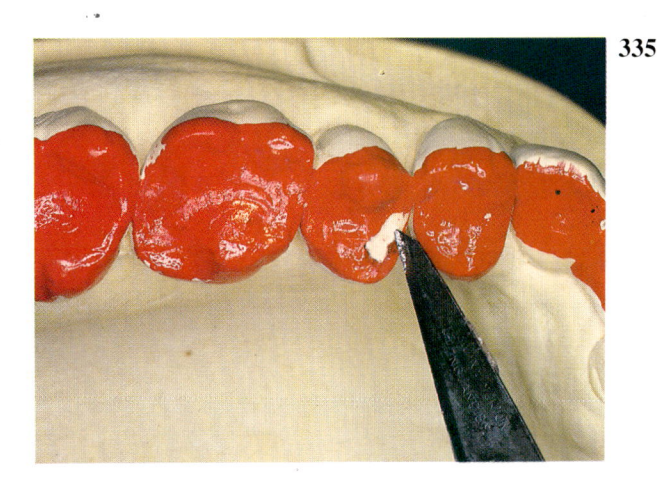

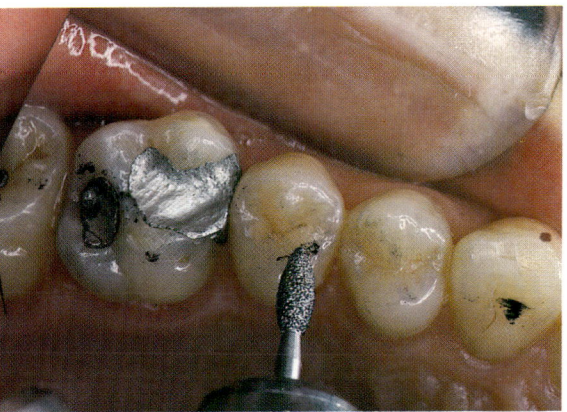

When equilibrating a patient's occlusion prior to carrying out extensive restorative dentistry, it is often advisable to allow the patient to function comfortably on the adjusted occlusion for several months prior to construction of definitive restorations. This is particularly true in patients prone to mandibular dysfunction, who have been wearing an occlusal splint.

In some cases, the post-occlusal splint RCP–ICP discrepancy will be too large for occlusal equilibration alone to correct. It may not be possible to establish anterior guidance and posterior stability without the occlusal splint, unless provisional restorations are employed.

(ii) The use of provisional restorations to re-establish anterior guidance and posterior stability

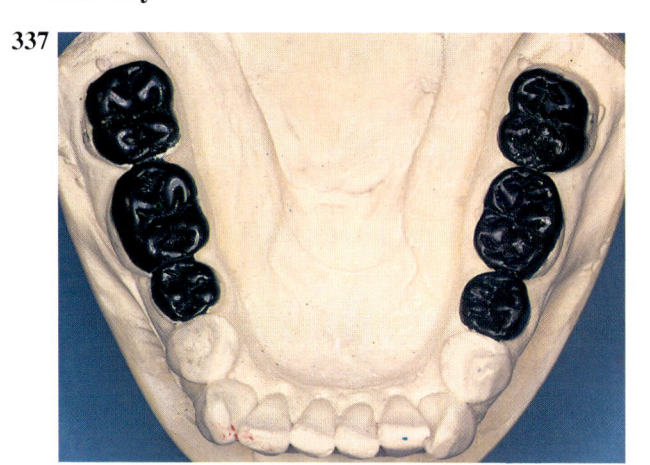

337 A diagnostic wax-up of the teeth to be restored is carried out on the equilibrated casts, in this case to restore posterior stability. This is used as a basis to determine the shape of the provisional restorations.

Posterior repositioning of the condyles in patients with a large horizontal RCP–ICP discrepancy may leave the anterior teeth out of contact, removing anterior guidance. If the anterior teeth are destined for restoration, they can be prepared and provisionals fitted, closing the space and providing immediate disclusion. If not, immediate disclusion may be provided by acid etch-retained guidance surfaces made on the equilibrated diagnostic casts. This technique is illustrated in Chapter 10.

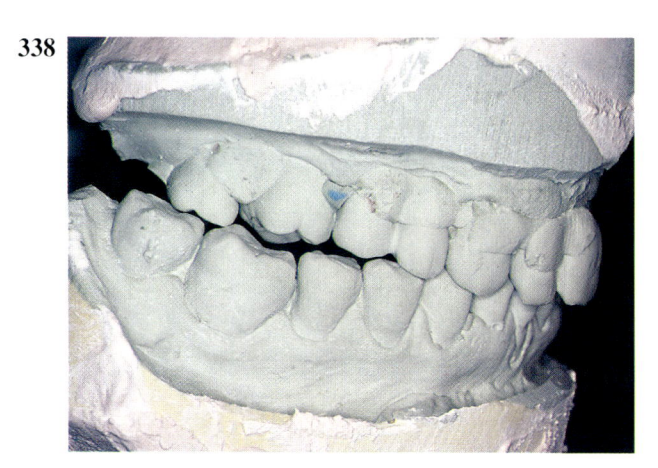

338, 339 An 84-year-old lady had suffered a condylar neck fracture which was left uncorrected. She presented with a posterior open bite and severe mandibular dysfunction. Occlusal splint therapy was carried out to alleviate her symptoms and achieve a stable jaw relation. Trial occlusal equilibration showed that it was impossible to bring the posterior teeth into stable contact to allow her to cease wearing the splint. A cobalt/chrome overlay partial denture was made as a long-term provisional restoration to fill this space and provide posterior occlusal stability. This carried the risk of increased wear of the opposing teeth; this would, however, have been of little consequence considering the patient's poor general health and age.

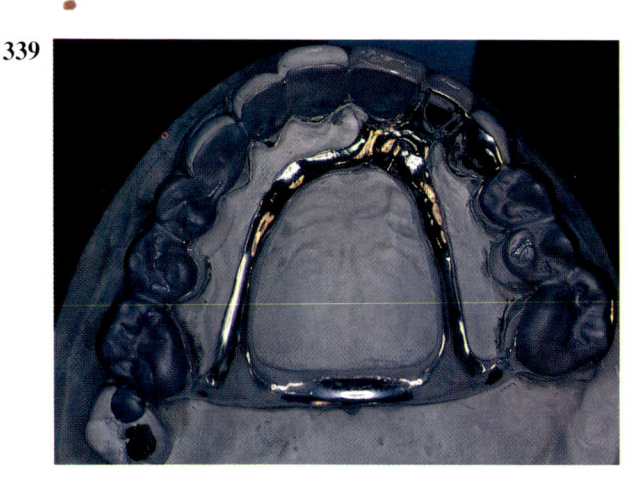

340, 341 This patient had a posterior reconstruction while suffering from an anteriorly displaced articular disc. She subsequently developed acute mandibular dysfunction and occlusal splint therapy was carried out which repositioned the disc. This opened up a space between the posterior restorations which could not be closed by the usual 'subtractive' occlusal adjustment. Provisional gold onlays were waxed on diagnostic casts of the existing restorations. These were cast in Type III gold and cemented onto the crown and bridgework with zinc phosphate cement, providing posterior stability. After a period of about six months, during which the temporary occlusion had remained stable and comfortable, the old restorations, which were poorly-fitting, were removed and replaced.
Courtesy of Dr J. Clayton.

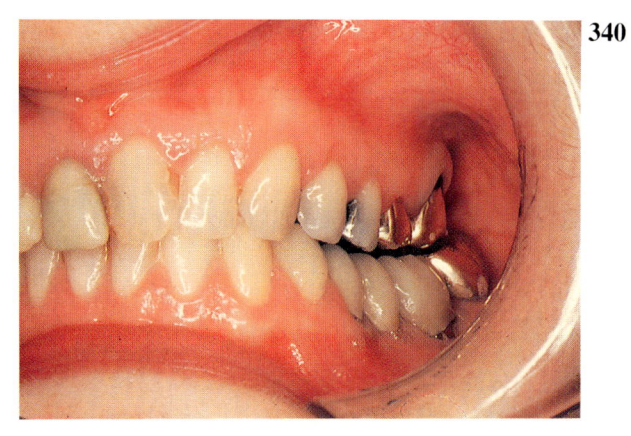

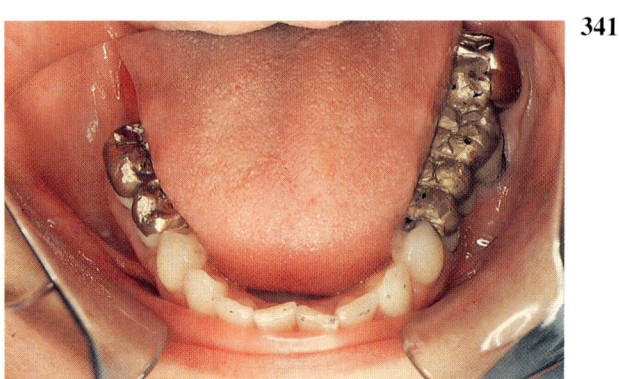

342 Indirectly-made polymethylmethacrylate provisional restorations are durable enough to be used for several months, provided they are of adequate thickness.

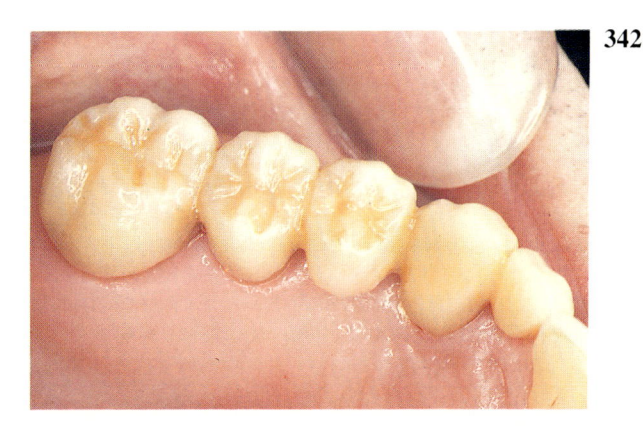

343 For longer periods of time, particularly in bruxers and where thinner, partial-coverage restorations are involved, the use of metal provisionals is advised. These are made of a silver containing alloy, which, although prone to tarnish, is less expensive than gold.

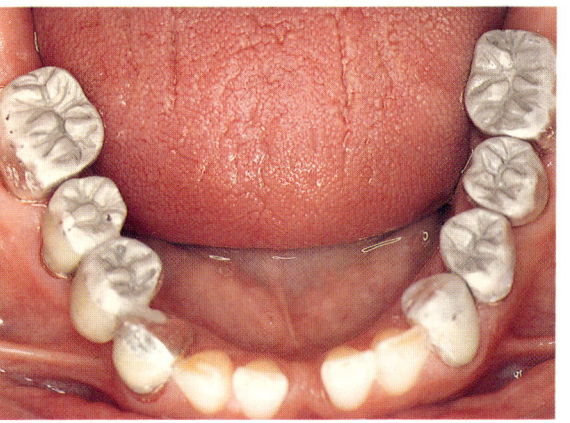

127

(iii) Reorganized orthodontics

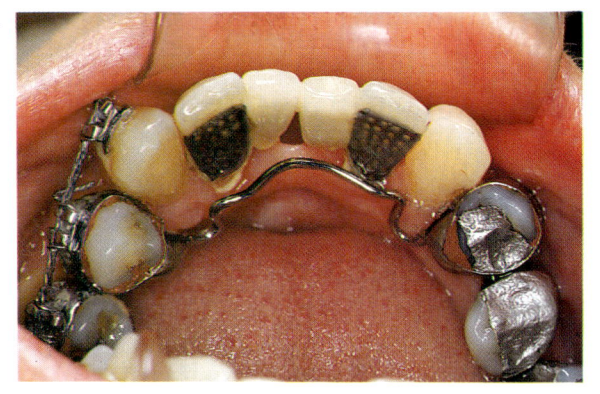

344 In the adult patient requiring restorative treatment, cast analysis may reveal a significant RCP–ICP discrepancy. If this cannot be eliminated by equilibration or by fitting provisional restorations, orthodontic tooth movement may be used. It is essential for the restorative dentist to provide the orthodontist with a cast set-up to indicate exactly where he would like the teeth moved. This patient had an acid etch-retained bridge placed to stabilize the lower labial segment, followed by orthodontic treatment to upright 35 & 38 and eliminate the RCP–ICP discrepancy prior to further restorative treatment.

(iv) Orthognathic surgery

345a, 345b Adult patients with severe skeletal base discrepancies and mutilated dentitions may require orthognathic surgery to permit the subsequent restoration of adequate anterior guidance and posterior stability. This rather drastic approach to treatment is only indicated if the patient presents with a severe functional disturbance due to the malocclusion, which cannot be treated in a more conservative way. This patient had straight-wire orthodontics (**345a**) to align the mandibular teeth, followed by a lower anterior segmental osteotomy to correct a Class II skeletal discrepancy (**345b**).

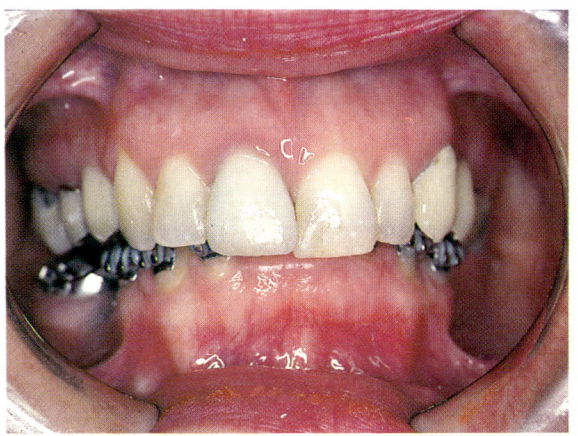

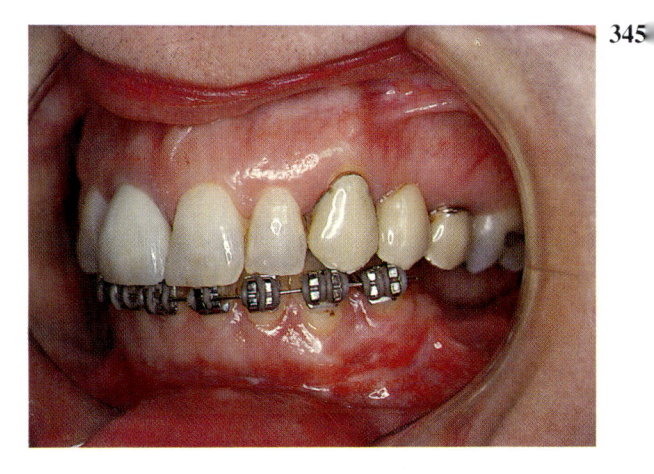

(v) Additions to existing dentures

Acrylic resin may be added to existing dentures with worn occlusal surfaces to restore ICP contacts prior to making a new prosthesis. In many situations this is not possible, as opposing teeth will have over-erupted, maintaining occlusal contact as the artificial teeth wear.

Conclusion

The treatment pathway for reorganizing occlusion has been illustrated; the next three chapters describe the practical techniques involved in the restoration of teeth.

Chapter 10: The restoration of anterior teeth

In the restoration of both anterior and posterior teeth, the restorations should either be made at the same time, or the anterior restorations first. Once anterior guidance has been established, restoration of posterior teeth is simplified because the extent of disclusion available, which will influence posterior cusp height, is a known factor.

General considerations in restoring anterior guidance

These include:

- Reproducing the correct maxillary lingual concavity.
- Occlusal considerations for tooth preparation.
- Establishing the anteroposterior jaw relation first.
- Metal coping design.
- Achieving stable ICP contacts.
- Choice of the type of guidance.

Reproducing the correct maxillary lingual concavity

346 A section through a cast of a maxillary central incisor demonstrates a palatal surface with a smooth, concave shape and flat cingulum, against which the lower incisors normally occlude in ICP.

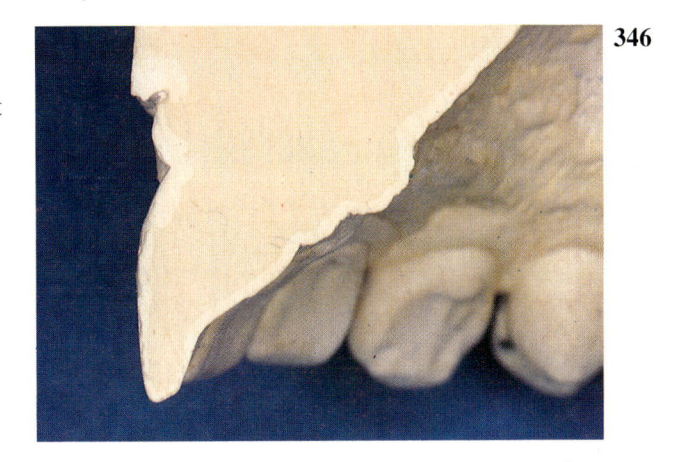

347 Both intra- and extra-coronal restorations should conform to this outline.

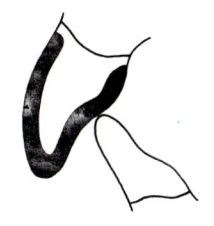

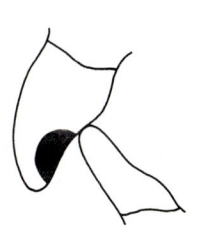

Occlusal considerations for tooth preparation

348

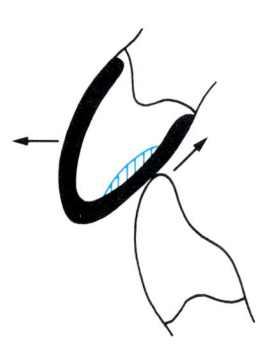

▩ Underprepared area

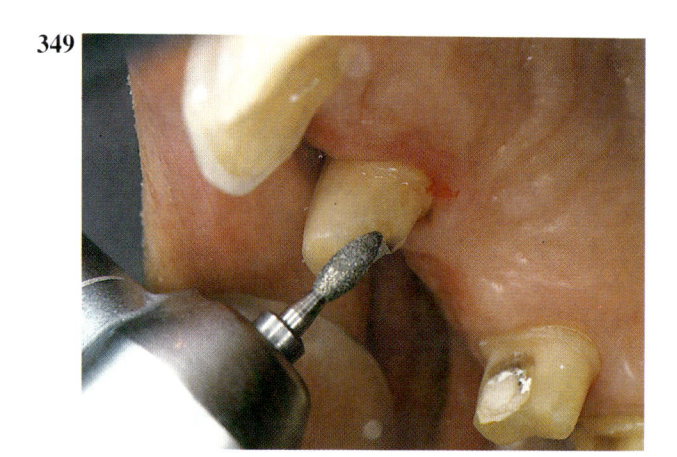

348 If restorations are placed whose palatal surfaces are too bulbous, the anterior guidance may become traumatic because excessive occlusal force may be applied to the restored teeth in protrusive or lateral excursions. This may result in labial drifting and hypermobility, hypersensitivity to cold and pressure, failure of the cement lute, fracture of the restorations and increased wear of the restored or opposing surfaces. A convex palatal surface will not reproduce a flat cingulum against which a stable ICP contact can be achieved. This may also result in the unfavourable direction of occlusal forces. A crown with an overcontoured palatal surface is often the result of under preparation.

349

349 The use of a rugby ball-shaped diamond stone will provide correctly shaped palatal reduction.

Establishing the anteroposterior jaw relation first

350a

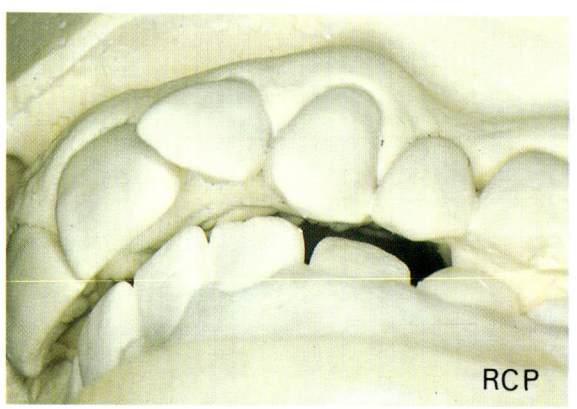

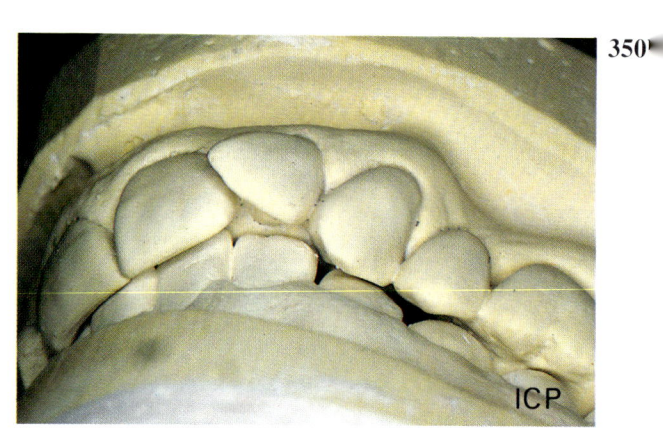

RCP

350b

ICP

350a, 350b The correct anteroposterior jaw relationship is established before assessment of the existing anterior guidance to decide whether modifications are necessary. If diagnostic cast analysis demonstrates a large horizontal discrepancy between RCP (**350a**) and ICP (**350b**), reorganizing the occlusion will alter this relationship.

Metal coping design

351, 352 It is advisable to restore guidance surfaces in porcelain, only when opposed by porcelain restorations. Porcelain is a potentially abrasive material which may cause increased wear of opposing teeth in patients prone to parafunction. Where porcelain is indicated, crowns should be designed with a narrow metal collar palatally. The ICP contact should be placed on porcelain, well away from the porcelain–metal junction.

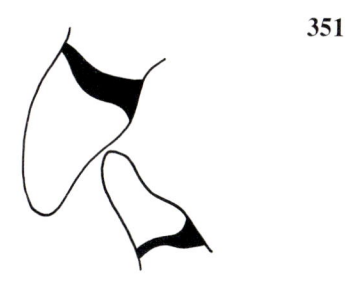

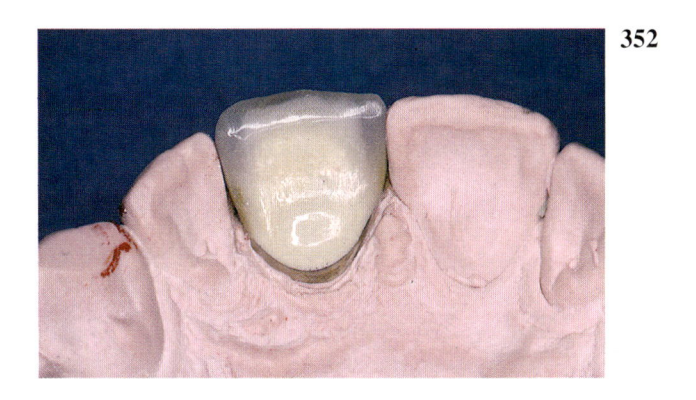

353, 354 It is advisable to restore the articulating surfaces of teeth in metal when they oppose unrestored teeth. Gold is a softer and more resilient material which wears at a similar rate to enamel. The location of the porcelain–metal junction must be judged individually. The ICP contact and first two millimetres of guidance should be on metal and the porcelain should be extended as far over the incisal edge as possible, for maximum bond strength to the metal coping.

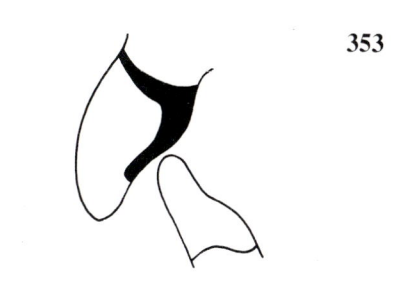

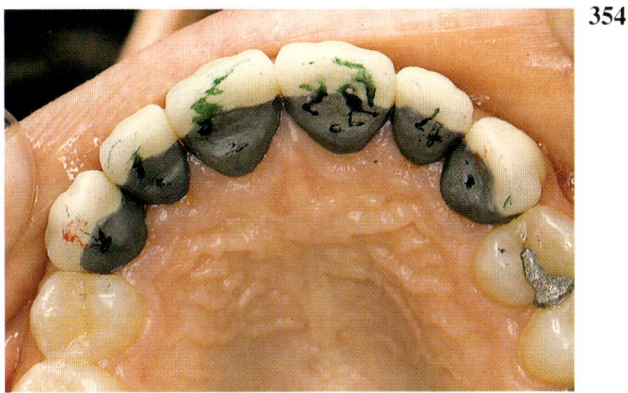

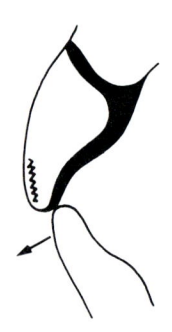

355 If the ICP contact is close to the incisal edge, it must be in porcelain. If the porcelain–metal junction is placed too far incisally, flexure of the thin metal edge under occlusal forces may fracture the porcelain facing.

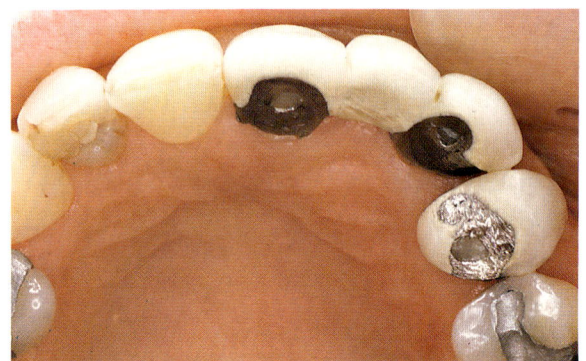

356 These restorations opposed unrestored mandibular teeth. The metal coping design and placement of porcelain–metal junctions is incorrect and inconsistent. The anterior guidance surfaces are overcontoured and have been roughly adjusted, resulting in the perforation of three castings. This may have resulted from lack of knowledge, planning and instructions to the technician.

Achieving stable ICP contacts and choice of the type of guidance

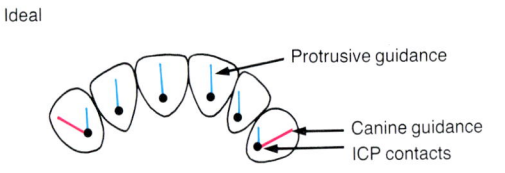

357 This diagram shows the ideal appearance of ICP contacts and anterior guidance marked on the palatal surfaces of maxillary anterior teeth with articulating paper. In an unrestored dentition in which the teeth have not been weakened by dental disease or the presence of restorations, the type of protrusive and lateral guidance is less important.

When restoring anterior teeth a choice has to be made as to which teeth will provide anterior guidance in protrusive and lateral excursions. Clinically, it is often difficult to achieve this ideal appearance owing to the relative positions of the maxillary and mandibular anterior teeth in ICP.

In ICP, ideally all anterior teeth should possess stable ICP contacts to distribute occlusal forces on closure axially, stabilizing tooth positions.

In protrusion, it is advisable to distribute the protrusive contacts evenly over as many teeth as possible, the only exception being the removal of protrusive contacts (but not ICP contacts) from teeth which have been weakened and which are less able to withstand lateral occlusal forces. These will include:

- Teeth restored with Class IV composite resins.
- Cantilevered pontics.
- Post crowns.
- Other endodontically treated teeth.
- Teeth with root fractures or resorption.
- Teeth with greatly reduced periodontal attachment.

In lateral excursion, when guidance teeth require restoration, a choice has to be made between canine guidance and group function. Various theoretical arguments have been put forward attempting to substantiate the use of these concepts of occlusion, none of which stands up to scientific scrutiny.

It is advisable to use canine guidance where possible, for the following practical reasons:

- The canine is a large, strong tooth near the front of the mouth with a naturally concave palatal surface which lends itself to providing smooth and adequately steep disclusion.
- It is only necessary to reproduce contact on the surface of one tooth outside ICP. Technically this is easy to achieve using a semi-adjustable articulator whose incisal guide table has been custom-moulded from casts of provisional restorations adjusted in the mouth to harmonize with condylar movements.

When the canines are not in contact in ICP, it becomes necessary to use other teeth to provide disclusion. The choice of which teeth to use is decided by those in the best position to provide adequate guidance and not by adherence to a fixed concept of occlusion. The use of multiple working side contacts such as group function is technically difficult to achieve and requires the use of a fully-adjustable articulator.

The same criteria for removing lateral contacts from weakened teeth in protrusion apply to lateral excursion.

Restoring anterior guidance

Techniques for restoring anterior guidance will be described under the following headings:

- Copying existing guidance.
- Altering existing guidance.
- Difficult situations.
- Occlusal considerations for acid etch-retained bridges.
- Partial denture occlusion when anterior teeth require replacement.

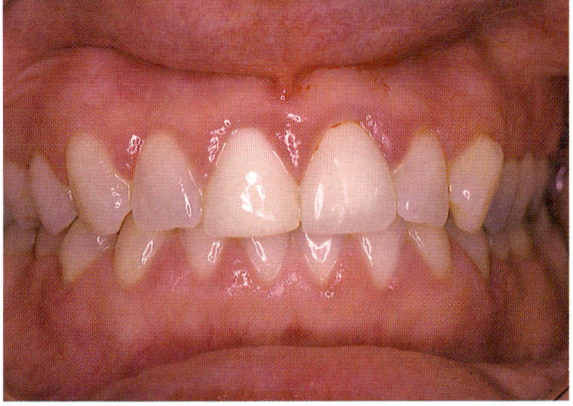

Copying existing guidance

358 This patient required replacement of porcelain jacket crowns on 11,21. The shape of 21 was satisfactory both aesthetically and functionally. It is advantageous to use a technique enabling this shape to be duplicated in the new restorations, and not to leave its determination to the technician.

358

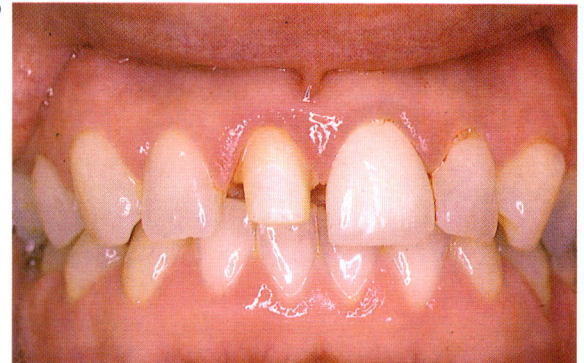

359, 360 11 was prepared and a working impression and cast were made.

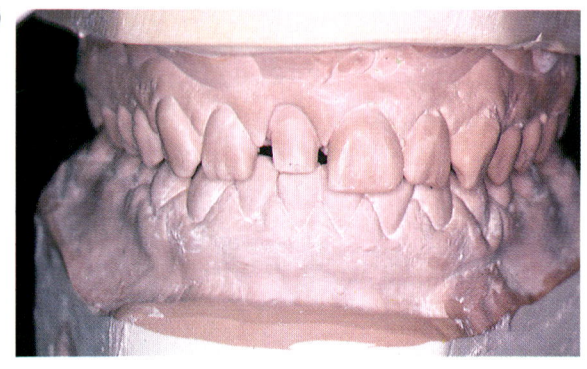

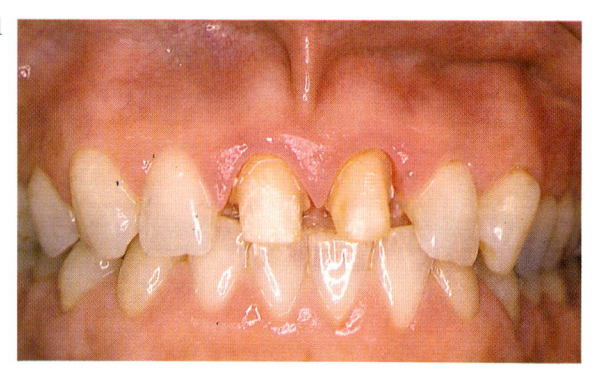

361, 362 21 was prepared, a second impression recording both preparations made, and the cast poured.

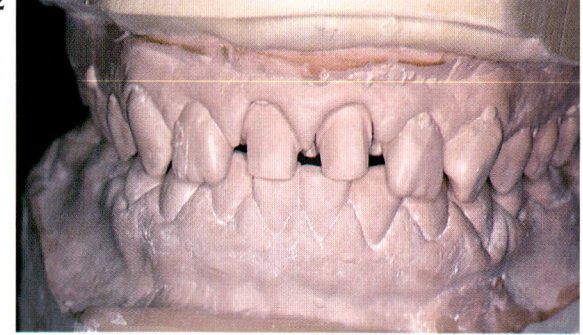

363, 364 A full contour wax pattern was made on the first cast, copying the shape of 21. The pattern was transferred to the second cast and used as a guide for waxing 11.

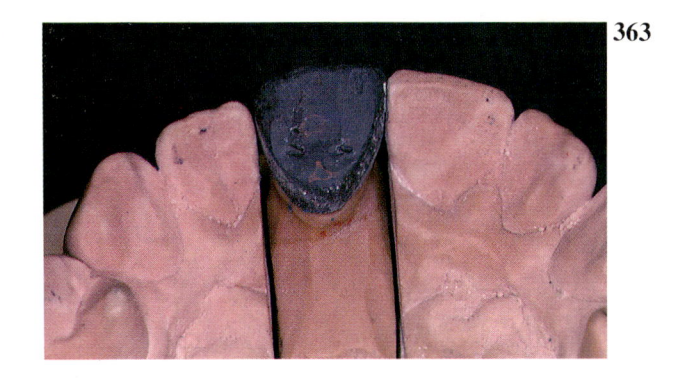

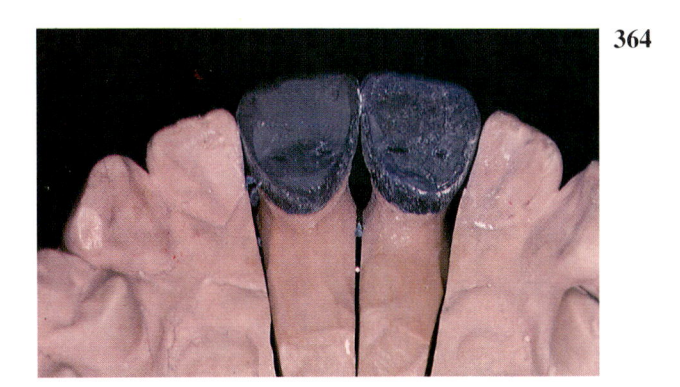

365, 366 The patterns were cut back, invested, cast and porcelain was applied. The final crowns were checked both labially and palatally by transferring 11 back to the first cast and comparing it to the stone model of the old crown on 21.

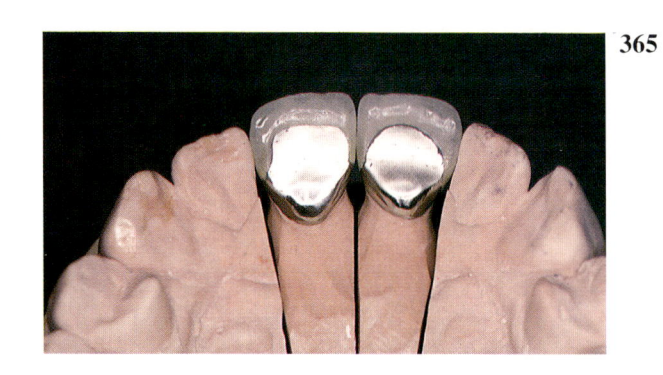

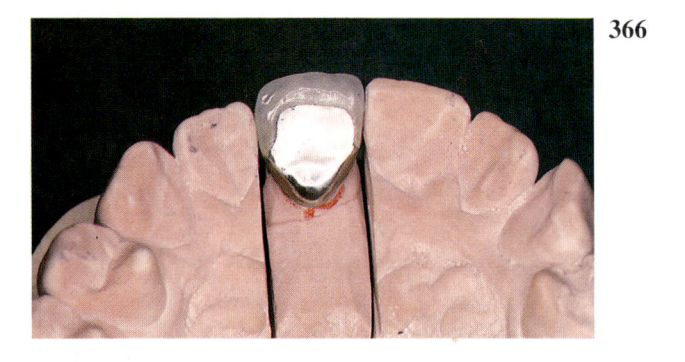

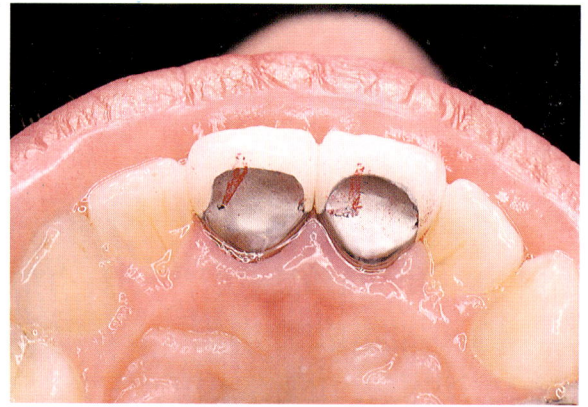

367, 368 The crowns were tried in and the ICP contacts marked in black and protrusive guidance in red. The matt finish on the metal surface, produced by blasting with glass beads, facilitated the marking of contacts with articulating paper. The palatal surfaces were smooth, concave and steep enough to disclude the posterior teeth. The technician had wrapped the porcelain around proximally to achieve greater translucency. This was inadvisable occlusally as it produced ICP contacts too close to the porcelain–metal junctions.

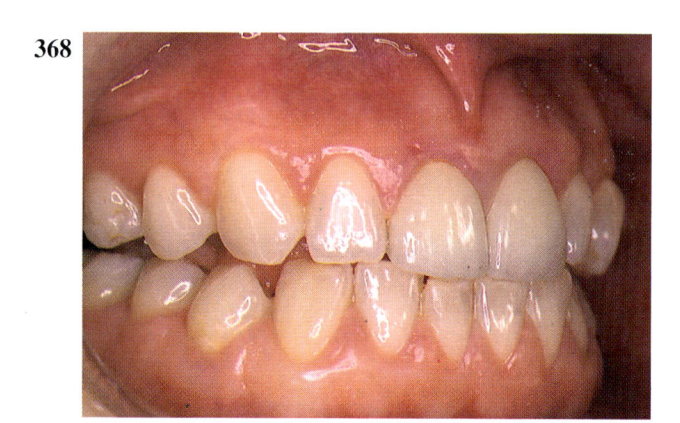

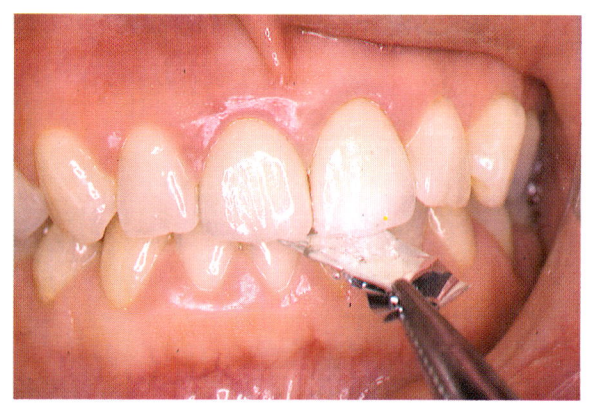

369, 370 The restorations and posterior teeth both held shimstock. When the patient tapped together in ICP, neither crown exhibited fremitus, which would have indicated heavy ICP contact.

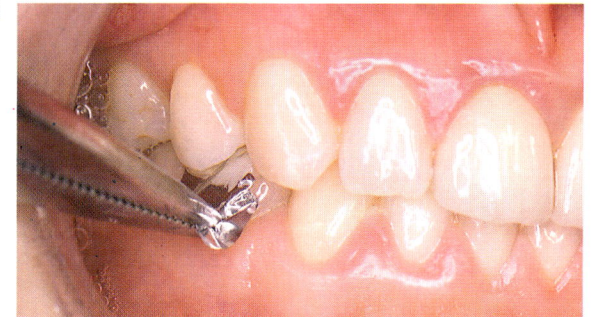

Altering existing guidance

371 This patient required restoration of both maxillary and mandibular anterior teeth. As the shape of the existing restorations was unsatisfactory, a technique was used which diagnosed the correct shape and then allowed it to be duplicated in the final restorations.

The shape of anterior teeth is governed by the following parameters:

- Aesthetics.
- Phonetics.
- The pathways of condylar movement.
- The need to disclude the posterior teeth.

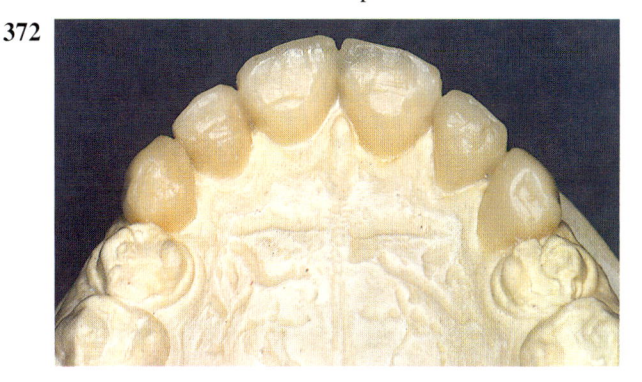

372, 373 A diagnostic wax-up was carried out on casts mounted on a semi-adjustable articulator. The palatal surfaces were shaped to be steep enough to disclude the posterior teeth, and to be in harmony with the path of lateral movement determined by the articulator. The teeth were prepared and a vacuform shell was made over a cast of the diagnostic wax-up, used to check if adequate reduction relative to the intended contour of the final restorations had been achieved.

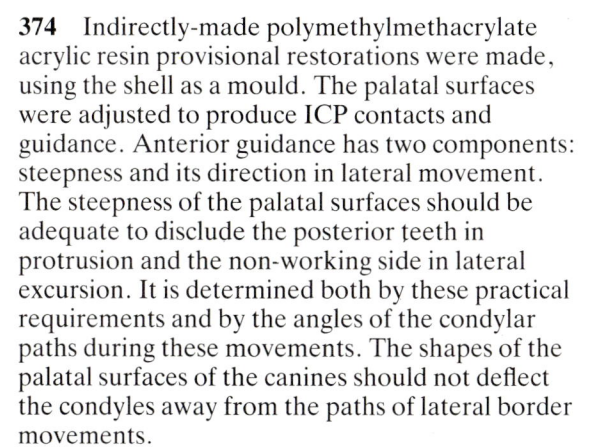

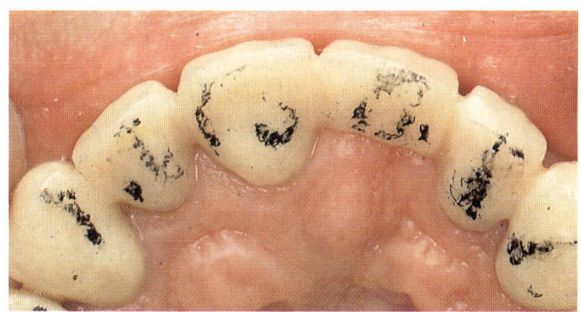

374 Indirectly-made polymethylmethacrylate acrylic resin provisional restorations were made, using the shell as a mould. The palatal surfaces were adjusted to produce ICP contacts and guidance. Anterior guidance has two components: steepness and its direction in lateral movement. The steepness of the palatal surfaces should be adequate to disclude the posterior teeth in protrusion and the non-working side in lateral excursion. It is determined both by these practical requirements and by the angles of the condylar paths during these movements. The shapes of the palatal surfaces of the canines should not deflect the condyles away from the paths of lateral border movements.

In the natural dentition, evidence linking the direction and steepness of anterior guidance to mandibular border movements is inconclusive. However, when restoring broken down anterior teeth, mandibular border movements, aesthetics and phonetics provide the only references from which to work.

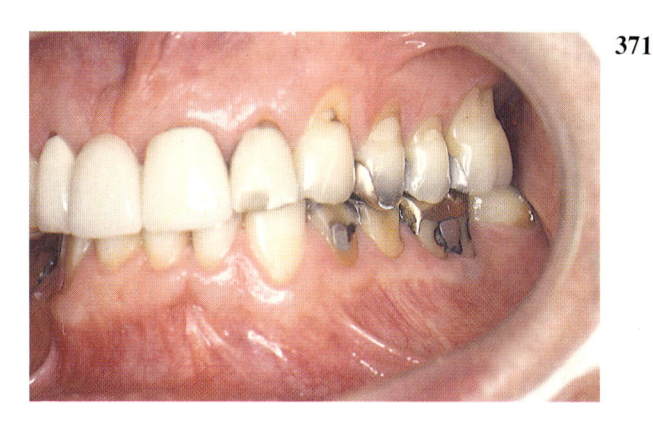

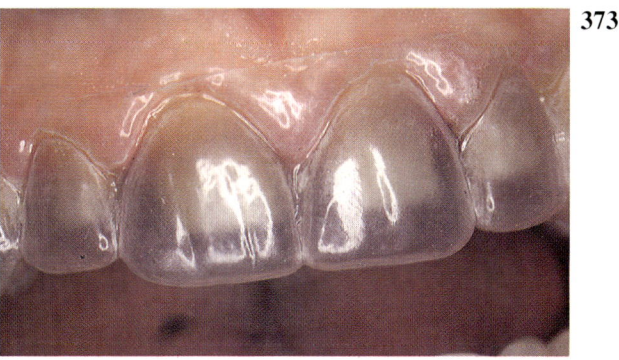

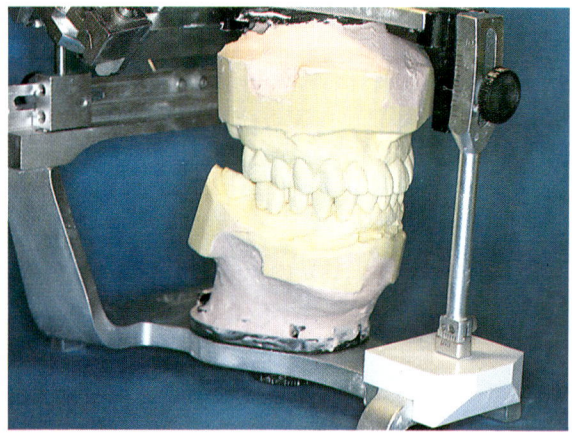

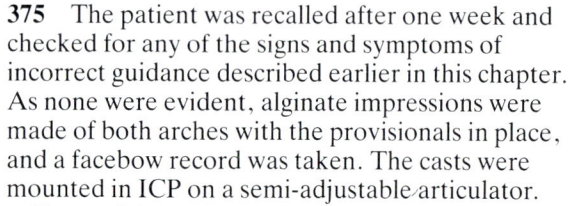

375 The patient was recalled after one week and checked for any of the signs and symptoms of incorrect guidance described earlier in this chapter. As none were evident, alginate impressions were made of both arches with the provisionals in place, and a facebow record was taken. The casts were mounted in ICP on a semi-adjustable articulator.

If any of these signs and symptoms had been present, the provisional restorations would have been readjusted and the patient dismissed for a further week.

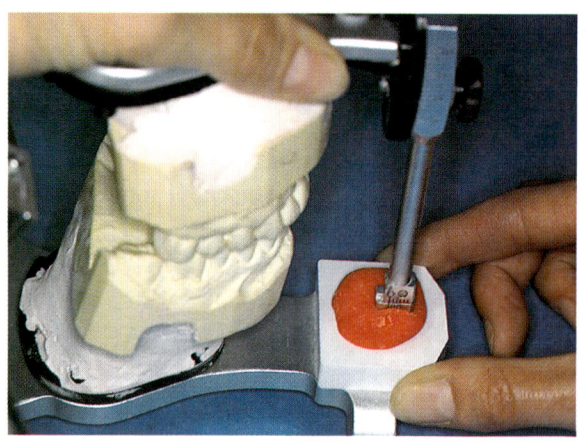

376 Duralay acrylic resin was applied to the plastic incisal guide table, and the casts moved into left and right lateral and protrusive excursions. The foot of the incisal pin carved out a shape which represented a magnified image of the lingual concavities produced in the maxillary provisional restorations.

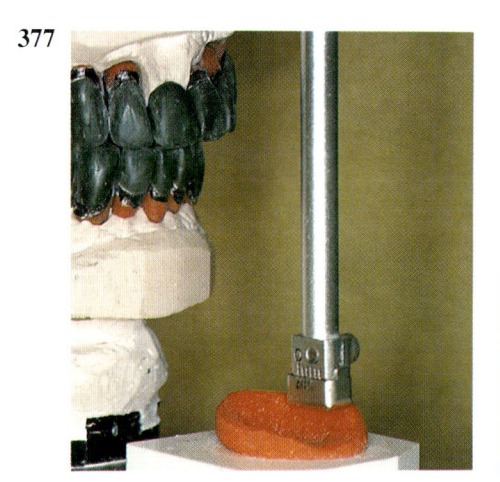

377 The restorations were waxed-up using the movement of the incisal pin over the custom-moulded table to determine the palatal contours.

378 After casting and porcelain application, the restorations were checked to ensure that as the incisal pin moved over the table, their articulating surfaces maintained contact, ensuring that the shape of the provisional restorations had been reproduced.

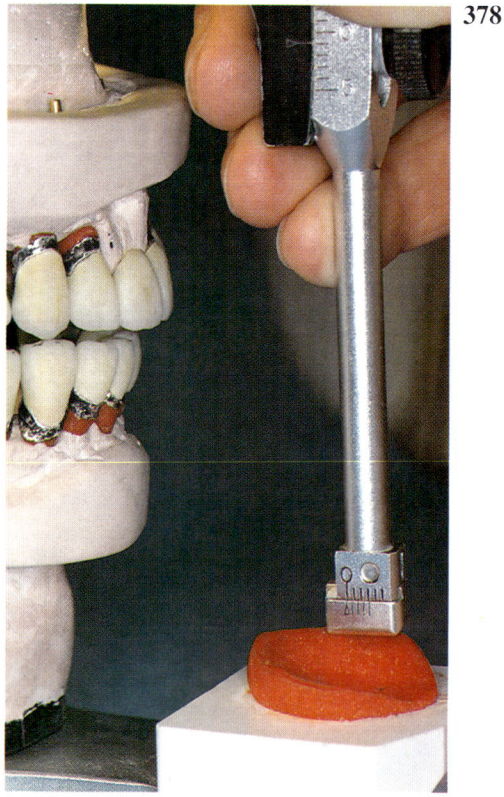

379 ICP contacts and canine guidance were marked on the palatal surfaces.

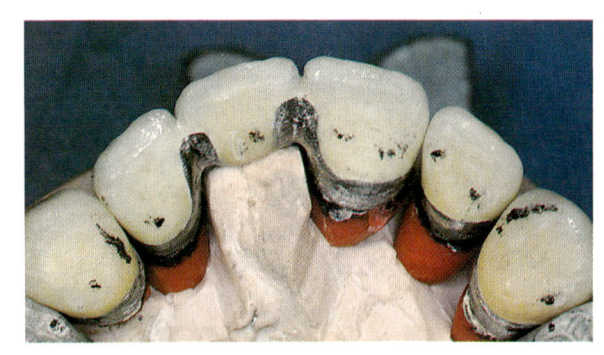

380 When the restorations were tried in, virtually no adjustment to the occlusion was needed. The use of this technique is important in ensuring that guidance is correctly reproduced. Positive errors may be adjusted by grinding, albeit at a risk of ruining the surface of the restoration. A negative error (the guidance being too shallow to provide disclusion) may require a remake. This may happen because the semi-adjustable articulator will not reproduce mandibular movements correctly.

This technique may be used whenever the shape of anterior teeth needs changing.

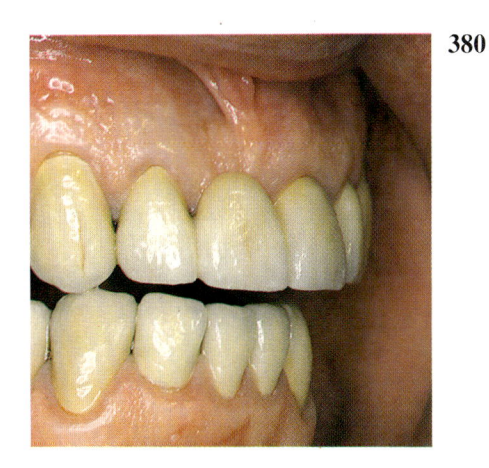

Difficult situations

(i) Cantilevered pontics

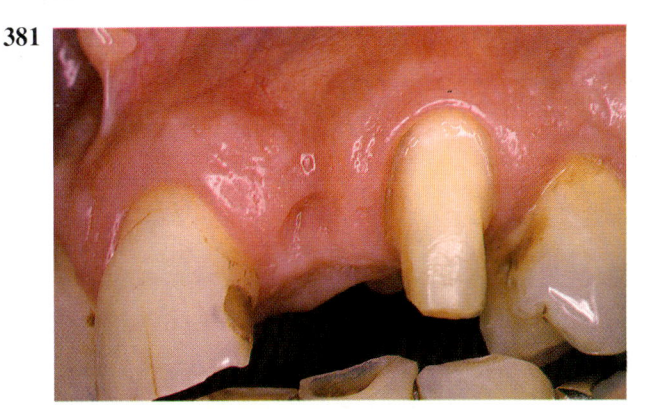

381 A missing maxillary lateral incisor may be replaced by a pontic cantilevered from the adjacent canine.

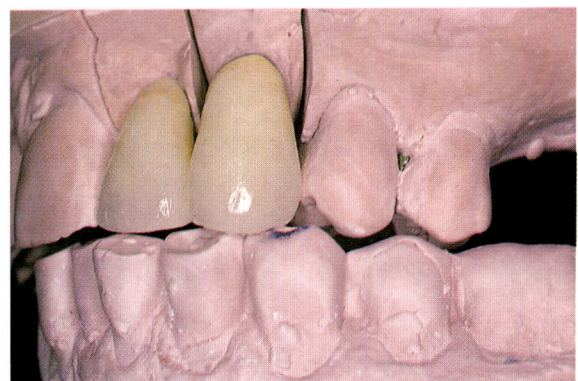

382 The use of a semi-adjustable articulator is advisable to ensure that no contact in lateral and protrusive movements falls on the pontic. In this situation, the canine was used to provide working side disclusion. It was important that both units possessed stable ICP contacts. If the pontic was left out of occlusion, the opposing tooth would over-erupt and lead to a less stable ICP contact than one which had been planned in the first instance.

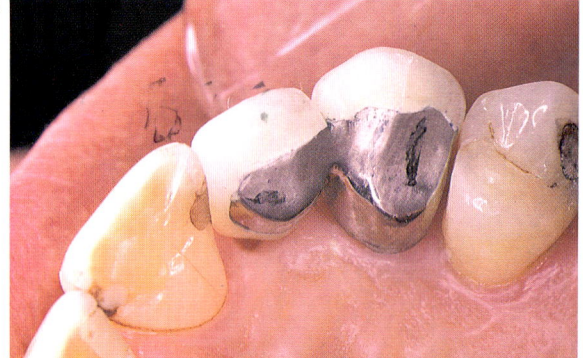

383 The bridge was tried in and the occlusal contacts marked. As the patient's condylar movements differed from those of the articulator, it was necessary to recheck that no contact outside ICP fell on the pontic and that the canine provided adequate disclusion.

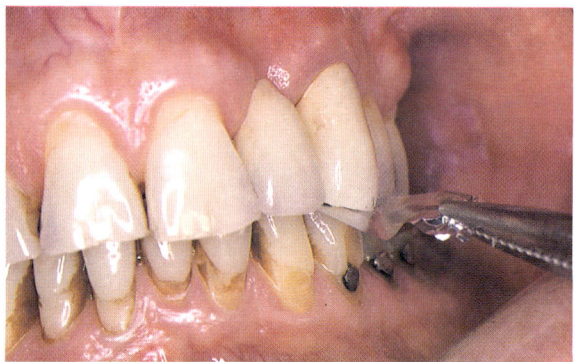

384 Shimstock was used to verify contact between the bridge and opposing teeth, and between adjacent unrestored teeth.

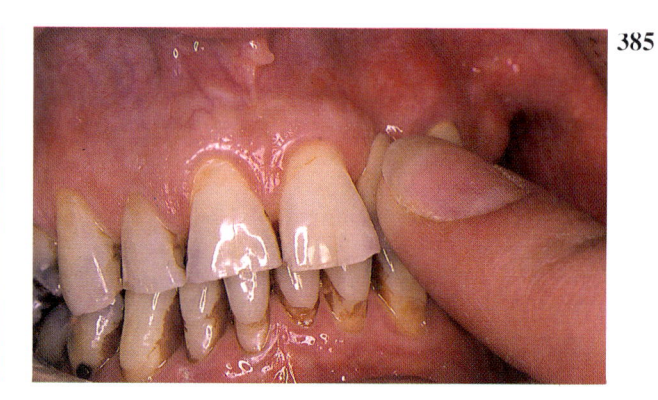

385 The patient was asked to tap together in ICP and the pontic was checked for fremitus, which, if present, would indicate a heavy ICP content.

(ii) Deep overbites

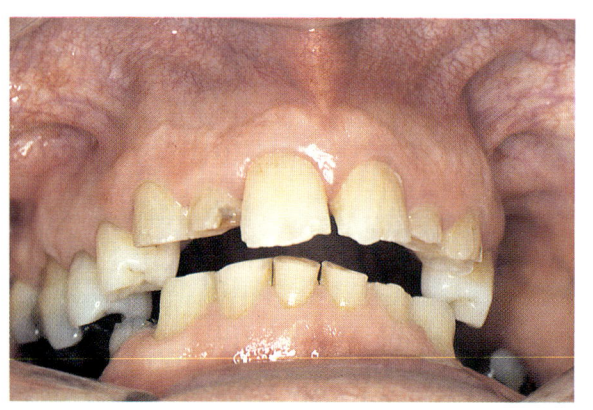

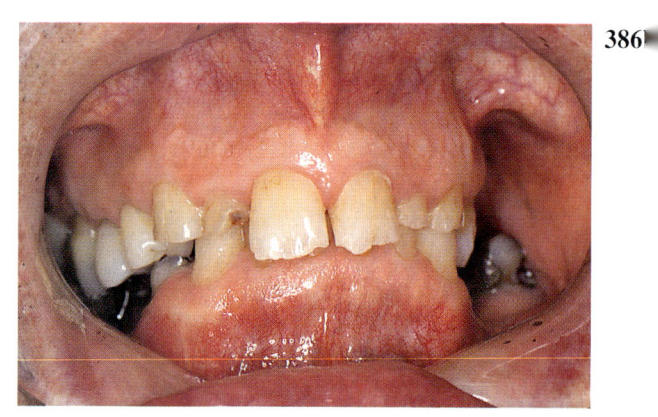

386a, 386b A deep overbite may create problems when anterior teeth need restoring, as there is often insufficient space in which to place the restorative materials. If there is a large horizontal discrepancy between RCP (**386a**) and ICP (**386b**) as in this patient, reorganizing the occlusion may provide the space required.

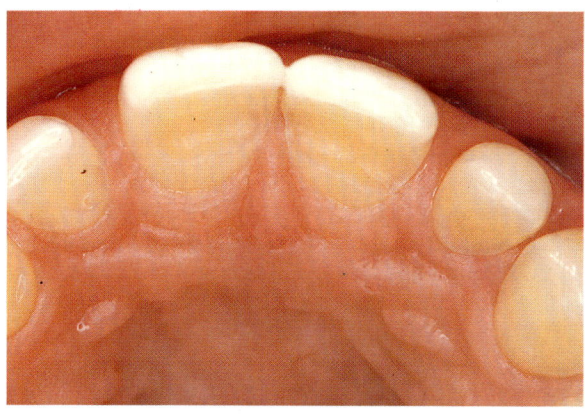

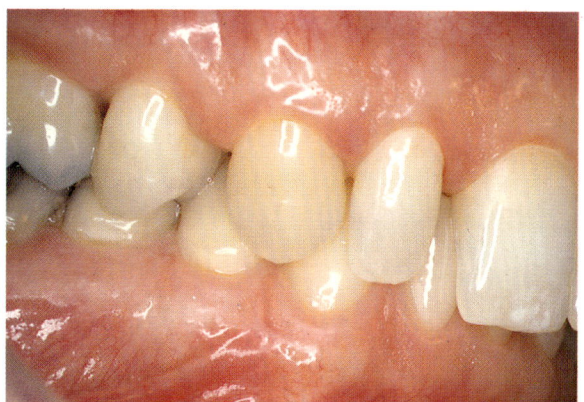

387a, 387b Extensive wear and erosion of the palatal surfaces of 12, 11, 21, 22 had occurred. These teeth required restoration to re-establish anterior guidance and prevent further damage (**387a**). There was a deep overbite and no discrepancy between RCP and ICP (**387b**), even after wearing an occlusal splint.

388 Lingual examination of diagnostic casts revealed a deep, complete overbite with no room available for restorations.

389 An alternative to shortening the mandibular anterior teeth to obtain space is to use a cobalt/chrome anterior biteplane (Dahl Appliance).

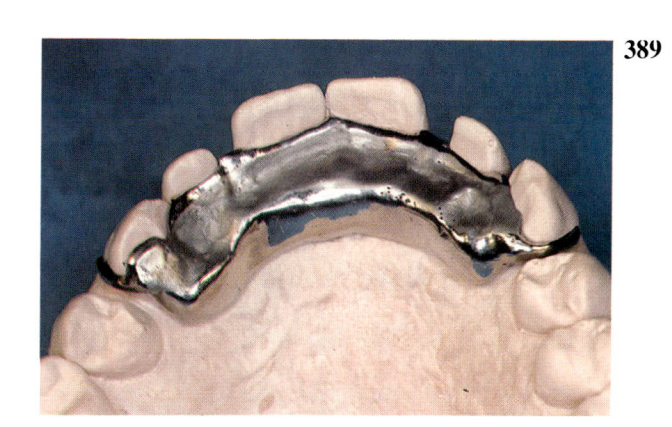

390 This prosthesis provides occlusal contacts in ICP with the mandibular incisors, separating the posterior teeth by several millimetres.

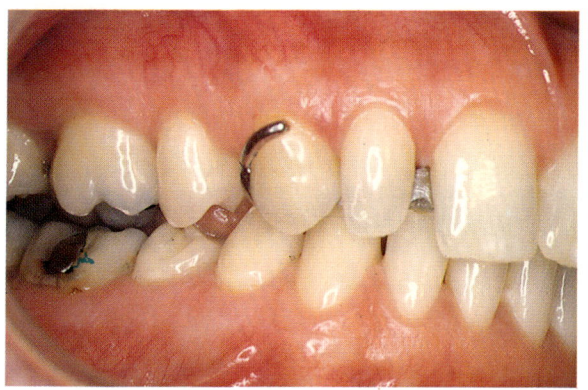

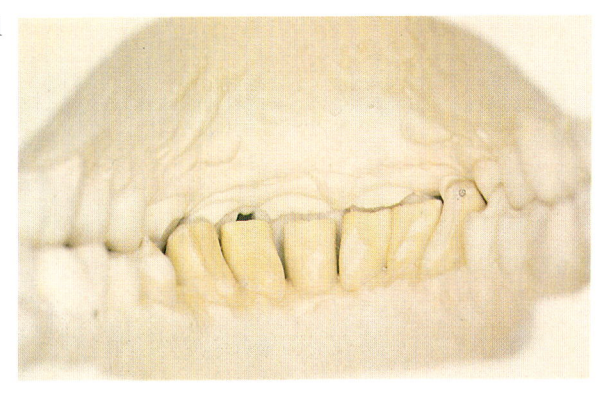

391 The biteplane was worn continuously for two and a half months, after which new diagnostic casts were made and mounted. The prosthesis caused the intrusion of the mandibular incisors and permitted over-eruption of the posterior teeth, creating enough space to restore the palatal surfaces of 12, 11, 21, 22. The final restorations were pinledges made from a type 3 gold alloy. Acid etch–retained restorations were not considered, as there remained insufficient palatal enamel to which they could be bonded.

(iii) Class 2 jaw relation

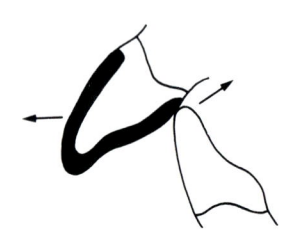

392 A Class 2 division I incisor relation may pose problems when restoring anterior or posterior teeth. An increased overjet and overbite may lead to the mandibular incisors occluding palatally to the cingulae of the maxillary anterior teeth. If maxillary restorations copy this relationship, it will be impossible to provide stable ICP contacts and correctly shaped anterior guidance. If there is no contact between the teeth in ICP, it is more difficult to disclude the posterior teeth.

393 To achieve stable ICP contacts, correct guidance and immediate disclusion, it is necessary to do two things: Firstly, the mandibular incisors may need shortening. Their edges should be reduced horizontally and not bevelled down labially, which would make it impossible to achieve stable contacts and avoid interference between the anterior teeth in protrusive movement. Secondly, the cingulum areas of the maxillary restorations are built out to form ledges against which the incisal edges of the lower teeth occlude. This permits smooth movements to be made forwards and laterally from ICP without increasing the steepness of the guidance.

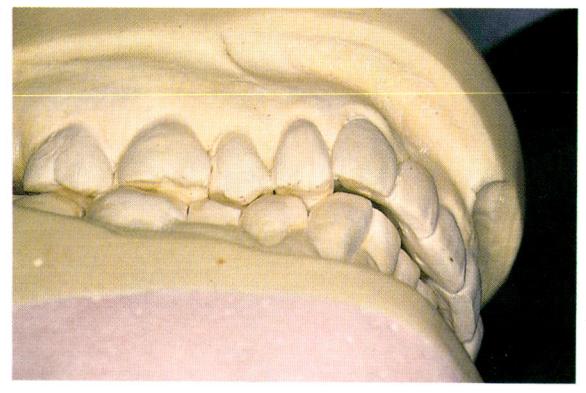

394 This patient required restoration of 13, 12, 11, and all maxillary posterior teeth. Diagnostic casts mounted in retruded revealed a large horizontal ICP–RCP discrepancy and no anterior contact.

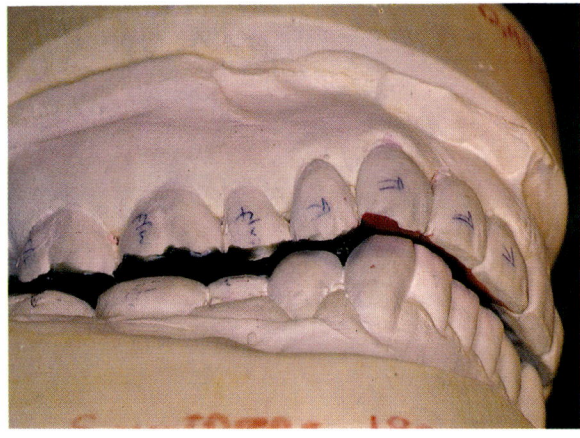

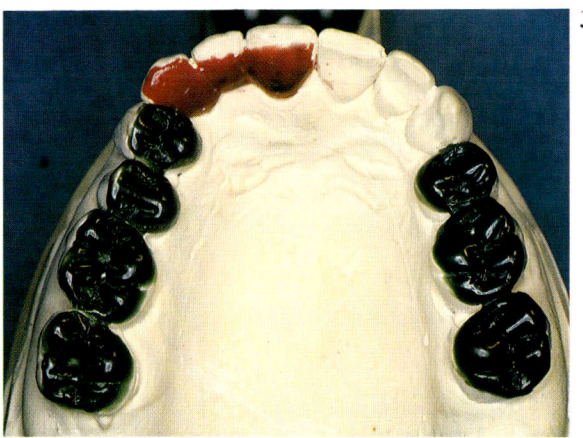

395, 396 A diagnostic wax-up built the palatal surfaces of 13, 12, 11 into contact with the lower teeth to provide an immediate disclusion.

397 The final restorations demonstrate these palatal ledges which patients tolerate well.

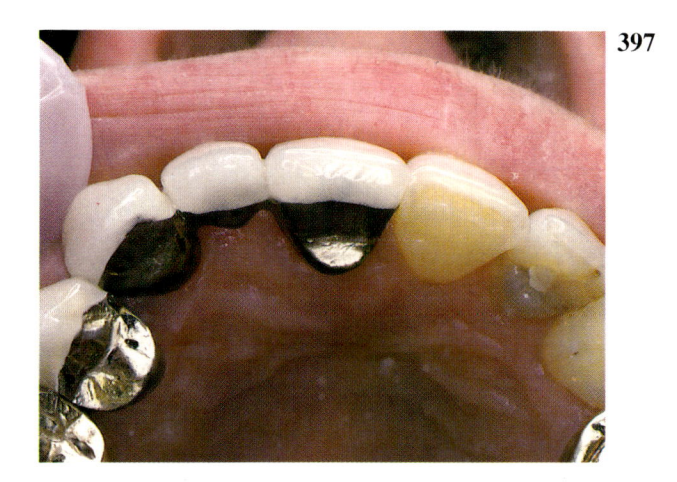

398 In another patient, diagnostic casts have been mounted after splint therapy and a trial occlusal equilibration carried out, leaving the anterior teeth, which do not require restoration, out of contact.

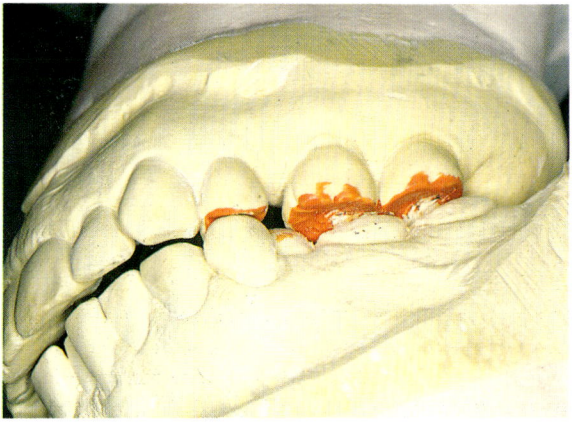

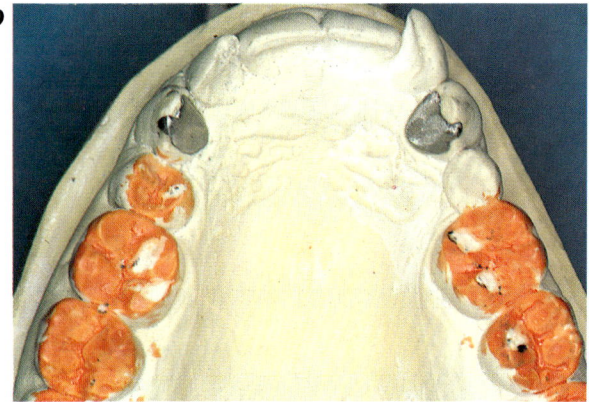

399, 400 This patient required equilibration but was not comfortable without immediate disclusion. Acid etch-retained canine guidance surfaces were bonded to the canines, providing contact in ICP with 43, 33, and canine guidance.

In the absence of anterior contact in ICP, posterior restorations should be waxed to a long centric. This permits even contacts to occur simultaneously on several posterior teeth in protrusion up to the point when anterior teeth contact and provide disclusion.

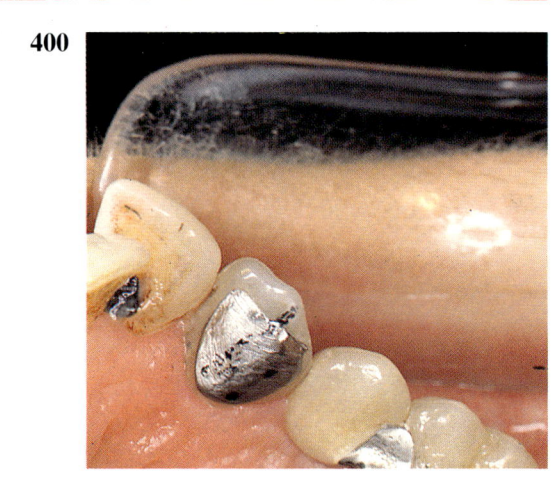

(iv) Class 3 jaw relation

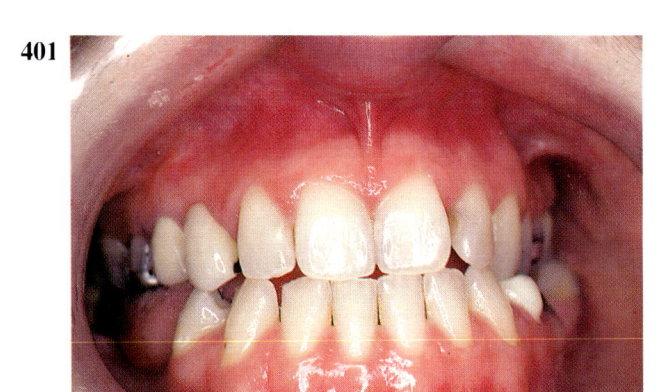

401 A Class 3 incisal and jaw relation also poses problems in obtaining adequate anterior guidance. This may be due to insufficient vertical overlap of the anterior teeth and the presence of anterior and posterior crossbites.

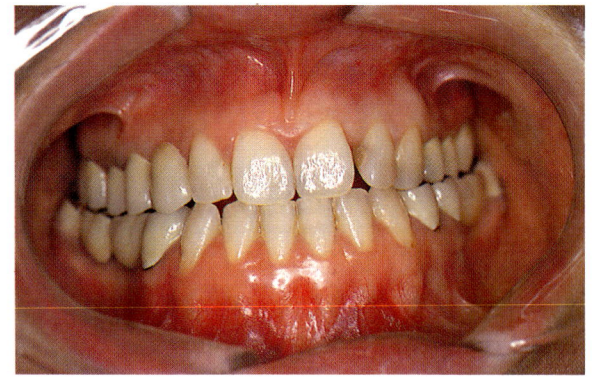

402 The posterior teeth have been restored; note the normal buccal segment relation on the right and the crossbite on the left. It was impossible to disclude the posterior teeth in protrusive, but care was taken to ensure that even, bilateral contacts were provided on the posterior restorations.

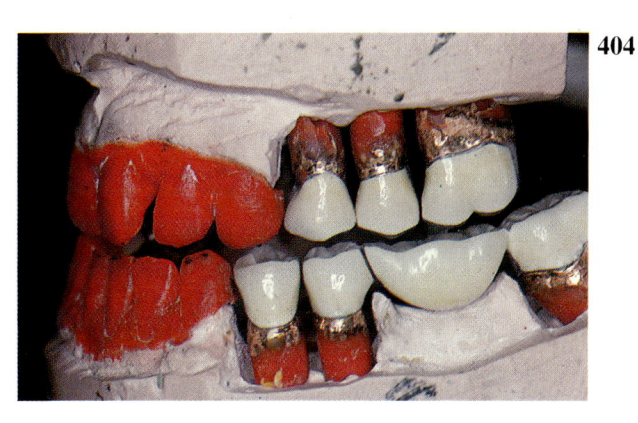

403 Working side guidance on the right side was provided by the maxillary first pre-molar and mandibular first molar. The situation was further complicated by 13 being a cantilevered pontic.

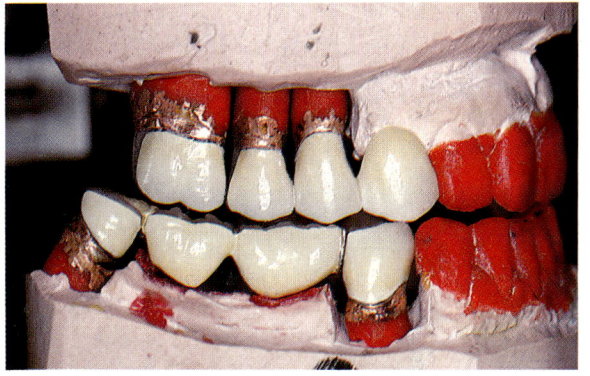

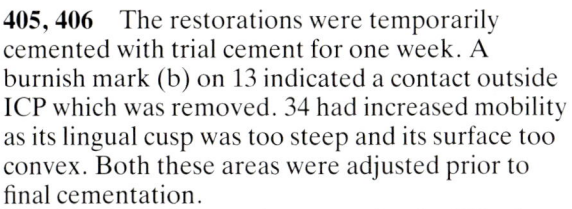

404 On the left side which was in crossbite, guidance was provided by 23 and the lingual cusp of 34.

405, 406 The restorations were temporarily cemented with trial cement for one week. A burnish mark (b) on 13 indicated a contact outside ICP which was removed. 34 had increased mobility as its lingual cusp was too steep and its surface too convex. Both these areas were adjusted prior to final cementation.

The use of temporary cementation in difficult cases is advisable as it permits castings to be removed and adjusted after a period of use.

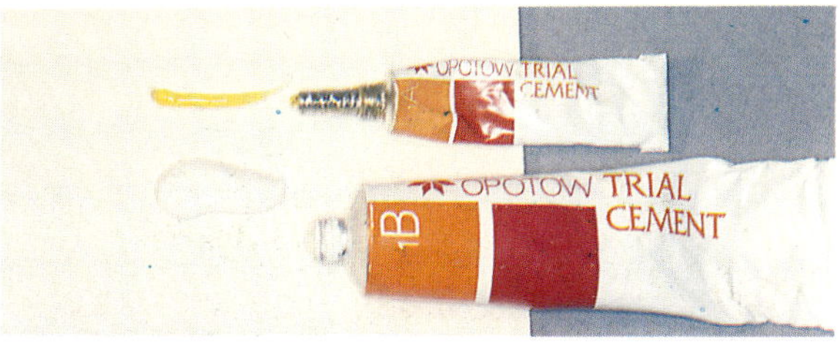

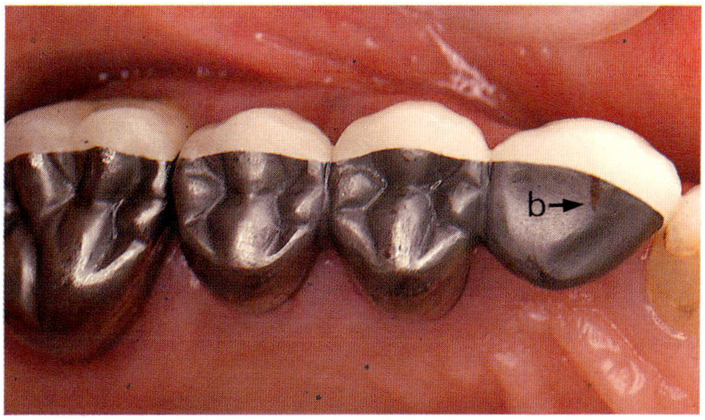

(v) Short clinical crowns

407 Inadequate clinical crown height makes the restoration of anterior teeth difficult.

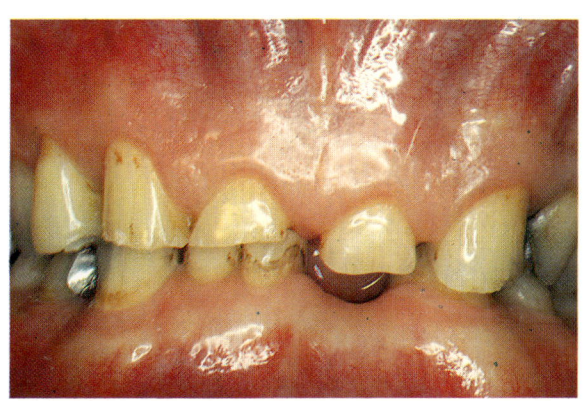

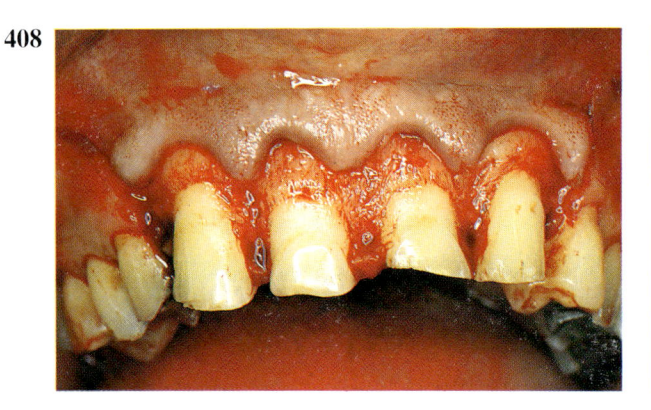

408 Periodontal surgery increases the length of clinical crown available for restoration.

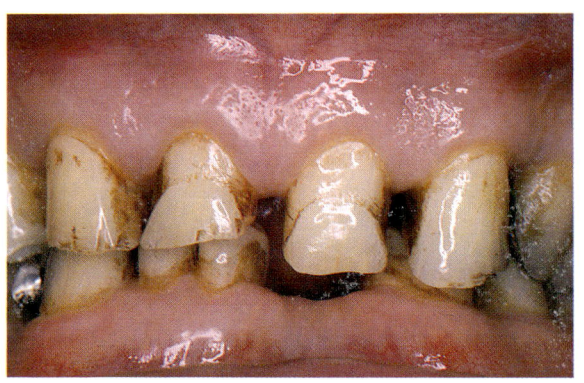

409 Two months after surgery, the teeth can be prepared, enabling adequate retention, aesthetics and anterior guidance to be achieved.

(vi) Malaligned guidance teeth

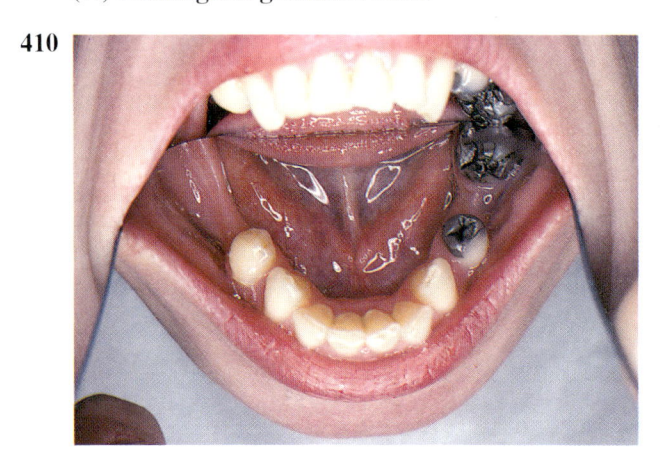

410, 411 This patient's mandibular anterior teeth were malaligned and the canines lingually inclined. The maxillary anterior teeth required restoration, but it was impossible to achieve stable ICP contacts and guidance with the teeth in their existing positions.

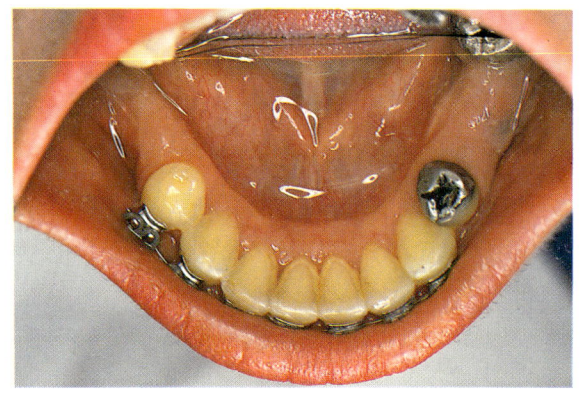

412 Simple orthodontic treatment realigned these teeth and proclined the canines, making it possible to achieve a correct occlusal relationship with the maxillary restorations.

Occlusal considerations for acid etch-retained bridges

413 Acid etch-retained bridges provide a conservative means of replacing missing anterior teeth. They are subject to the same occlusal requirements as conventional fixed prostheses. It is often necessary to create space for maxillary palatal retainers by shortening the opposing teeth horizontally, not bevelling the edges.

414 This diagram illustrates the ideal design of a bridge to replace 12 with the occlusal contacts marked. The following features are important:

- Stable ICP contacts on all units.
- Protrusive guidance on 11, 21.
- Canine guidance on 13, 23.
- Smooth, shallow guidance surfaces.

Maximum coverage of the abutment teeth by the retainers ensures a large area of bonding, and by wrapping around the mesial and distal aspects of the abutments provides greater resistance to lateral displacement. It also ensures that both the ICP contact and guidance occur on the retainer. If a lower tooth is able to rub over the junction between retainer and tooth, it will push the tooth out from under the bridge and cause bond failure. This can happen more easily if the edge of the retainer is not extended right up to the incisal edge.

Acid etch-retained bridges are useful in replacing missing teeth in many situations.

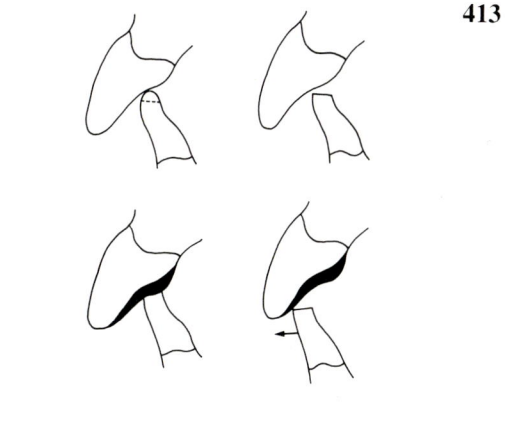

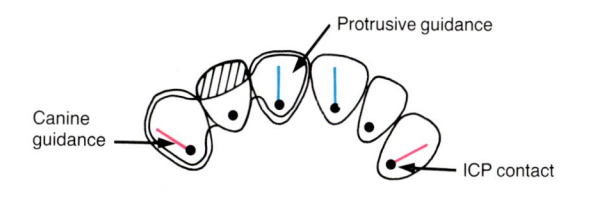

(i) Treatment of hypodontia

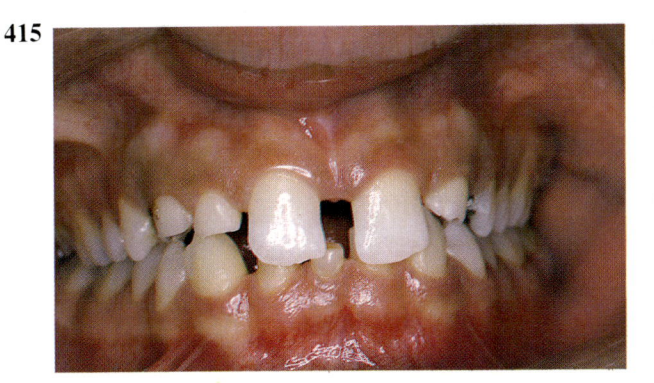

415 This patient is missing 12, 11, 21, 22, 31, 41; the deciduous teeth are mobile and of poor prognosis. The treatment plan involved replacing these teeth with acid etch-retained bridges. However, the potential abutments are poorly positioned, aesthetically and functionally.

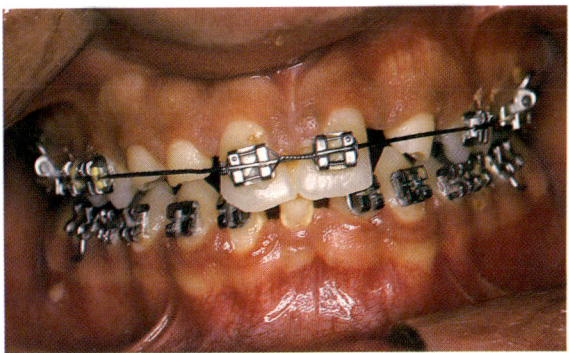

416 Orthodontic treatment was carried out to approximate 11, 21 and to bring 13, 23, 33, 31, 41, 43 into a functional relationship. The deciduous teeth were then extracted.

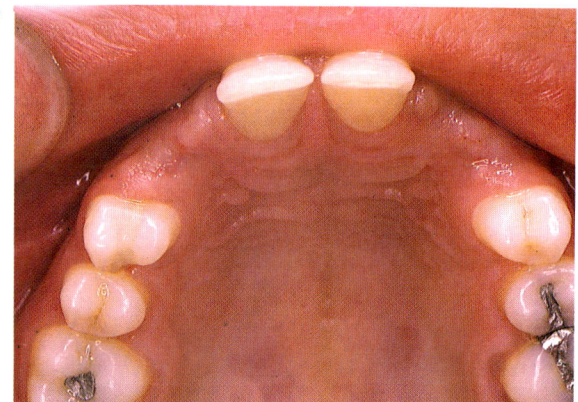

417 Once orthodontic treatment had been completed, guide planes and occlusal rests were prepared on 14, 11, 21, 33, and impressions were made for construction of the prostheses, which was carried out on a semi-adjustable articulator.

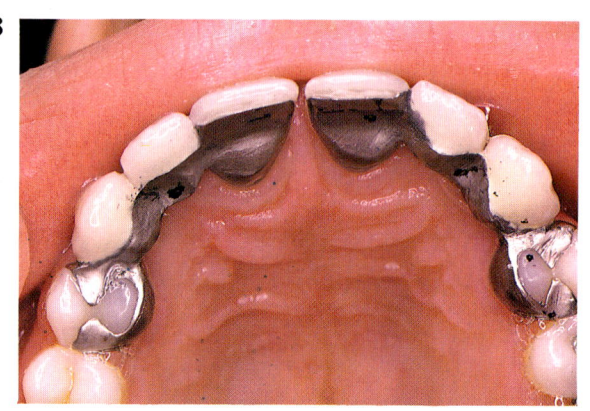

418 The finished maxillary bridges with occlusal contacts and guidances marked. Note the large area of coverage of the abutment teeth and correctly designed anterior guidance. Lateral disclusion was provided by the canines.

(ii) Replacement of teeth lost through trauma or resorption

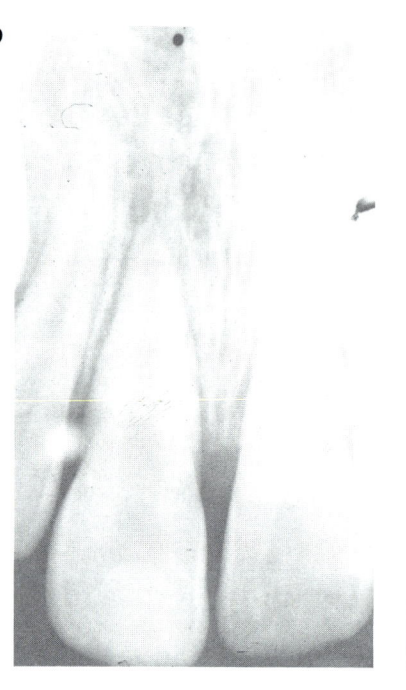

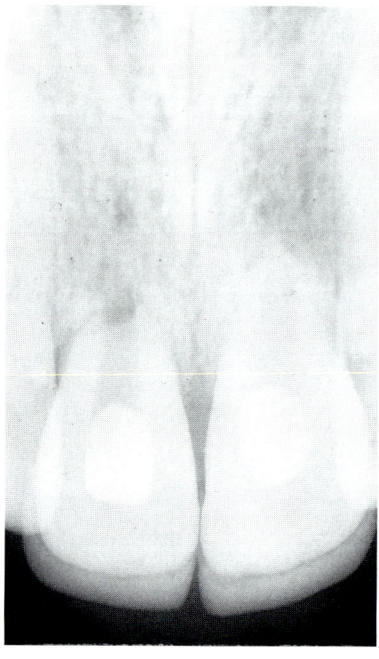

419, 420 This young girl lost 12, 21 through inflammatory resorption which had destroyed most of the roots of these teeth over a period of six years, despite endodontic treatment.
Courtesy of Mr S. Cunnington.

421 She had an incomplete overbite and edge-to-edge incisal relation.

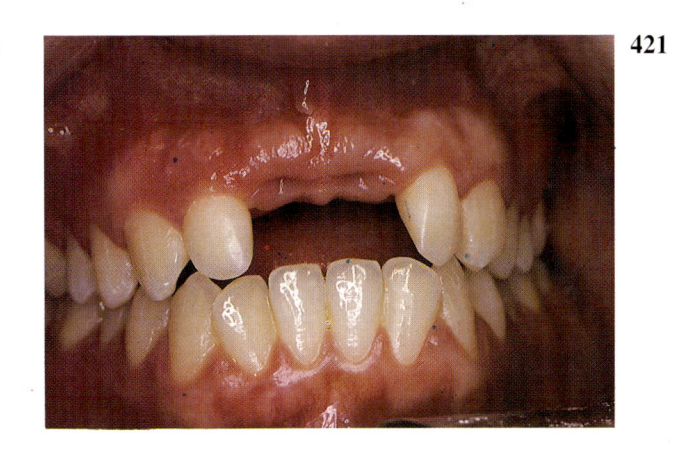

422, 423 The central incisors were replaced with an acid etch–retained bridge. As with conventional bridgework there is no need to double abut, providing the occlusion is managed correctly. The ICP contacts were close to the incisal edges and so it was necessary to cover the palatal surfaces with porcelain. Where possible, such contacts should be placed on metal as with conventional crown and bridgework.

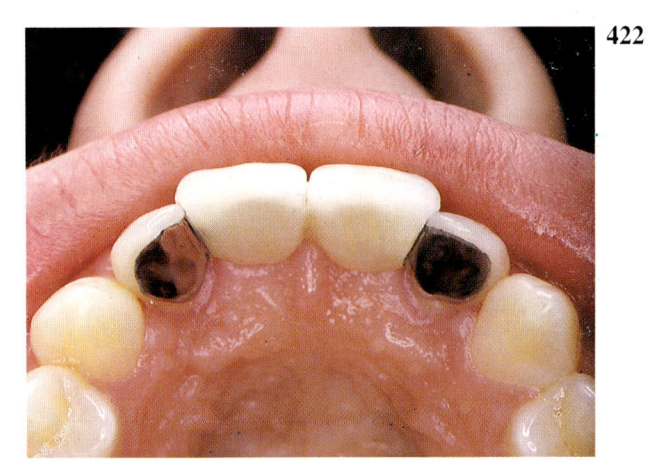

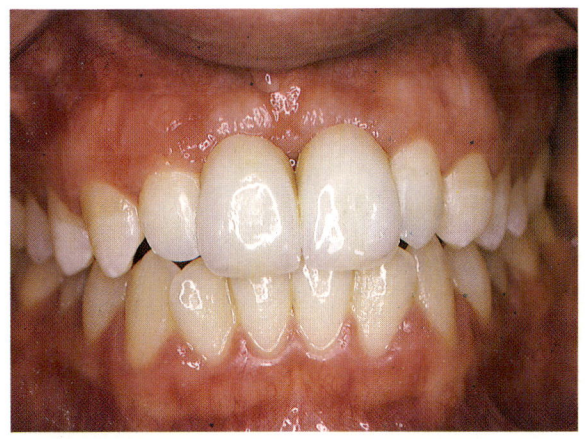

(iii) Post-orthodontic and periodontal retainers

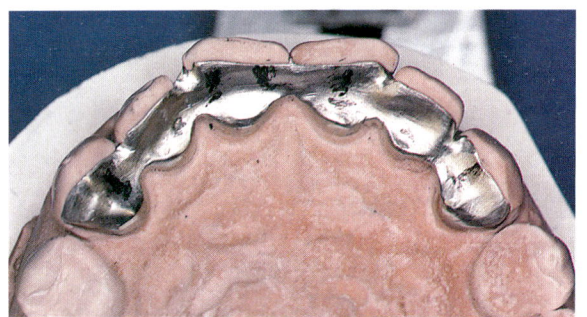

424 Acid etch-retained prostheses may be used as splints to retain tooth position after orthodontic or periodontal treatment in adults. Once again it is important that the design incorporates all the occlusal guidelines described in relation to crown and bridgework.

(iv) Failures

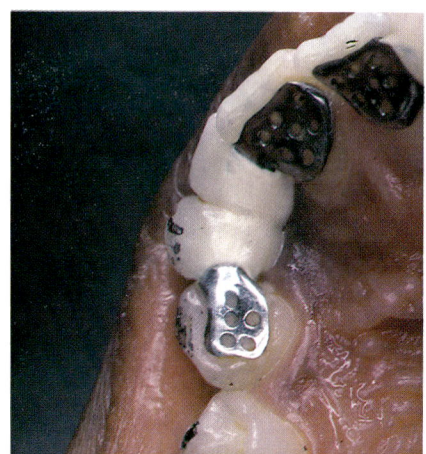

425 This bridge has failed owing to poor design, the retainer on 13 becoming uncemented. Note the small area of abutment coverage and the occlusal contact on 13 which had pushed the tooth out from under the bridge, causing bond failure.

Partial denture occlusion when anterior teeth require replacement

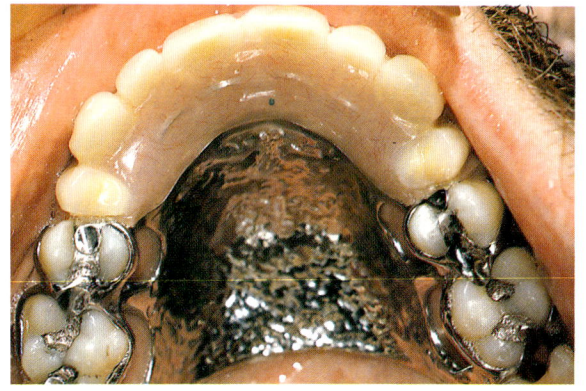

426 Where maxillary anterior teeth are to be replaced (Kennedy Classification IV), it is important to achieve contact with the opposing mandibular teeth in ICP, along with stable posterior tooth contacts. Anterior guidance should be provided by the natural teeth, if possible. This removes lateral displacing forces from the removable prosthesis.

Conclusion

The basic principles in restoring anterior teeth have been illustrated. It is important that a patient possesses a stable posterior occlusion before the restoration of anterior teeth is undertaken.

Chapter 11: The restoration of posterior teeth

This chapter describes the principles involved in restoring posterior occlusion. These principles apply to all types of posterior restorations from conventional fixed and removable prostheses to the newer types of adhesive restorations, including acid etch-retained bridges and indirect porcelain and composite inlays and onlays.

The treatment of four patients in which these principles have been applied, in situations of differing complexity, is illustrated.

General considerations in restoring posterior teeth

These include:

- The influence of the anterior and posterior determinants.
- The maintenance and reproduction of stable ICP contacts.
- The importance of levelling the occlusal plane.
- The absence of anterior tooth contact in ICP.
- Materials for restoring occlusal surfaces.
- The occlusal aspects of tooth preparation.
- The principles of mounting working casts.

The influence of the anterior and posterior determinants

This involves the influence of the anterior guidance and inclination of the condylar pathways on the morphology of the occlusal surfaces of posterior teeth and restorations.

The occlusal objective when restoring posterior teeth is to restore posterior stability. To achieve this, steep cusps and well-defined ridges and grooves are necessary, providing ICP contacts, yet discluding in protrusive and lateral excursions. The ability to disclude posterior restorations depends upon a patient possessing adequately steep anterior guidance. It is also dependent upon the cusps being positioned to avoid each other rather than interfering during mandibular movements.

When a patient possesses steep anterior guidance it is possible to provide steep cusps and still disclude them. This applies even if the restorations are made on a semi-adjustable articulator which does not accurately duplicate mandibular movements. The shallower the anterior guidance, the more critical becomes the influence of the condylar pathways. If restorations are made on a semi-adjustable articulator, their occlusal surfaces must be kept relatively flat to avoid interferences. If a fully-adjustable articulator is used, which copies mandibular movements accurately, it is possible to provide steeper posterior cusps. They will be correctly positioned relative to the direction of movement and so disclude where required.

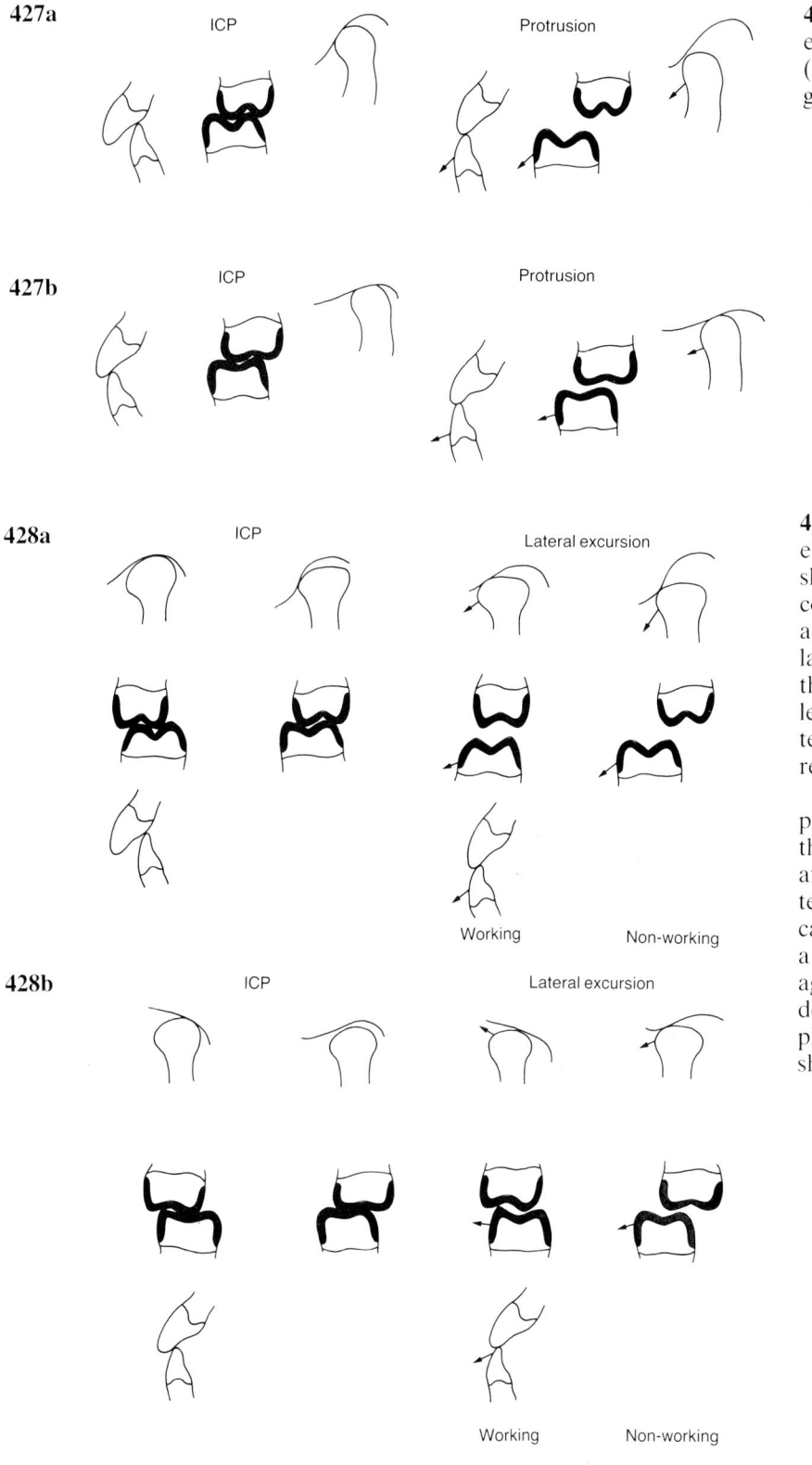

427a, 427b Illustration of the effect of steep (**427a**) and shallow (**427b**) anterior and condylar guidance during protrusion.

428a, 428b Illustration of the effects in lateral excursion. It should be noted that the working condyle in (**a**) moves laterally and downwards, and in (**b**) laterally and upwards. This has the effect of causing greater and lesser disclusion of the posterior teeth on the working side respectively.

In the horizontal plane, the paths of condylar movement and the intercondylar distance will affect the angle at which the teeth pass over each other. This can only be accurately copied by a fully-adjustable articulator and again becomes critical in determining correct cusp placement in patients with shallow anterior guidance.

The maintenance and reproduction of stable ICP contacts

429 Stable ICP contacts on posterior restorations may be achieved in two ways:

a) Each supporting cusp makes three small points of contact with the opposing tooth. These points suspend the cusp above a fossa and prevent contact of the cusp tip. This occlusal scheme is called tripodization and is the most stable. It is technically difficult to produce and its application lies in the restoration of opposing teeth. The multiple small points of contact and lack of cusp tip contact are supposed to reduce wear.

b) The second type involves contact between supporting cusp tips and fossae. This is a simplified approach suited to the fabrication of restorations against an existing occlusion.

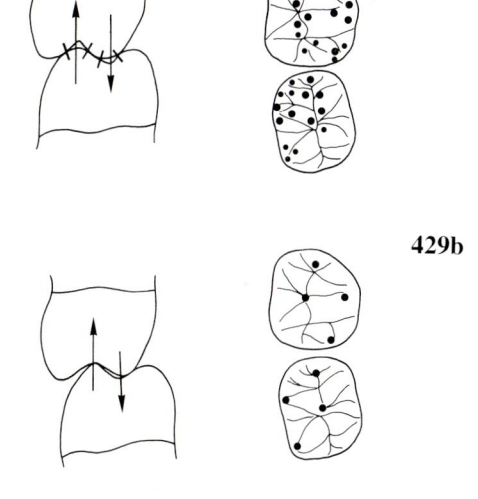

430 Once removed, it is difficult to restore stable ICP contacts owing to the difficulties of manipulating restorative materials, and the problems of differential wear.

It is advisable to mark existing ICP contacts prior to cavity preparation for intra-coronal restorations. If possible, the cavity outline for a small Class 2 restoration in 14 should avoid these points of contact, leaving them on enamel.

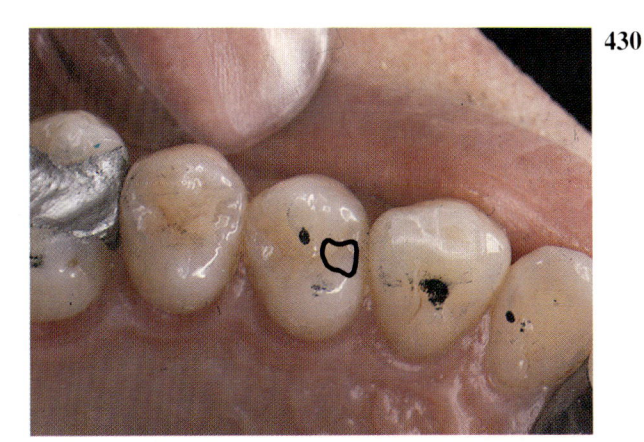

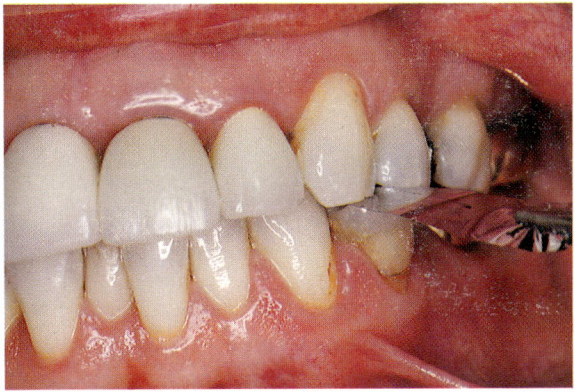

431, 432 The use of the articulating paper and shimstock foil to mark and verify contacts pre-operatively, during all laboratory stages and on completion or try-in of a restoration is important. The paper should mark the position of contacts and the foil should ensure that the restoration is neither high nor low.

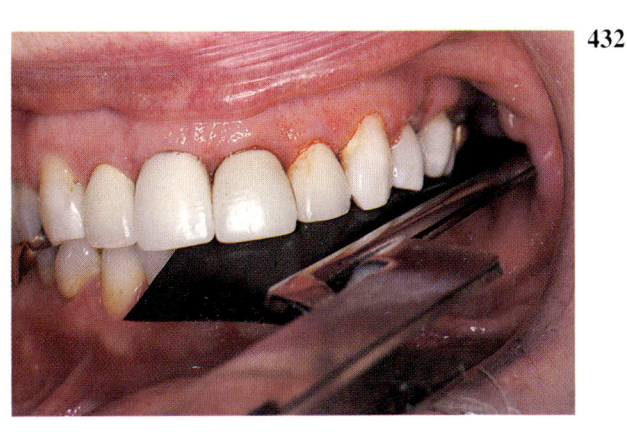

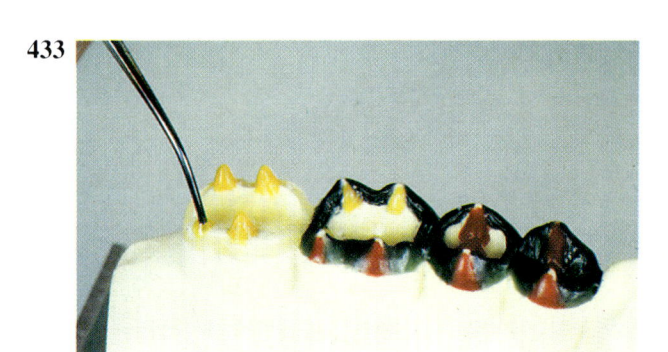

433 To reproduce correct occlusal anatomy it is advantageous to use a wax-added technique in the laboratory. This enables each element of the occlusal surface to be accurately positioned with respect to its antagonist, and ICP contacts to be precisely located for maximum stability. Building up and carving down an excess of wax makes these objectives very difficult to achieve.

The importance of levelling the occlusal plane

434 One of the objectives when restoring posterior teeth is to level the occlusal plane. This makes interferences between posterior teeth less likely (**a**). A steep curve of Spee (**b**), over-erupted unopposed teeth (**c**), or tilted molars (**d**) are more likely to lead to interferences in lateral and protrusive movements. These features should be noted during diagnostic procedures and corrected prior to restoring the teeth involved.

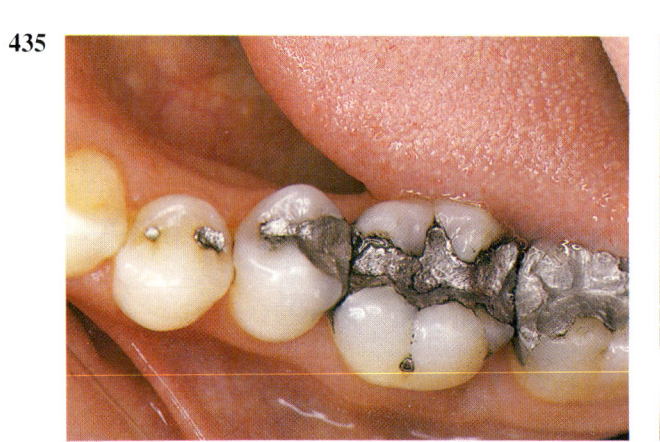

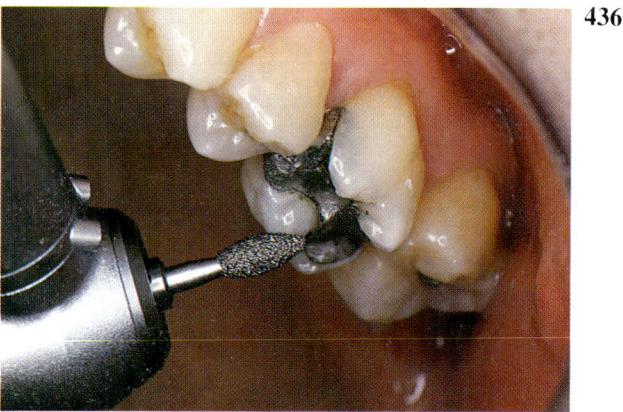

435, 436 The localized over-eruption of a tooth opposed by an undercontoured amalgam should be corrected by adjustment prior to replacing the amalgam. This adjustment should not flatten the palatal cusp but reduce it in height, maintaining its original shape.

437 Making restorations with stable contacts to occlude against uneven opposing teeth is difficult. If restorations are required in both arches it is advisable to make them together. This gives the technician greater control over their occlusal anatomy.

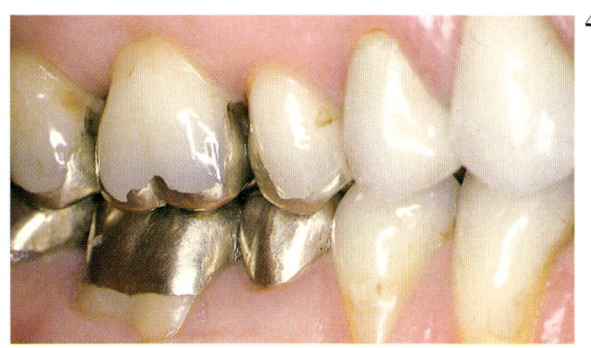

When there is no anterior tooth contact in ICP

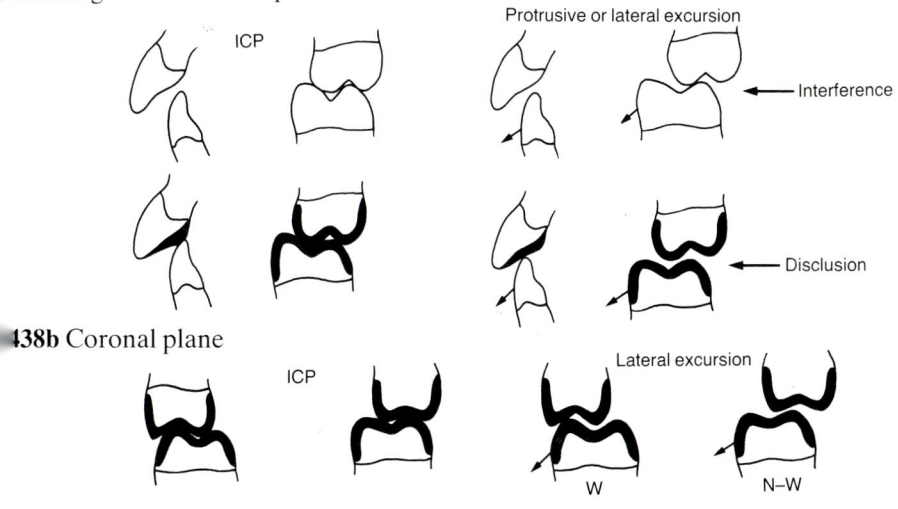

438a Sagittal or coronal planes

438b Coronal plane

Group function in lateral excursion

438 A lack of anterior tooth contact in ICP complicates the restoration of posterior teeth as it makes their disclusion outside ICP more difficult to achieve.

There are three solutions to this problem:

a) The anterior teeth are restored, building them into contact in ICP and providing immediate disclusion.

b) Guidance in protrusive is obtained from bilateral contacts on the posterior teeth. In lateral excursion the restorations are shaped to provide group function.

c) Posterior restorations are designed to provide a long or wide centric, permitting them to rub smoothly over each other until the anterior teeth contact and provide disclusion. This occlusal scheme is difficult to achieve as it involves the production of simultaneous, multiple tooth contacts outside ICP. This can only be achieved using a fully-adjustable articulator.

Sagittal plane (long centric) or coronal plane (wide centric) **438c**

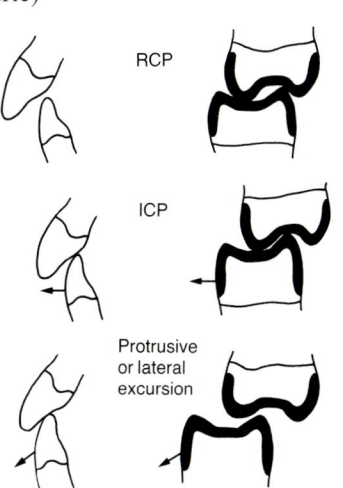

Materials for restoring occlusal surfaces

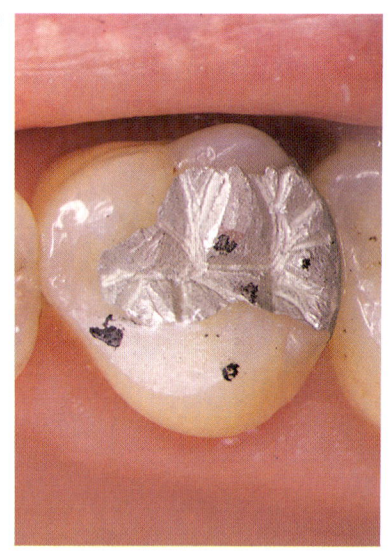

439 Amalgam should still be regarded as the plastic material of choice for restoring posterior teeth. It is relatively easy to manipulate and can be carved to provide reasonable ICP contacts and contours. The high copper alloys exhibit adequate longevity provided they are used correctly.

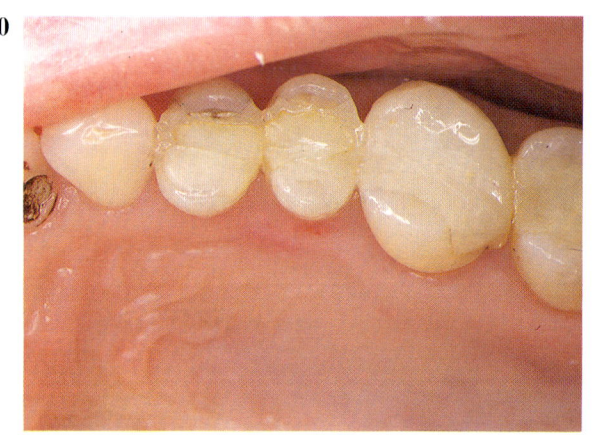

440 Direct posterior composite resins are not ideal materials for restoring anything but minimal cavities in posterior teeth. They are difficult to condense and obtain adequate contour, proximal and occlusal contact. There is some evidence that even when packed incrementally, their polymerization shrinkage may cause cracking of the enamel and dentine in adjacent cusps, as well as marginal leakage. They are highly abrasive materials likely to cause increased wear of opposing teeth in patients with group function.

This patient had all her large posterior amalgams replaced with composite resin after reading about alleged amalgam toxicity. The new restorations were poorly contoured and lacked adequate occlusal anatomy and stable occlusal contacts. The patient had lost posterior stability, started fracturing cusps and required removal of the composite resin and crowning of the affected teeth.

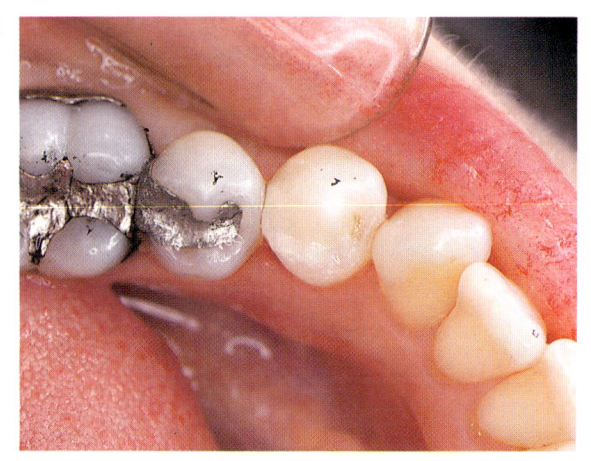

441 A small Class 2 composite resin has been placed in 34, for aesthetic reasons. A minimal restoration, playing no part in restoring the occlusion, is one of the few indications for posterior composites. In this situation, the tooth's only ICP contact remained on the tip of the buccal cusp.

442 Recent advances in the area of adhesion have made it possible to make indirect restorations from ceramic and composite materials, which can be bonded to posterior teeth. This is an example of an indirect composite onlay on 46. The indirect method of fabrication avoids some of the problems associated with direct composite resins. Restoration of adequate contour and occlusion can be achieved, although doubts must remain regarding their durability, marginal integrity and the possibility of wearing the opposing teeth. They are not advised in patients with group function and those who show evidence of parafunction. In such situations, excess lateral forces are more likely to cause mechanical failure of the restoration.

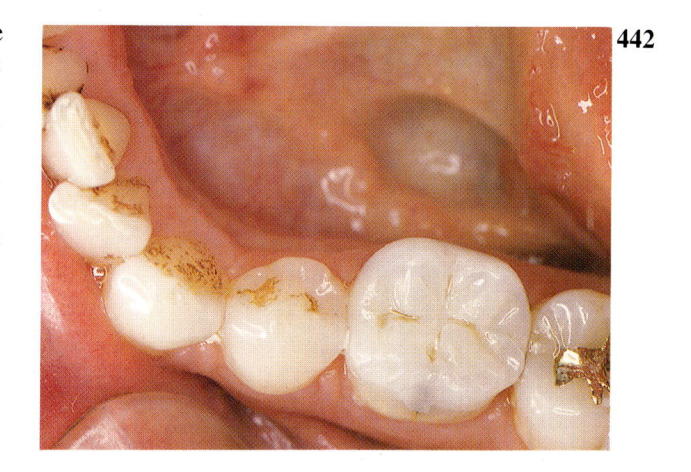

443 Type 3 gold is the material of choice for restoring occlusal surfaces where aesthetics is not the overriding factor. The use of partial coverage restorations permits control of the occlusion in conjunction with conservative tooth preparation. This allows the retention of sound tooth structure rather than its removal during the more radical preparation required for a porcelain-fused-to-metal crown. Type 3 gold is durable, permits the restoration of stable ICP contacts, and wears at about the same rate as enamel.

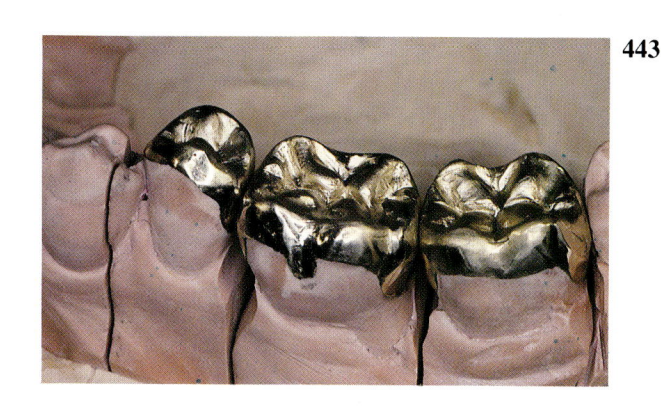

Porcelain-fused-to-metal crowns are the most common cast restorations for posterior teeth. A choice has to be made between porcelain and metal occlusal surfaces.

Indications for gold v porcelain occlusal surfaces

Age of patient. The more radical tooth preparation required for porcelain occlusion is more likely to cause pulpal damage in young patients. The use of gold occlusion or partial coverage is more sensible.

Extent of restoration of the tooth. If the tooth requiring preparation consists largely of amalgam or some other core material, there is less merit in being conservative with tooth preparation. If the tooth is less heavily restored, but required as a bridge abutment, the use of gold occlusion or partial coverage is again advised.

The anterior guidance. It is safer to use porcelain occlusals in patients with immediate disclusion and canine guidance. If used with group function, there is more chance of the porcelain fracturing and causing increased wear of the opposing teeth.

Evidence of parafunction. It is safer to use gold occlusal surfaces which are more durable and less likely to cause increased wear of the opposing teeth. Heavy occlusal contacts will show up as burnish marks on the sandblasted gold surfaces, and can be adjusted. Porcelain has a shiny surface on which it is difficult to mark occlusal contacts.

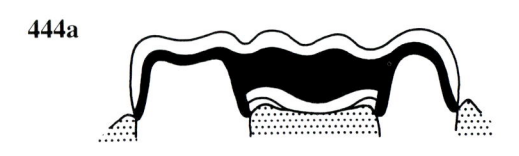

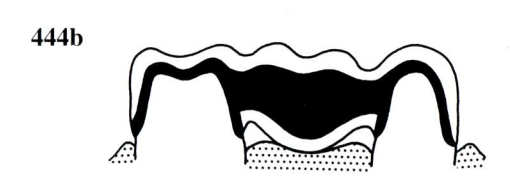

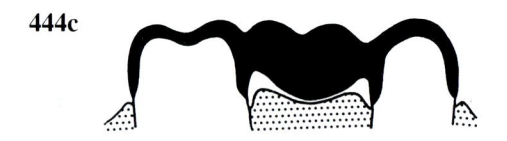

444a–444c Clinical crown height available. This illustrates the problems of using porcelain occlusal surfaces on short teeth. The extra vertical space needed for layers of both porcelain and gold, occlusally and in the region of the solder joints, causes two problems: firstly, greater occlusal reduction is needed, which reduces the height of the preparation and hence decreases retention; secondly, to maintain adequate solder joint height for strength, the proximal embrasures are unacceptably closed, making the maintenance of adequate plaque control difficult (**444a**). This problem may be resolved by surgical crown lengthening (**444b**). If gold occlusal surfaces are used the problems may be avoided (**444c**).

Aesthetics. The aesthetic demands of the patient should not override the criteria already discussed. There is much to be said for using gold occlusals wherever they will be accepted.

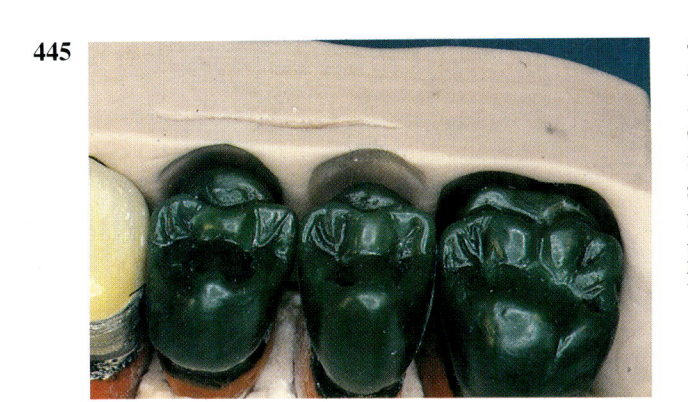

445, 446 Wax-ups for porcelain-fused-to-metal crowns should always be carried out to full contour. A matrix is made over the buccal surfaces which can be used as a guide for cutting back the patterns to ensure adequate space for porcelain. The metal substructure is designed so that all occlusal contacts fall on the metal surface, well away from the porcelain–metal junction. This is the typical design for maxillary crowns.

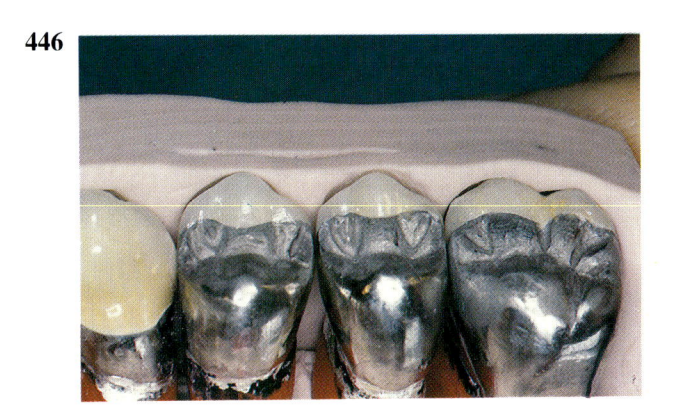

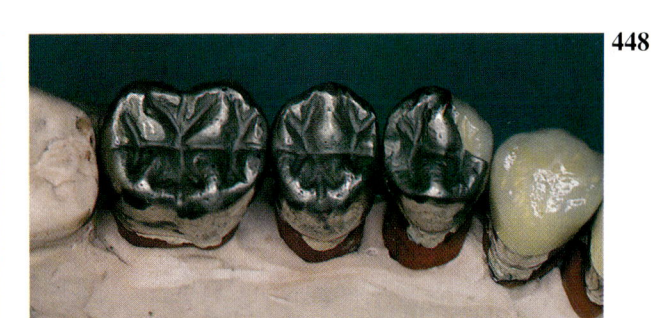

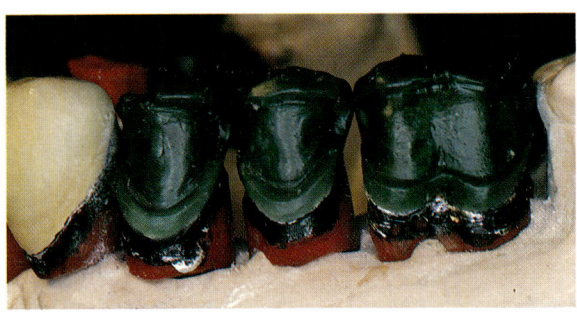

447, 448 To achieve the same objectives in the mandibular arch it is necessary to cover the whole occlusal surface and extend the metal over the tips of the buccal cusps.

449 Wax patterns for crowns with porcelain occlusals should also be waxed to full contour, the occlusal contacts being developed on the wax.

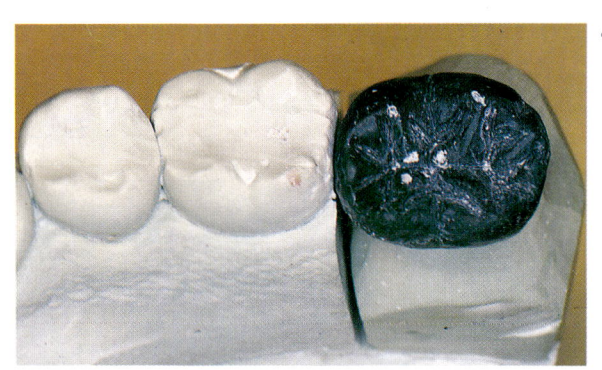

450 A matrix is then made over the wax-up, which can be cut back and cast, ensuring adequate space for the porcelain to be applied. It also ensures that the porcelain is adequately supported by the metal underneath. This is achieved by waxing the final coping to mirror the contours of the finished restoration, building up where necessary to ensure an even thickness of porcelain of no more than 2 mm.

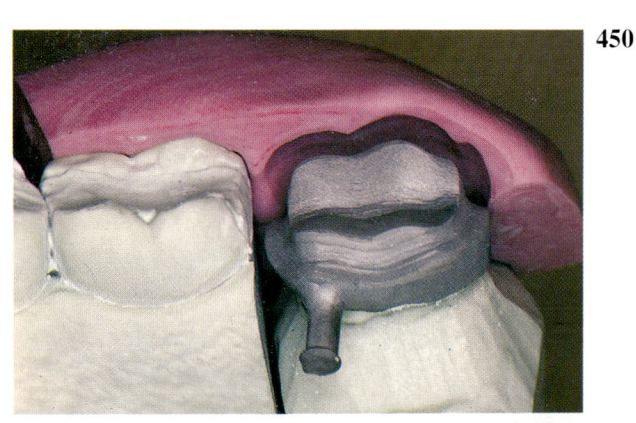

451 The final occlusal contacts are refined on the porcelain surface.

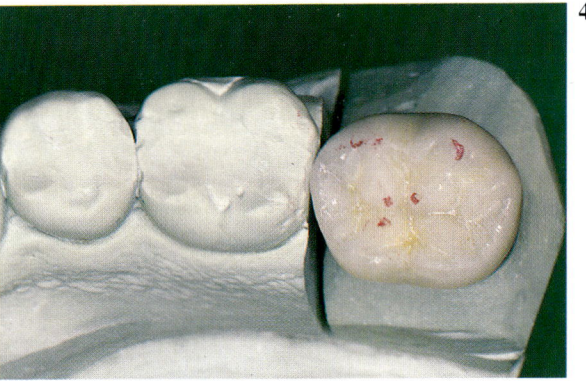

The occlusal aspects of tooth preparation

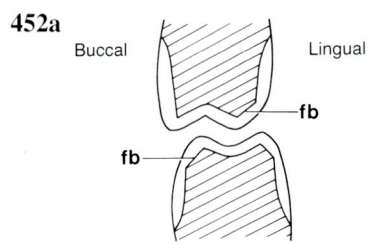

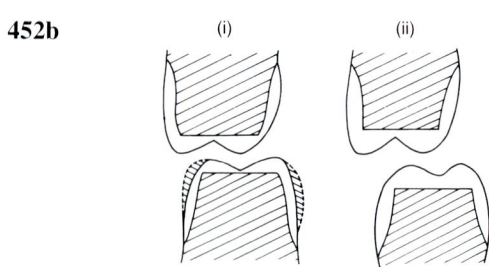

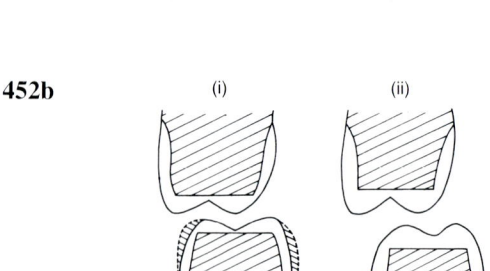

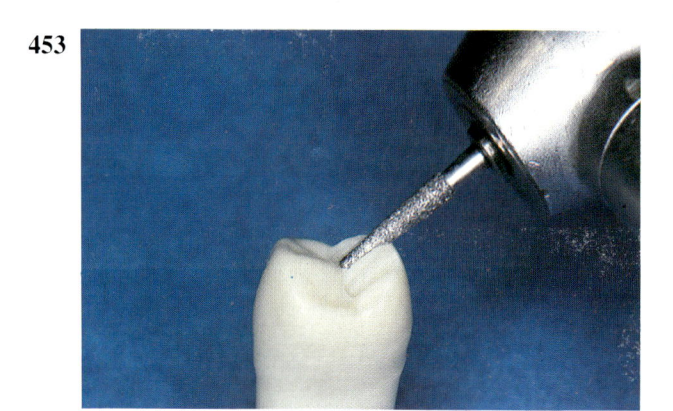

452a, 452b Preparations should have maximum height and minimal taper, for optimum resistance and retention form. To achieve this, and to permit an even and adequate thickness of restorative materials without overcontour, the surface of the preparation should mimic that of the intended restoration, both occlusally and axially (**452a**). This involves the preparation of a functional cusp bevel (fb) on the outer aspect of the supporting cusps.

If these guidelines are not followed, problems may occur (**452b**): in order to maintain adequate preparation height, insufficient reduction will be provided in the central fossa and on the occlusoaxial line angles. This will result in inadequate strength and poor aesthetics, and buccal and lingual overcontour respectively (**i**). If sufficient reduction is provided in these areas, the preparation will be excessively short and tapering (**ii**).

453 Depth cuts with a bur of known dimensions provide an easy way of judging the amount of reduction. They are only useful when the shape of the restoration is very similar to that of the original tooth.

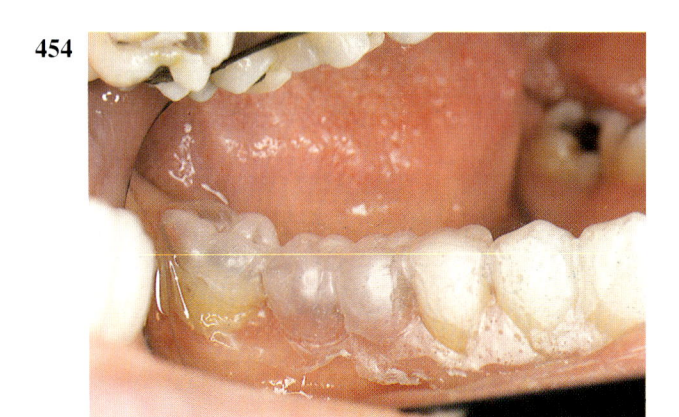

454 When the shape of the restoration is different from that of the original tooth, a vacuform shell made over a cast of the diagnostic wax-up is more useful.

The principles of mounting working casts

These differ from those used to mount diagnostic casts, the interocclusal record being taken at the intended vertical dimension of occlusion with any unprepared teeth in contact in ICP. Equilibration required to create a new ICP is performed first, followed by tooth preparation. An interocclusal record is only required if there are insufficient unprepared posterior teeth to enable the casts to be accurately located for the purpose of mounting on an articulator. An interocclusal record serves merely as an index in ensuring accurate cast location.

Making the interocclusal record at the VDO allows an average axis facebow to be used. If it were necessary to alter vertical dimension on the articulator (as when removing the interocclusal record and closing diagnostic casts into ICP), the error in tooth contacts produced by closing on an average axis would be unacceptable for working cast mounting.

The restoration of posterior teeth

The treatment of four patients requiring posterior restorations of varying complexity is described below; these restorations include:

- A single-unit porcelain-fused-to-metal crown (conformative).
- A three-unit bridge with a cantilevered pontic (conformative).
- A four-unit bridge where restoration of an over-erupted opposing tooth was necessary (reorganized).
- Restoration of opposing quadrants (reorganized).

A single unit porcelain-fused-to-metal crown

455 15 required restoration with a porcelain-fused-to-metal crown. The tooth was built up with a fast-setting amalgam core prior to crown preparation. The posterior occlusion was stable and so the crown was made to conform to the existing ICP.

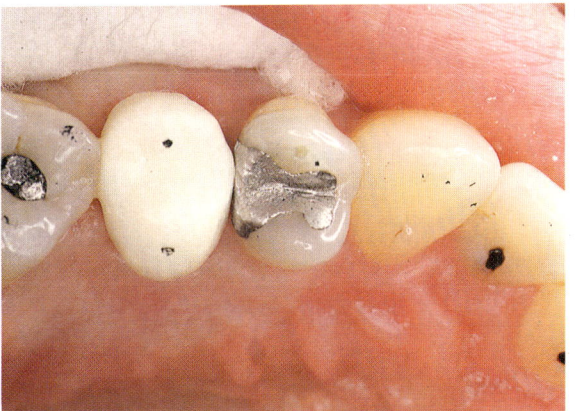

456 The temporary restoration provided ICP contacts to prevent over-eruption of the opposing tooth, between preparation and fitting the final crown.

457

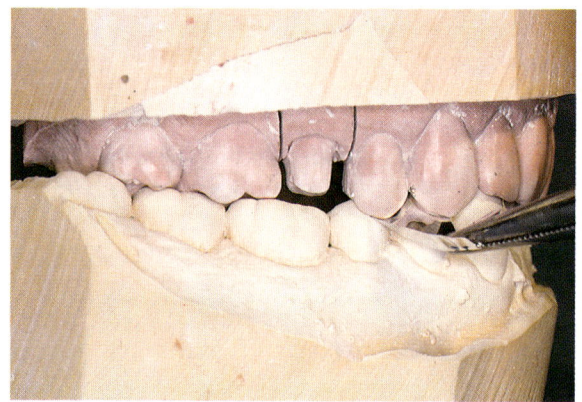

457 It was acceptable to mount the working casts on a hinge as the patient had steep anterior guidance. If the crown is to be involved in providing group function contact, the casts need mounting on a semi-adjustable articulator. Hand-held casts make the accurate restoration of the occlusion very difficult. The mandibular cast was mounted in ICP, no record being needed, and the occlusal contacts were checked with shimstock and compared to those observed in the mouth. If the two sets of contacts are the same, the casts have been mounted accurately.

458a

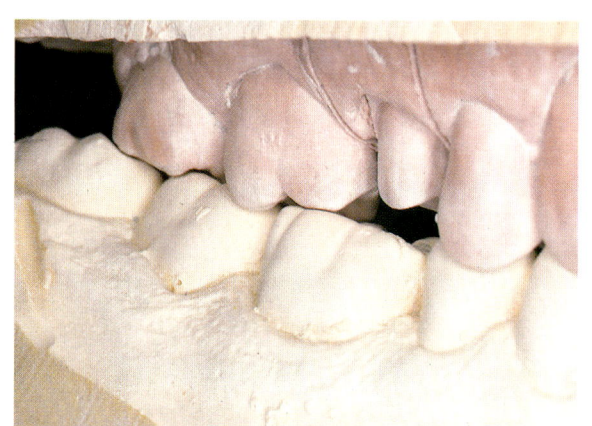

458a, 458b 46 was almost in crossbite which would make it difficult to achieve stable ICP contacts (**458a**). The outer aspect of the mesiobuccal cusp of 46 was reshaped, moving the cusp tip lingually (**458b**). This enabled the ICP contacts to be kept away from the porcelain–metal junction.

458b

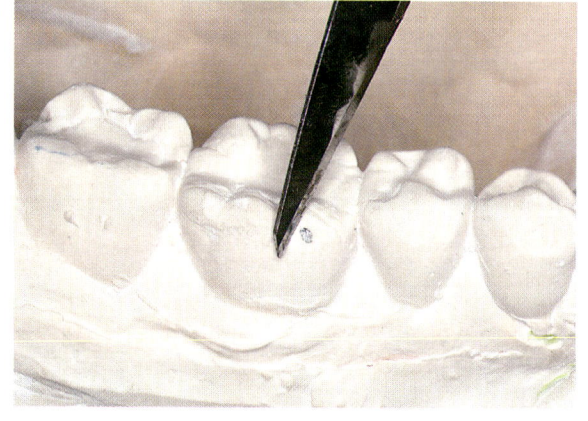

459a, 459b The ICP contacts were marked with articulating paper prior to starting the wax-up. The intended positions of the contact between the crown and the mesiobuccal cusp and mesial fossa of 46 are marked with a black pen (**459a**). The penmarks serve as a guide in locating the cusp cone for the supporting cusp of 15 (**459b**).

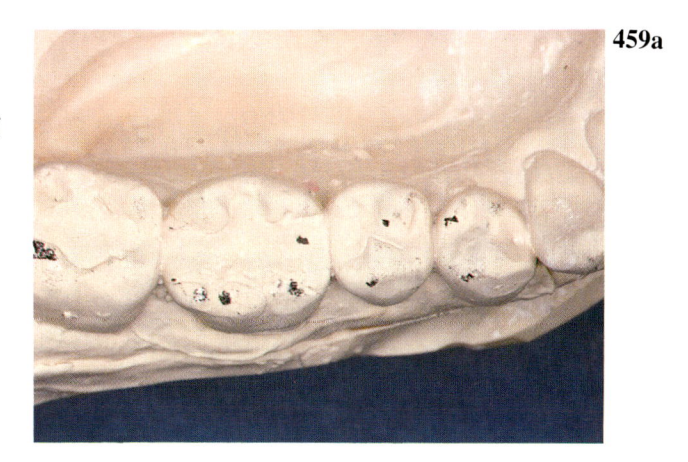

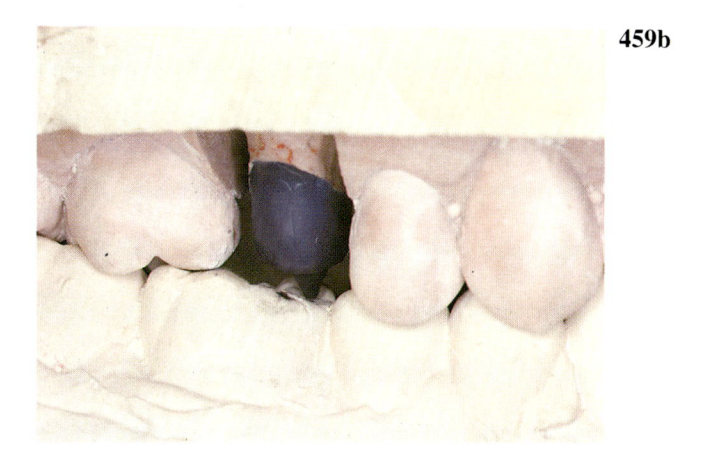

459a

459b

460 The finished restoration on the cast showing the ICP contacts on the buccal triangular ridge and palatal cusp tip. They are not ideally placed, their positions being influenced by the morphology of the opposing tooth.

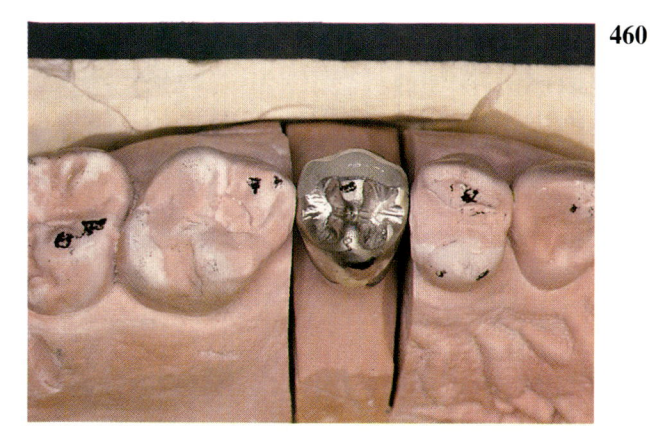

460

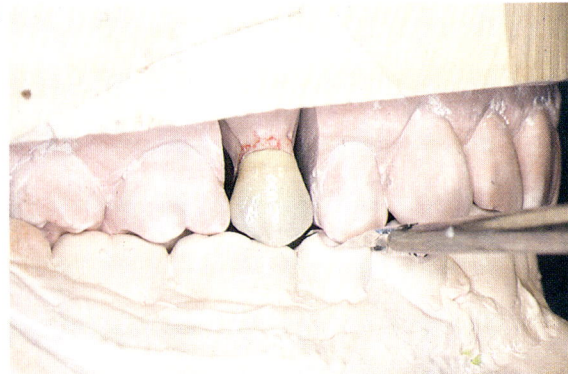

461, 462 Before the patient arrived shimstock was used to verify that the crown was neither high nor low in relation to the adjacent teeth.

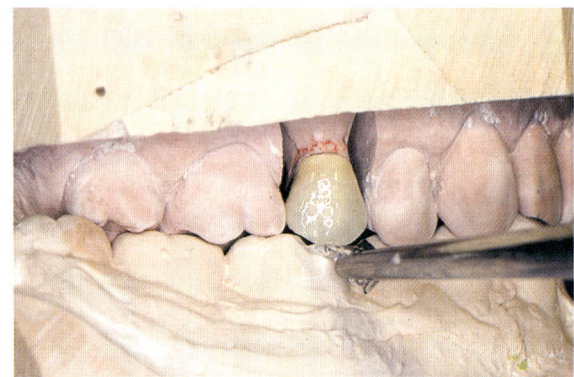

463, 464 The restoration was tried in and shimstock again used to verify contacts between the crown and 46 and between adjacent teeth. Very little adjustment was needed.

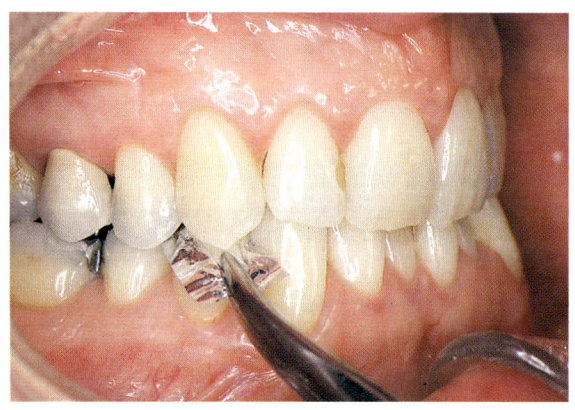

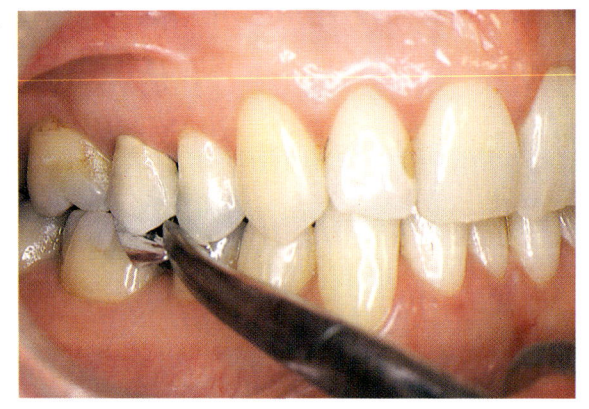

465 The restoration was checked in lateral excursion to ensure disclusion. This patient had steep anterior guidance and so no adjustment was needed. Had this not been the case, any contacts in lateral or protrusive excursion would have been marked and removed, care being taken to preserve the ICP contacts.

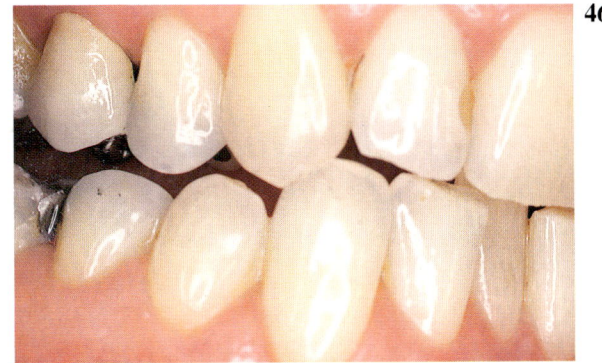

A three-unit bridge with a cantilevered pontic

466 This patient required a three-unit bridge, replacing 26 with a pontic, cantilevered from porcelain-fused-to-metal crowns on 24, 25.

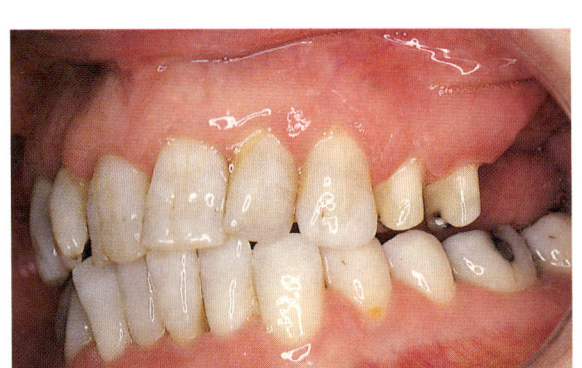

467, 468 As the posterior occlusion appeared stable, the bridge was made to conform to the existing ICP. After tooth preparation and impression making, interocclusal and face-bow records were required to mount the working casts on a semi-adjustable articulator. When using stone dies the interocclusal record may be made with a small piece of extra-hard wax held in forceps. The wax was softened in a water bath, placed between the teeth and the patient closed into ICP. Once the wax hardened it was removed and used to locate the mandibular cast, as there were insufficient unprepared teeth for a stable location. After mounting, shimstock contacts were verified between the other teeth and compared to those observed in the mouth.

An alternative type of record may be made when making restorations with porcelain occlusal surfaces. The metal substructure was tried in, and small beads of acrylic resin applied to its occlusal surface, into which the patient closed. Once set, contact between the acrylic resin record and mandibular teeth and between adjacent unprepared teeth in ICP was verified. The record was then used to mount the mandibular cast, and the mounting verified in the usual way.

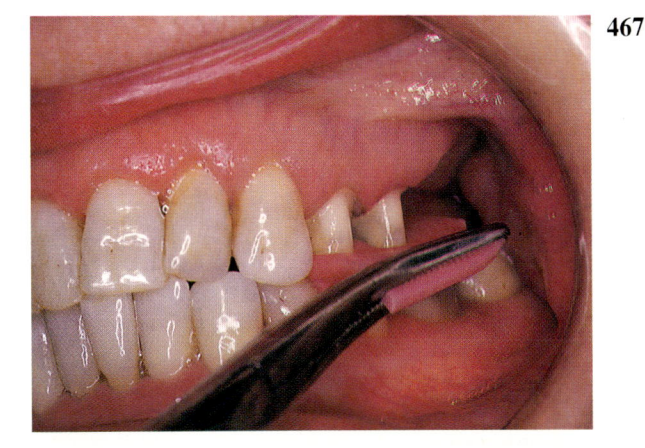

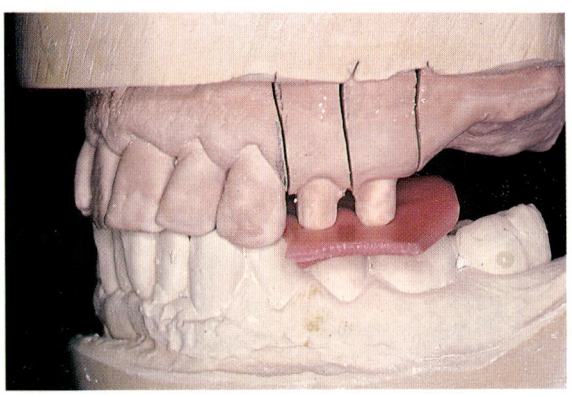

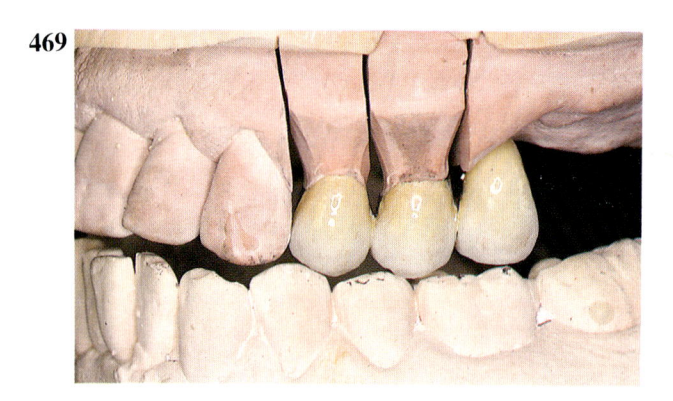

469, 470 It was important that all three units possessed stable ICP contacts, and that all lateral contact on the pontic was avoided. This patient required group function, with contacts on the buccal cusps of 24, 25 providing disclusion. The bridge was made on a semi-adjustable articulator and so some adjustment of the contacts in lateral and protrusive excursions was necessary when the restoration was tried in.

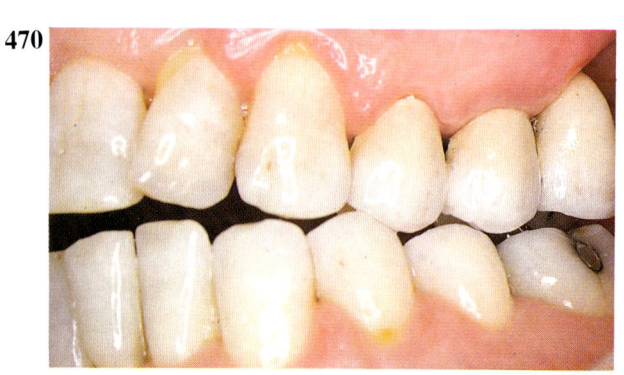

A four-unit bridge where restoration of an over-erupted opposing tooth was necessary

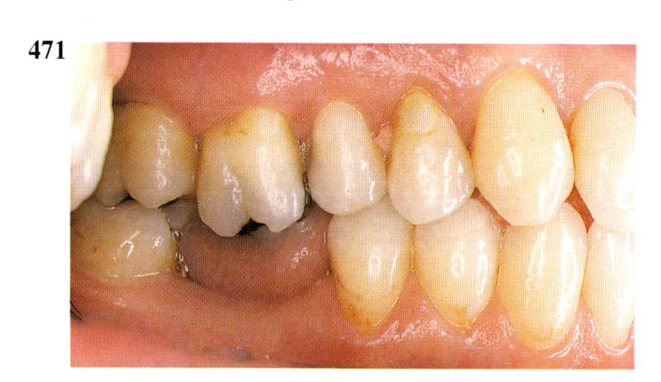

471 This patient required a four-unit fixed–movable bridge to replace 47, 46. 16 was occlusally unopposed and had over-erupted.

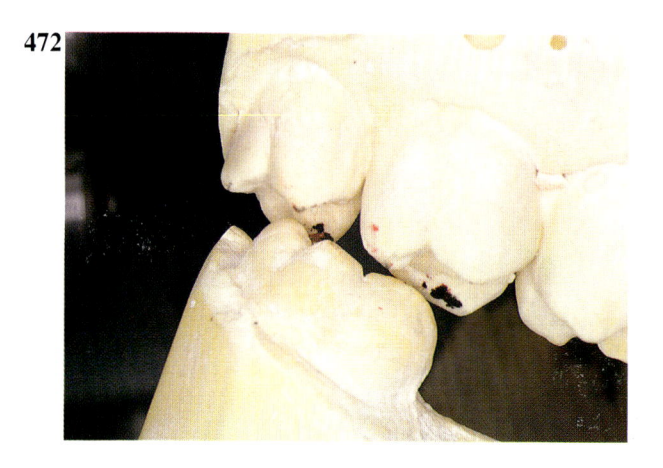

472 Diagnostic cast examination revealed a large vertical, small horizontal discrepancy between RCP and ICP, with the RCP contact between 18 & 48.

473, 474 48 had tipped mesially and there was a non-working side interference between 18 and 48 which passed through the supporting cusp tips. It was necessary to remove both the RCP contact and the non-working side interference from the distal bridge abutment prior to tooth preparation. In view of this, and because a trial equilibration of the diagnostic casts revealed that it would be easy to remove the RCP–ICP slide and preserve anterior tooth contact, it was decided to reorganize the occlusion prior to making the bridge.

A week after carrying out an occlusal equilibration, 48 and 45 were prepared and a working impression made. In order to level the occlusal plane, the distal aspect of 48 was heavily prepared and the prominent palatal cusps of 18, 17 were reduced. The over-eruption of 16 could not be corrected by occlusal adjustment, so it was prepared for a ¾ crown. Heavy occlusal reduction was carried out to bring it into line with the adjacent teeth, and a vacuform shell made over a cast of the diagnostic wax-up used to verify adequate reduction.

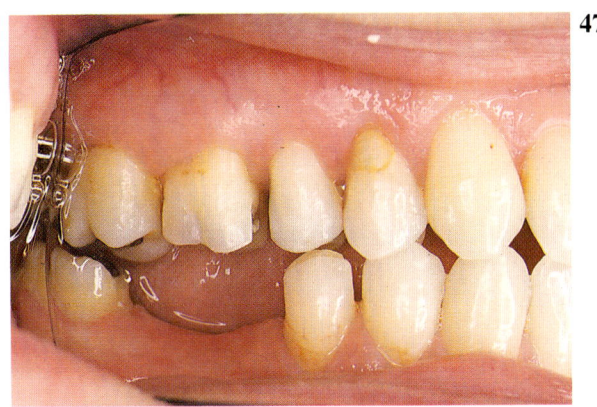

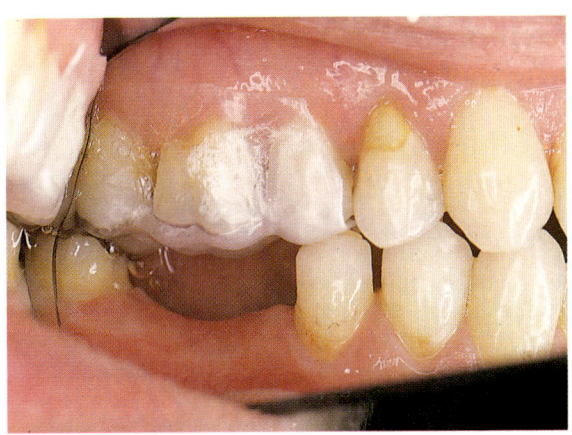

475 The maxillary working cast was mounted on a semi-adjustable articulator using an average axis facebow record.

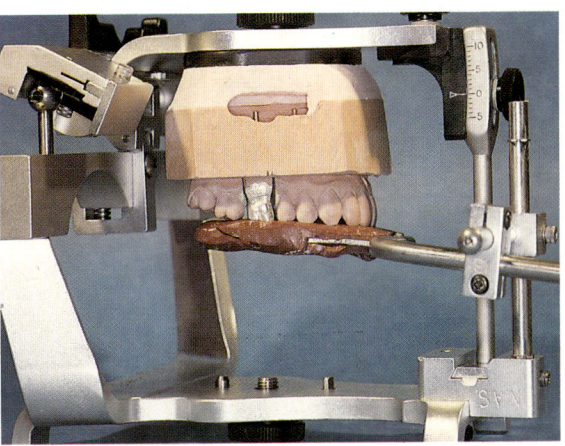

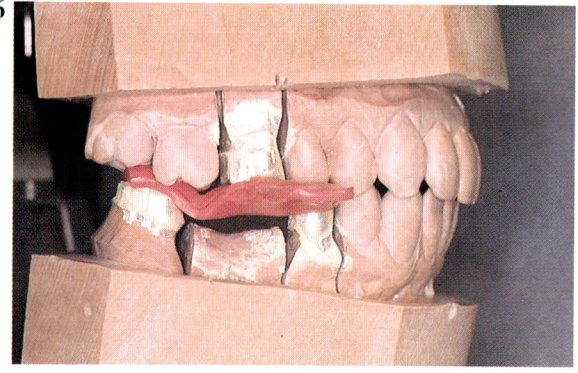

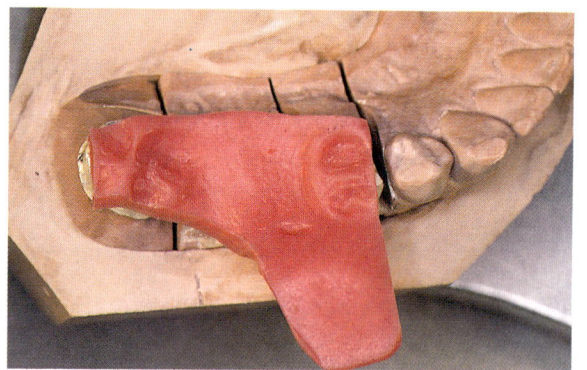

476, 477 A hard wax interocclusal record was required to stabilize the mandibular cast in ICP during mounting on the articulator.

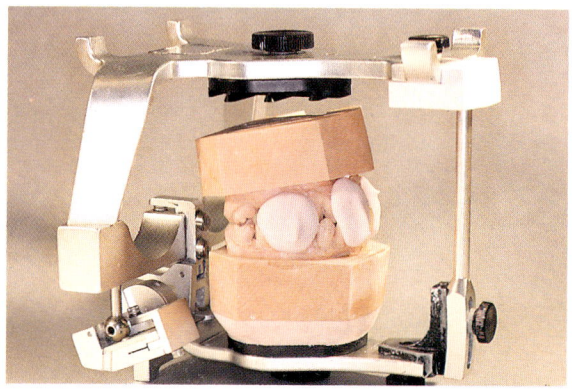

478 It is important to lock the casts together before attaching the mandibular cast to the lower member of the articulator. This may be achieved using impression plaster applied to areas of the casts coated with a separating medium.

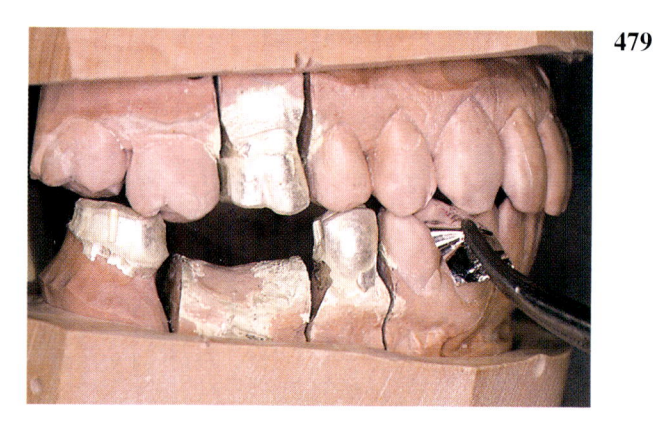

479 Once the mounting plaster had set, the record was removed and shimstock contacts were verified between the unprepared teeth and compared to those observed in the mouth.

There is an alternative way of making an interocclusal record when using silver-plated dies. An acrylic resin (Duralay) coping is made on the die of 48. It is tried in the mouth and adjusted so as to be just out of contact in ICP with the opposing tooth. A small increment of acrylic resin is placed on the coping with a brush and the patient closed into ICP, the opposing palatal cusp indenting the resin. Once set, the teeth are parted and shimstock contacts between the resin record and opposing cusp and between the unprepared teeth are verified. The coping is then removed, placed on the die and the casts located and attached to the articulator. Shimstock contact between the coping and opposing teeth is verified after mounting.

480, 481 Copings were waxed on the dies and pontic areas, on which cusp cones were built, designating the positions of the supporting cusps. White dots were placed on the surface of the copings to aid location of the tips of the supporting cusp cones in stable positions. The cusp cones were then checked in lateral and protrusive excursions to ensure disclusion.

The achievement of tripod contacts between restorations and existing occlusal surfaces is unrealistic. The main objective was to position the supporting cusp tips close to the central fossae of the opposing teeth, the precise nature of the ICP contacts being a combination of cusp tip to fossa and opposing incline planes, depending upon the morphology of the opposing occlusal surfaces.

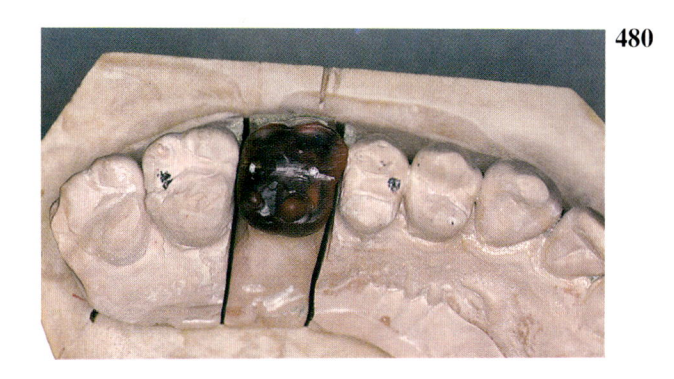

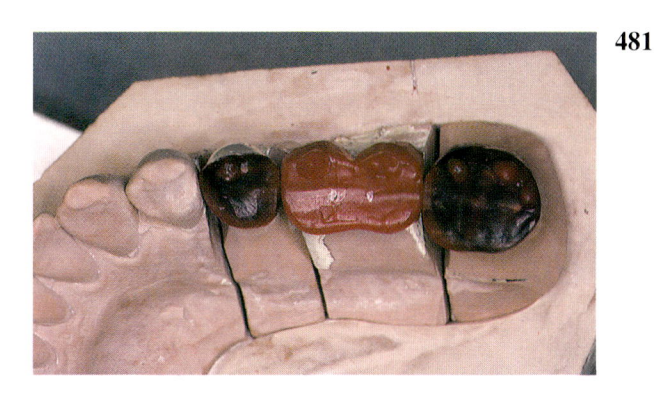

482, 483 The finished wax patterns, the ICP contacts having been marked with white articulating paper.

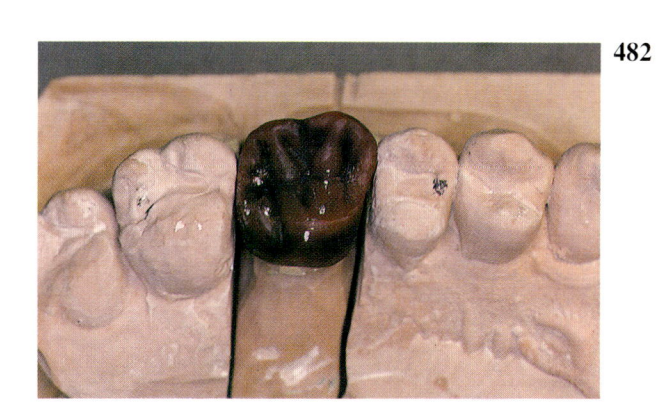

169

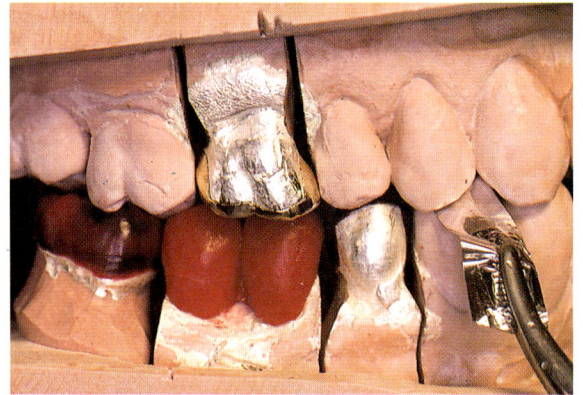

484 When opposing restorations are made it is advisable to wax them together, cast them in one arch and seat them on their respective dies first. The opposing wax-ups can then be refined against the surface of the finished restorations. This minimizes the occlusal errors produced during the technical procedures. In this case, the ¾ crown on 16 was cast and finished and the mandibular wax patterns were subsequently refined.

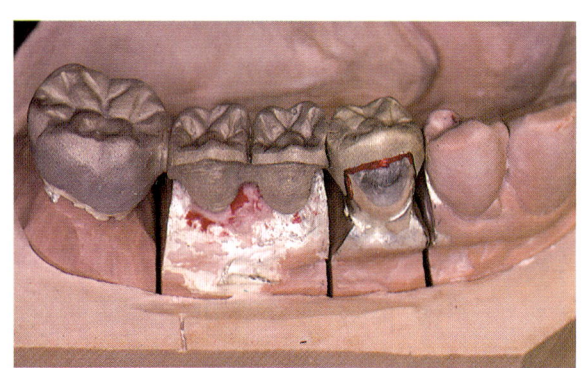

485 The completed casting for the mandibular bridge. The occlusal and axial surfaces should be completely finished in the wax-up stage. Extensive finishing of occlusal surfaces subsequent to casting will destroy the occlusal contacts created during waxing. Note the metalwork design with coverage of the supporting cusps.

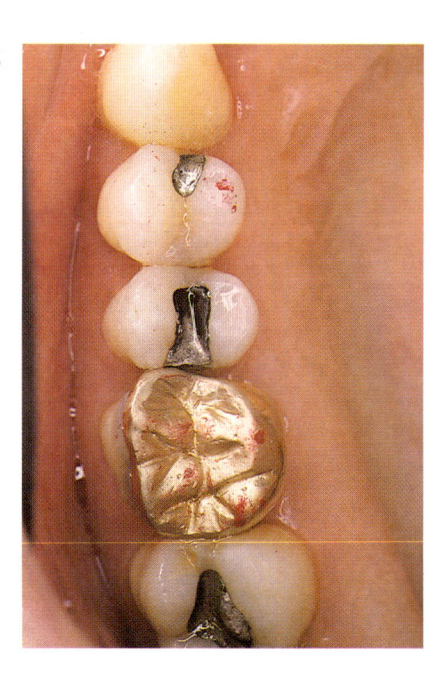

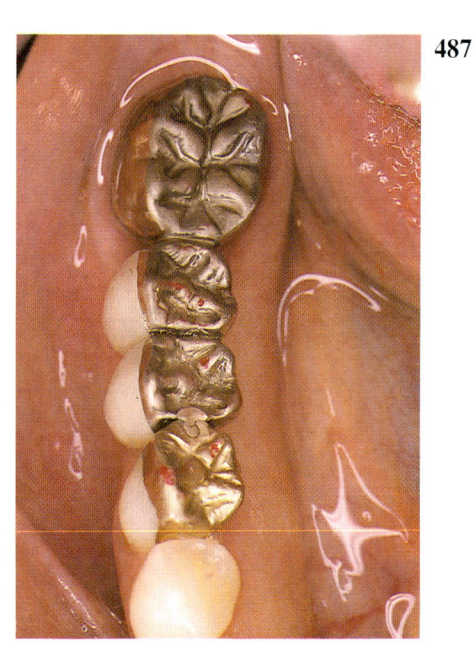

486, 487 The finished restorations were tried in the mouth and ICP contacts were marked and checked with shimstock. The restorations were checked for disclusion in protrusive and lateral excursions and then temporarily cemented for two weeks. At the following appointment the occlusal surfaces were checked for any burnish marks indicative of heavy contacts and the restorations were finally cemented with zinc phosphate cement.

Restoration of opposing quadrants

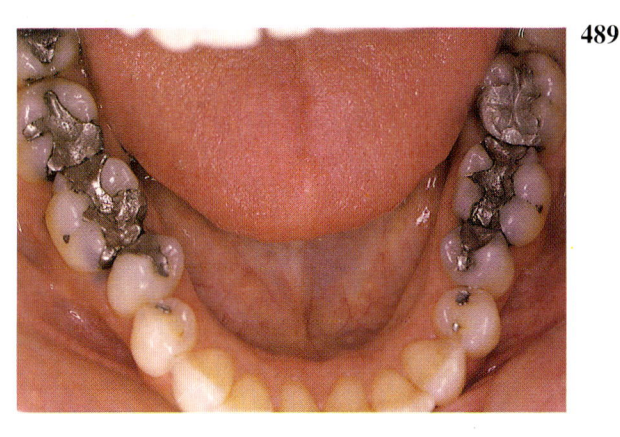

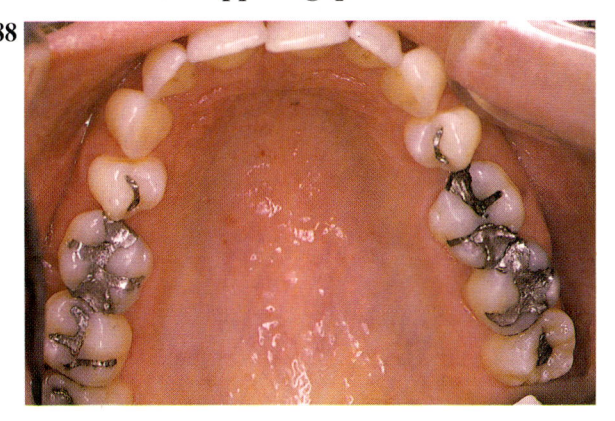

488, 489 This patient presented with a history of repeated fracture of teeth and restorations. Clinical examination revealed a number of large, poorly contoured amalgam fillings, a fractured mesiolingual cusp of 46, a loss of posterior stability and numerous working and non-working side interferences. There was a small discrepancy between RCP and ICP, which was mainly vertical in direction.

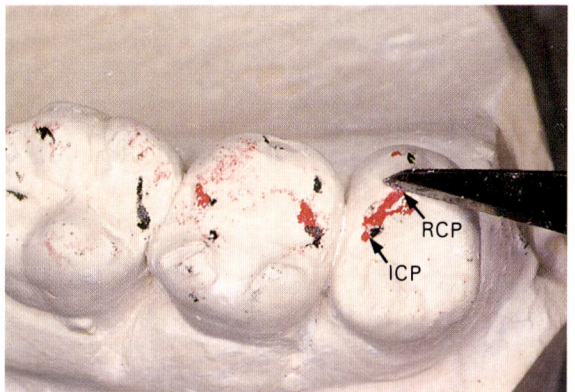

490 A maxillary occlusal splint was fitted and worn for a period of one month before the RCP contacts had stabilized, indicating a stable retruded position.

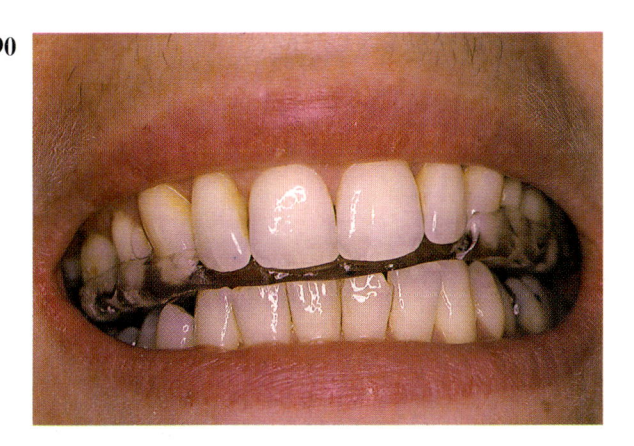

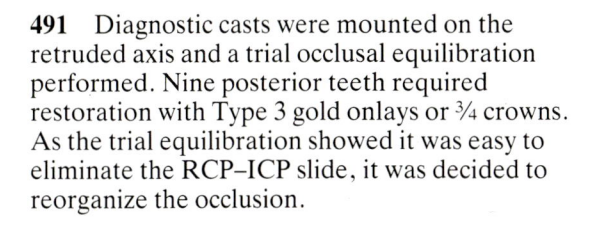

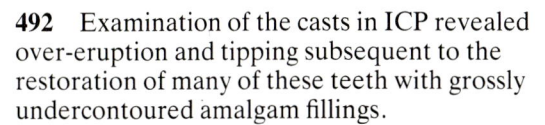

491 Diagnostic casts were mounted on the retruded axis and a trial occlusal equilibration performed. Nine posterior teeth required restoration with Type 3 gold onlays or ¾ crowns. As the trial equilibration showed it was easy to eliminate the RCP–ICP slide, it was decided to reorganize the occlusion.

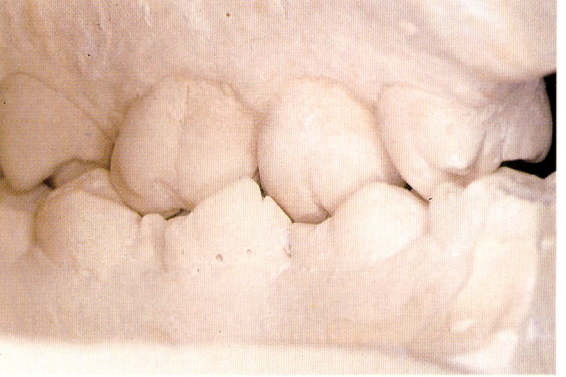

492 Examination of the casts in ICP revealed over-eruption and tipping subsequent to the restoration of many of these teeth with grossly undercontoured amalgam fillings.

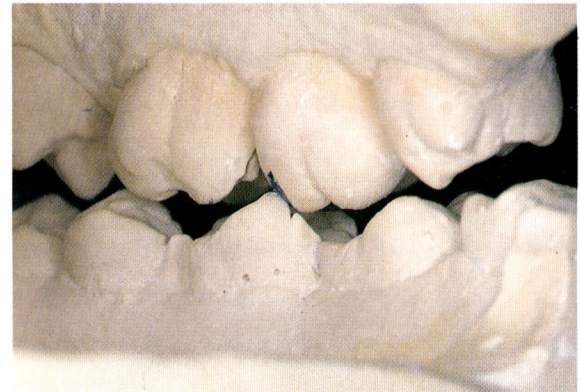

493 In lateral excursions there were several large working and non-working side interferences which had contributed to the fracture of cusps.

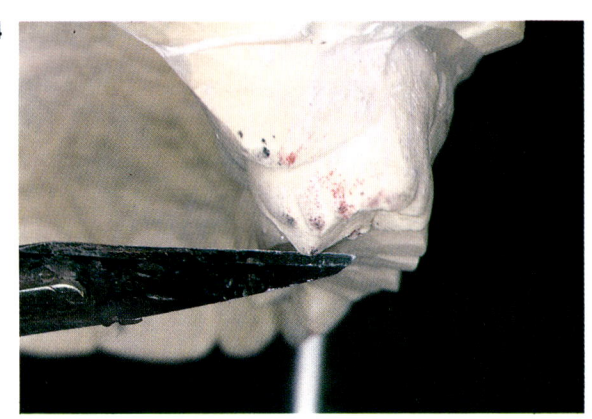

494 It was essential that the final restorations did not duplicate these interferences. Prominent cusps and over-erupted and tilted teeth not destined for restoration were reduced on the casts and a note was made to do the same in the mouth at the time of tooth preparation.

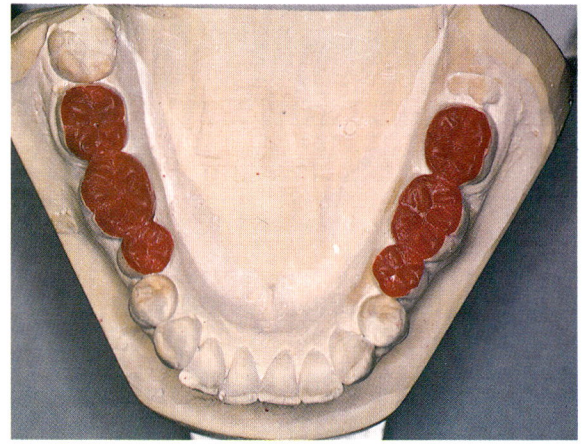

495, 496 A diagnostic wax-up was carried out in which the malalignment of the teeth requiring castings was corrected, and a level occlusal plane, with stable ICP contacts and posterior disclusion, was established. It is important for the clinician to carry out the diagnostic wax-up rather than delegating it to the technician. Only by doing this can all the diagnostic information, regarding modifications of the opposing occlusion during preparation, be obtained.

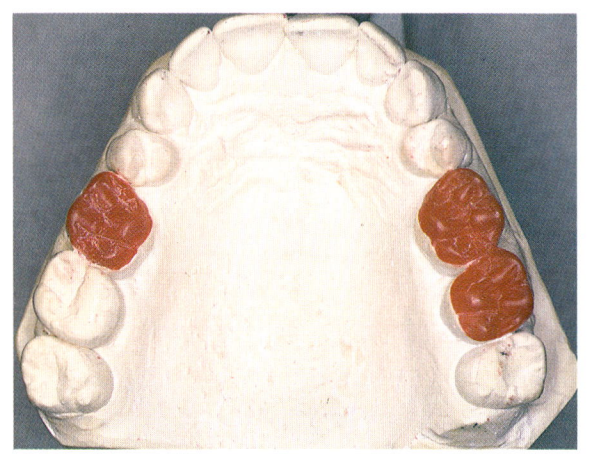

497 Alginate impressions made from the diagnostic wax-up were poured in yellow stone, and the casts used to make vacuformed shells. These served both as moulds for the construction of provisional restorations, and as tooth preparation guides.

After completion of splint therapy the patient's occlusion was equilibrated so that RCP–ICP and the anterior teeth were in contact, providing an immediate disclusion with canine guidance. At four subsequent appointments the posterior teeth were prepared, prominent opposing cusps reduced, and reversible hydrocolloid impressions made of both arches. These were poured in stone to produce maxillary and mandibular working casts.

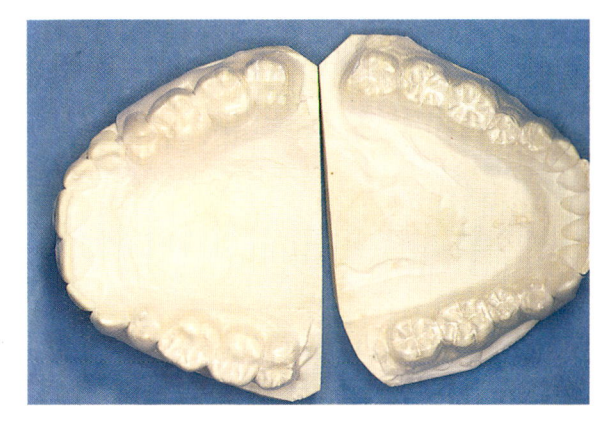

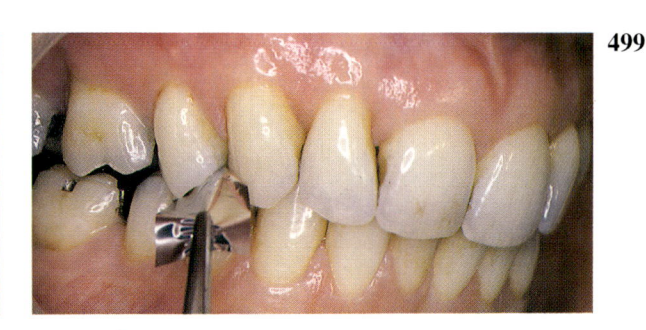

498, 499 An interocclusal record made from hard wax was taken with the unprepared teeth in ICP contact. Shimstock was used to verify these contacts so that the accuracy of cast mounting could be verified in the laboratory.

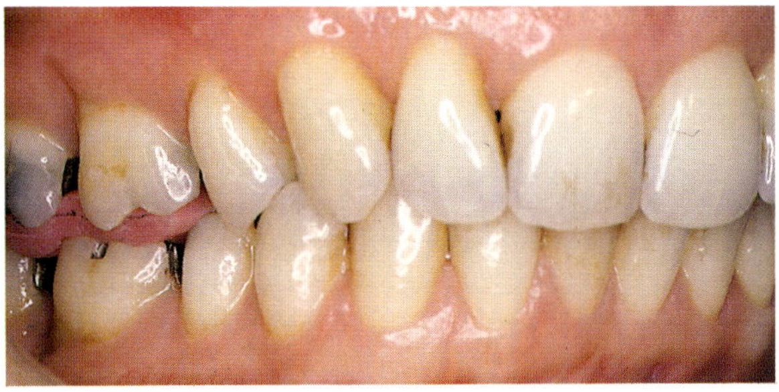

500, 501 The maxillary cast was mounted with an average axis facebow, on a fully-adjustable articulator set from pantographic tracings. This patient possessed good anterior guidance and so the use of a semi-adjustable articulator would have been acceptable. This might have resulted in the need to adjust the castings in protrusive and lateral excursions when they were tried in.

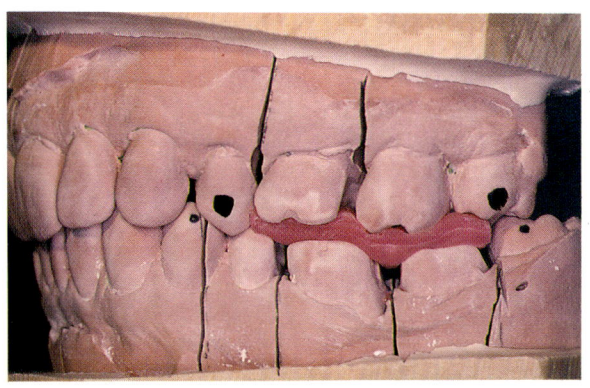

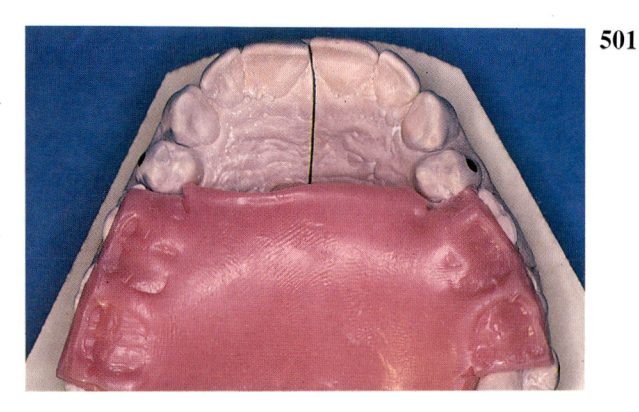

This is reasonable for a small number of units, but less so in more complex cases in which it is advantageous to be able to carry out the adjustments at the wax-up stage on an articulator which correctly reproduces mandibular movements.

The mounting of working casts should be carried out by the clinician as soon after record taking as possible, to give the materials less chance to distort. It is helpful to mark the unprepared teeth which hold shimstock in the mouth as a guide for the technician during waxing and finishing procedures.

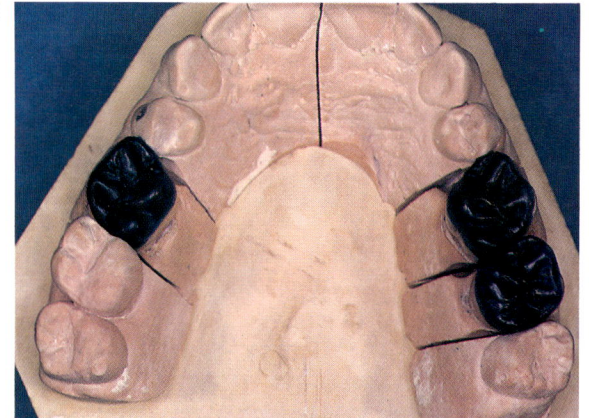

502, 503 The wax patterns were completed using a wax additive technique to establish stable contacts.

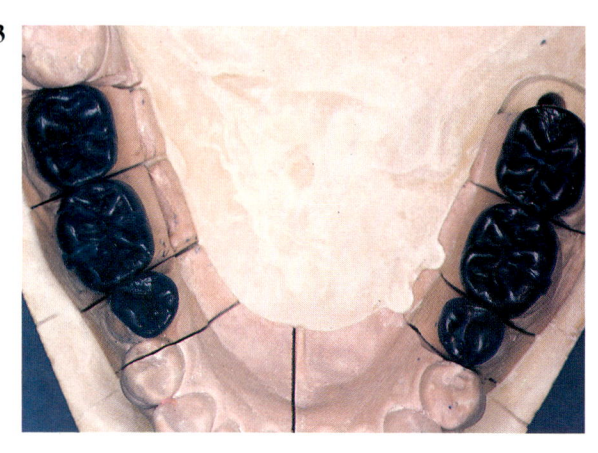

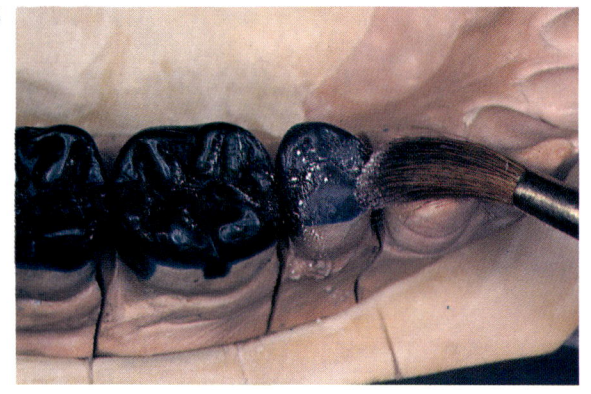

504, 505 Zinc stearate powder was dusted over the occlusal surfaces which were tapped together, revealing the points of contact as shiny spots. These were adjusted as necessary.

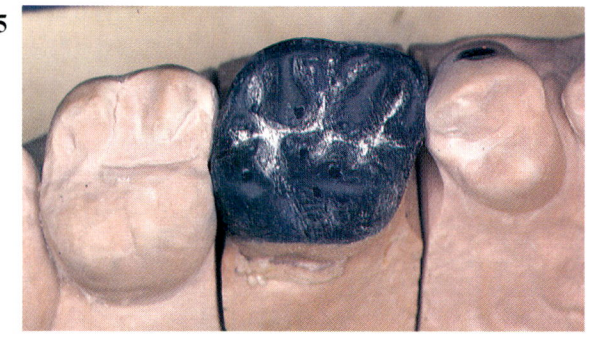

506 Shimstock was used between unprepared teeth to ensure that the wax patterns were not high.

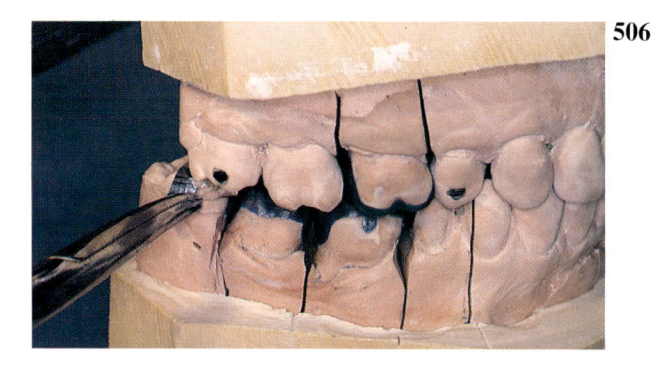

507, 508 After casting and devesting, the fit surface of each casting was examined under a binocular microscope and any small casting defects or air bubbles were removed. This was carried out before trying the castings on the dies and is important because incomplete seating of restorations causes errors in the occlusion, as well as lack of marginal adaptation.

After seating the castings on the dies, very little finishing of the occlusal surfaces should be necessary.

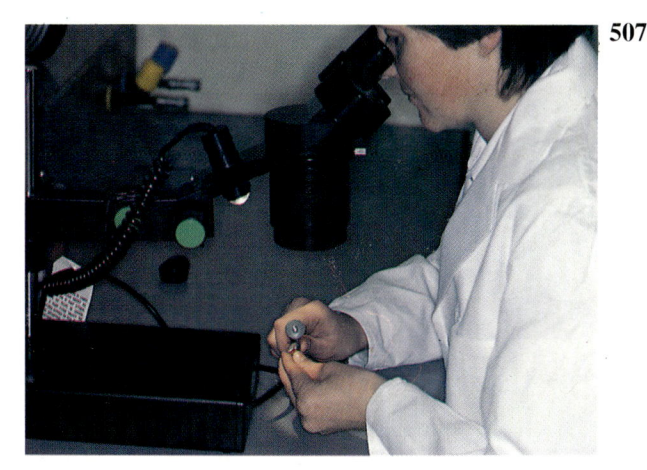

509 The occlusal surfaces were blasted with glass beads to impart a matt finish which facilitates the marking of occlusal contacts.

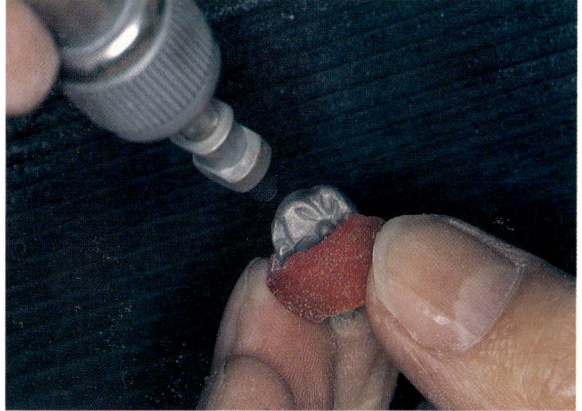

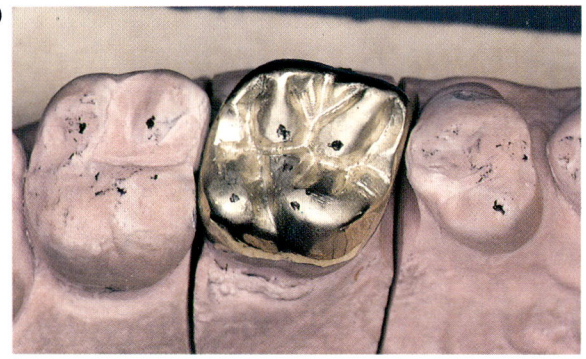

510 Articulating paper was used to mark the occlusal contacts so that any minor final adjustments could be carried out.

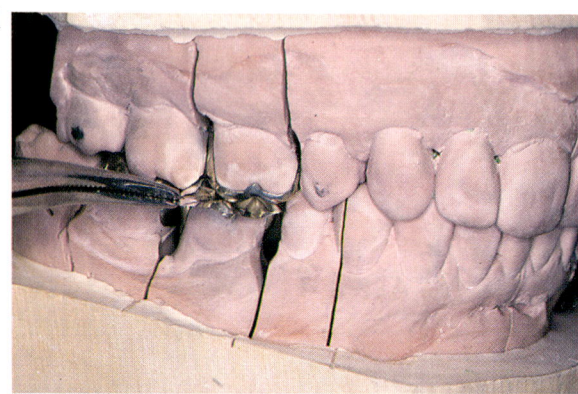

511, 512 Shimstock was used to verify that the restorations were in tight contact but not so high as to separate the unprepared teeth.

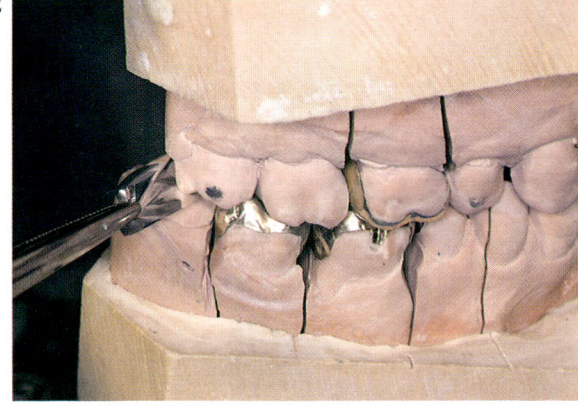

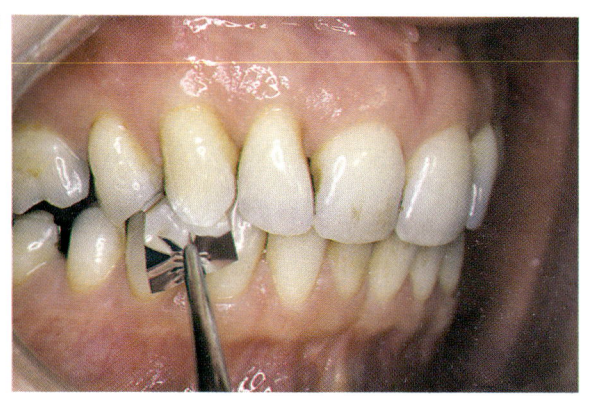

513 The provisional restorations were removed and the ICP contacts between unprepared teeth verified.

514–516 The restorations were tried in and shimstock was employed to check the ICP contacts, using those between the unprepared teeth as a baseline. Articulating paper was used to mark contacts and to check for any working or non-working side interferences which should be eliminated. If a discrepancy is found between the occlusion on the articulator and that in the mouth, the source of error must be located. It may arise from:

- Castings not seating.
- Prepared teeth having moved owing to inadequate provisional restorations.
- Inaccuracy in the master casts.
- Inaccurate mounting of the mandibular cast.
- The patient's condylar position having changed owing to a lack of stability of the provisional restorations, or a dysfunctional problem.

If the cause is an inaccurate jaw relation record, it is more sensible to make a new record, remount the lower cast and adjust the occlusion on the articulator rather than attempt to adjust multiple castings in the mouth.

When the marginal adaptation, contours, proximal contacts and occlusion had been deemed satisfactory, the restorations were temporarily cemented for two weeks.

Prior to final cementation, a wire wheel may be used to impart a shiny occlusal surface without polishing away the occlusal contacts. Rubber polishing wheels or polishing compound are too abrasive and will result in the loss of contacts. It is advisable to leave the crowns with a matt finish, making it easier to monitor the occlusion at subsequent recall appointments.

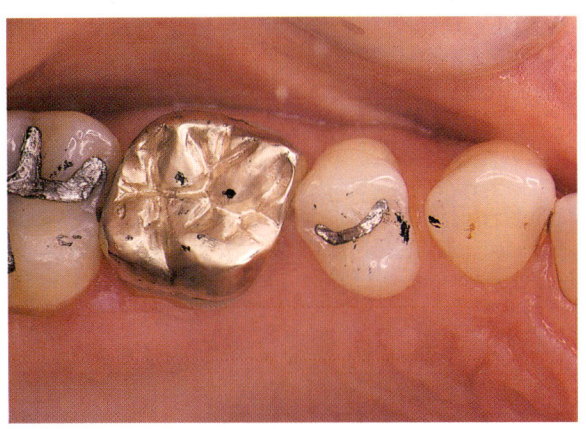

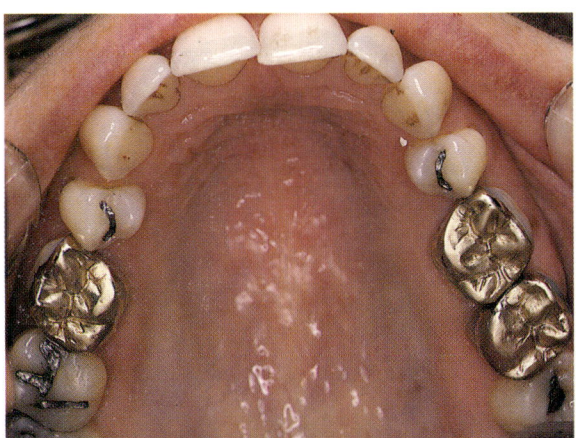

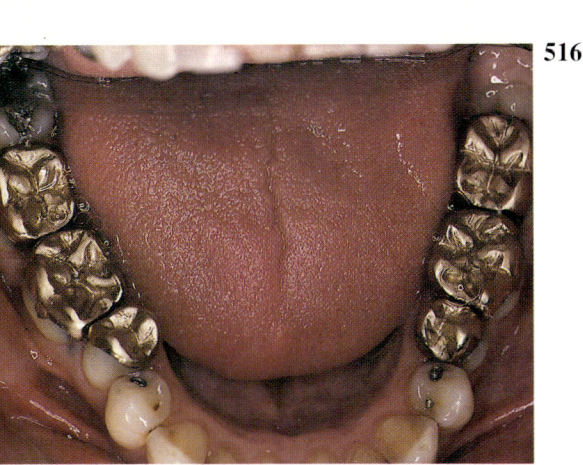

Partial denture occlusion when posterior teeth require replacement

The occlusal requirements for partial dentures replacing posterior teeth are very similar to those for fixed restorations. It is important that artificial posterior teeth provide stable contacts in the intercuspal position, and that anterior guidance and ICP contacts are provided by the remaining natural teeth. Although acrylic resin teeth are usually used in partial dentures, they have poor resistance to wear and rapidly lose stable ICP contacts. This may cause the denture to wear out of occlusion or allow a gradual over-eruption of the opposing teeth.

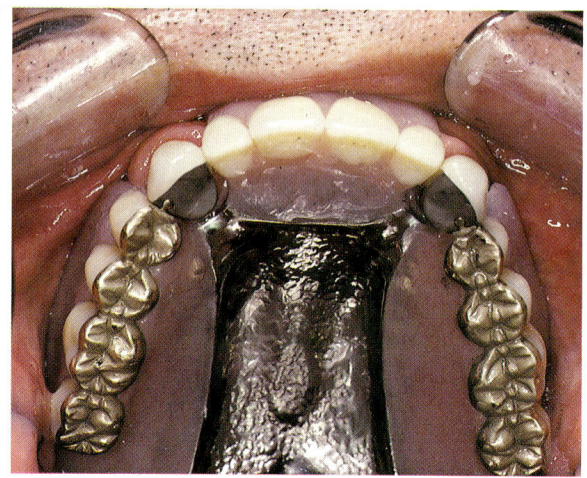

517 The use of more durable materials will provide a more stable posterior occlusion. Custom-waxed gold occlusal surfaces were used in this partial denture.

518, 519 Porcelain denture teeth may be used where they oppose the porcelain occlusal surfaces of fixed or removable restorations.

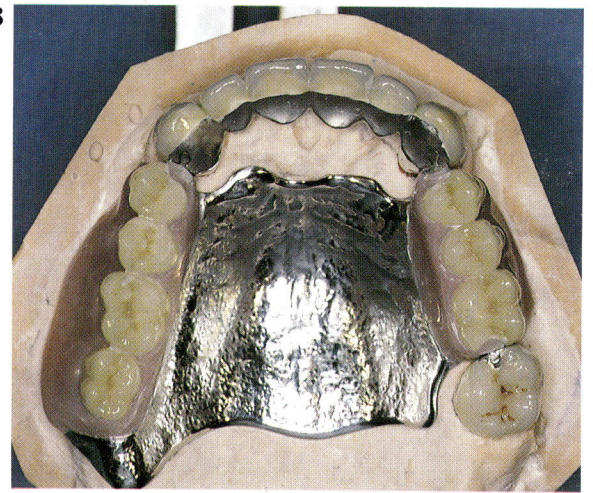

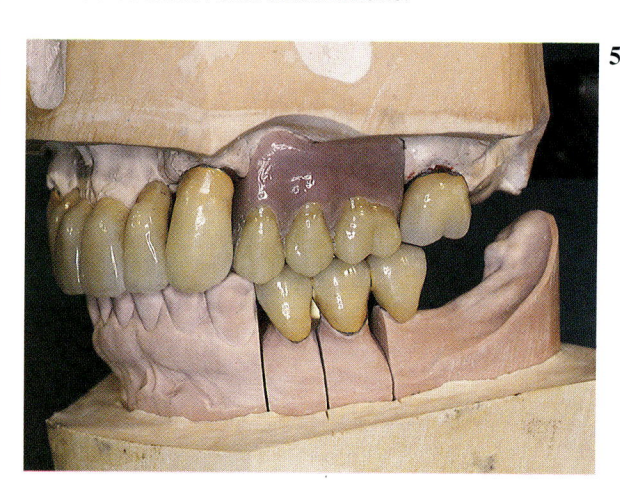

Conclusion

The basic principles involved in the restoration of posterior teeth have been described. They apply equally when conforming or reorganizing.

Chapter 12: The restoration of anterior and posterior teeth

If a patient requires full mouth restorations, it is often possible to divide the treatment plan into a number of stages:

- Occlusal splint therapy.
- Equilibration so that RCP=ICP.
- Restoration of anterior guidance.
- Restoration of the posterior teeth which may be carried out all at one time or split, restoring opposing quadrants on one side first and then on the other side at a later date.

Dividing complex treatment into several stages spread over a period of time has several advantages:

- It is less tiring for both clinician and patient.
- It may be easier for a patient to afford the time necessary for treatment.
- It spreads the cost over a longer period.
- It is easier to control technical procedures.

Provided the treatment plan is divided in this way the end result should not be compromised. If individual quadrants are restored against an existing occlusion, it is more difficult to produce ideal occlusal anatomy and posterior stability.

There are a few occasions when it is impossible to plan treatment in this way, and all the restorations must be made together. Clinical and technical procedures become more demanding as preparation of all a patient's teeth removes landmarks with respect to tooth position, contour and occlusion. It is important to use well-made provisional restorations to establish the correct appearance, tooth positions and occlusal relations. This information can be supplied to the technician for incorporation into the final restorations.

The principles of restoring anterior and posterior teeth, which have already been described, apply in these cases. This chapter illustrates the two main situations in which full-mouth reconstruction carried out at one time is the best treatment plan. It also describes some of the practical techniques used in the treatment of such cases, which have not been covered in other parts of this book.

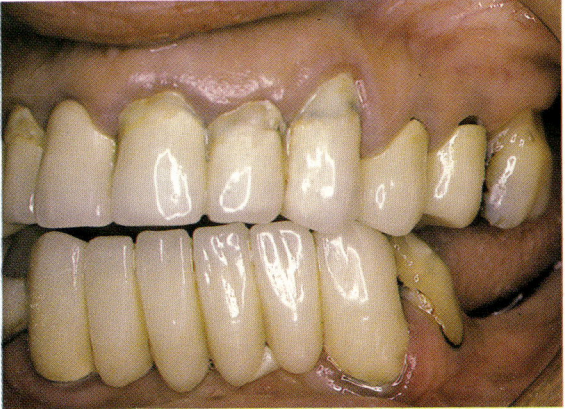

520 This patient required replacement of all her old restorations which were ill-fitting, poorly contoured and lacking in posterior stability and anterior guidance. There was no alternative but to remake all the restorations together.

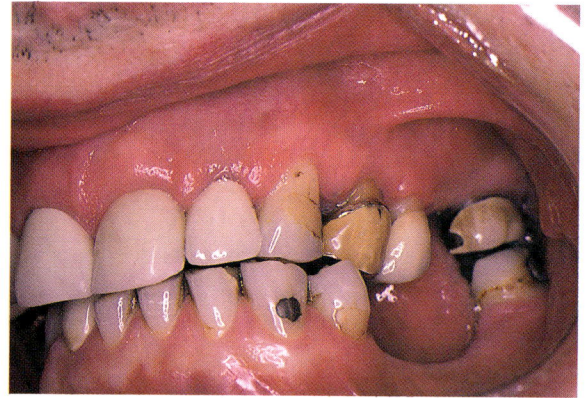

521, 522 The second situation in which simultaneous restoration of both anterior and posterior teeth is required is when it is necessary to increase the vertical dimension of occlusion. This patient, showing increased wear of many teeth, particularly the lower incisors and left canine, required full-mouth reconstruction. The right canine had been restored with a porcelain-fused-to-metal crown several years before. Increasing the vertical dimension of occlusion enabled occlusal reduction of the teeth during preparation to be avoided. This preserved maximum clinical crown height, avoiding the need for surgical crown lengthening. It also increased the vertical space available for bridge connectors, whilst maintaining open embrasures for plaque control, and increased tooth length, thus providing a better appearance.

Wearing an occlusal splint is important to achieve muscle relaxation and to enable a correct and stable retruded jaw relation to be established. The splint is not necessary for testing increases in vertical dimension which are easily accommodated, provided the occlusion is correctly managed.

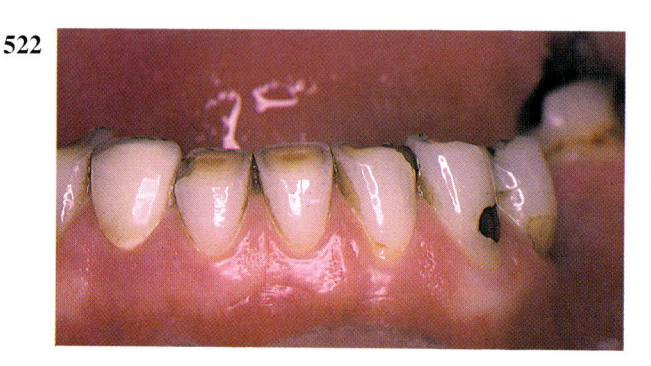

523 It is helpful to carry out both diagnostic and treatment procedures on a fully-adjustable articulator, set from pantographic tracings. A diagnostic pantograph will show whether a reproducible retruded position can be obtained. In the absence of both anterior guidance and a stable ICP, the only reproducible reference positions available are the mandibular border positions (posterior determinants of occlusion). The occlusal surfaces of the restorations can be made to harmonize rather than interfere with the border movements.

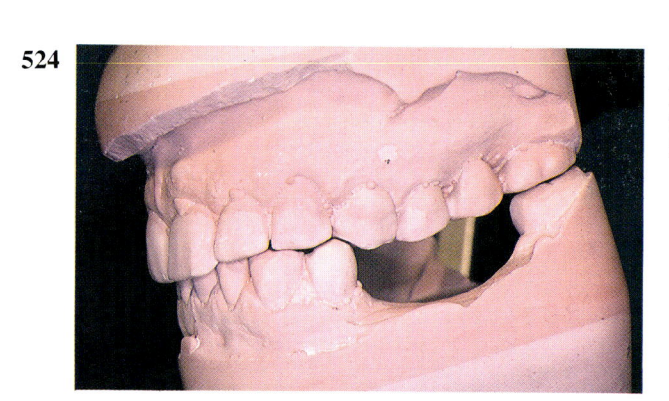

524 Once the articulator had been set from a pantographic survey, diagnostic casts were mounted using an average axis facebow and wax interocclusal records.

525 The incisal pin was opened, increasing the VDO to provide enough space for the restorative materials without needing to carry out any occlusal reduction.

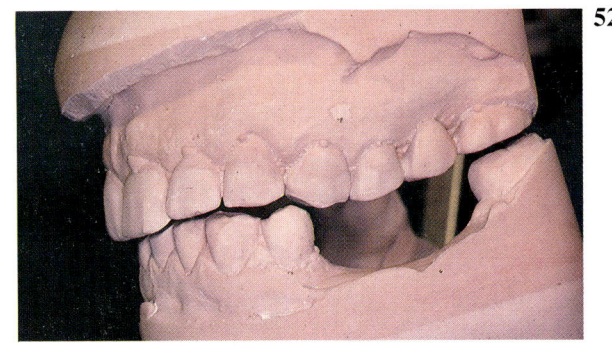

526 A full-mouth diagnostic wax-up was carried out to this new VDO, the angle of the anterior guidance being determined by the condylar movements of the articulator (and hence of the patient), and its steepness by the need to disclude the posterior teeth.

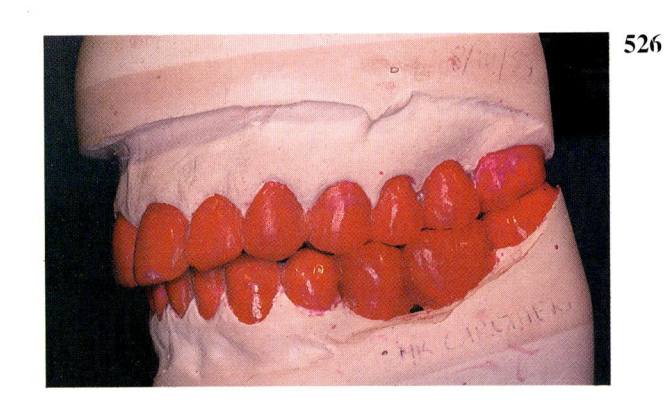

527 The teeth were prepared and indirect acrylic resin provisional restorations fitted. They were fabricated using moulds made over the diagnostic wax-up which determined the VDO, occlusal plane, tooth positions and shape and anterior guidance. The patient wore the provisional restorations for at least one month, during which time their appearance and occlusion were checked and altered as necessary.

When the shape of the provisional restorations was satisfactory, impressions were made and study casts poured and given to the technician who used them as a guide when waxing the final restorations. The anterior determinants of occlusion were transferred to the articulator by custom-moulding the incisal guide table.

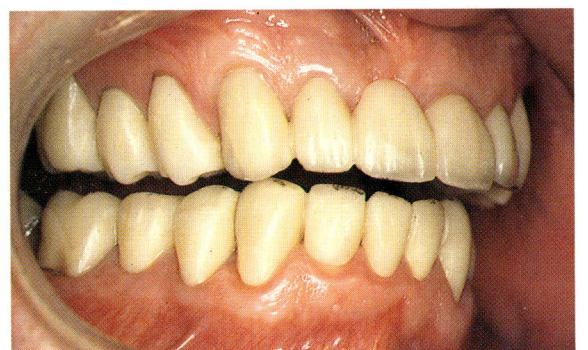

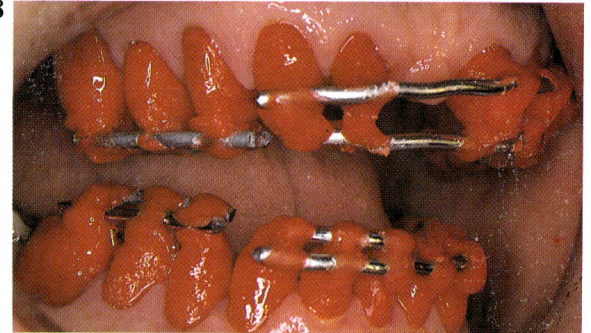

528, 529 To avoid having to make full-arch impressions of the preparations, a transfer coping pickup technique may be used. Tooth preparation is carried out during six appointments. On each occasion, a quadrant of teeth is prepared, a working impression is made and indirect provisional restorations are fitted. The impressions are silver-plated and individual dies and acrylic resin copings (Duralay) are made. After completion of tooth preparation, the provisional restorations are removed, the copings are tried on the teeth and their accuracy of fit is checked as an indication of the adequacy of the original impressions. Groups of copings are joined together using wire and acrylic resin, and maxillary and mandibular full-arch impressions are made, pulling the copings out of the mouth. The dies are placed into their respective copings, sealed in position with sticky wax, and the casts are poured in die stone.

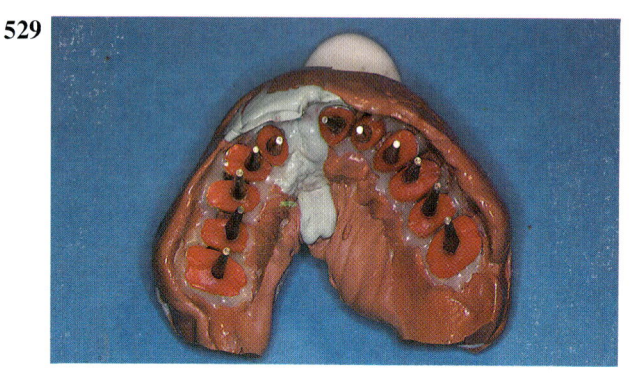

530, 531 Errors in the occlusion of the final restorations may result from inaccuracies in the position of the dies within the working casts. This is particularly so if a transfer coping pickup technique has been used to make full-arch casts. It is important to verify that the casts are accurate prior to taking the jaw relation records. A compound bitefork lined with zinc oxide-eugenol paste was made over the occlusal surfaces of the preparations. This was used as an index into which the working casts were seated to ascertain whether any dies were out of position.

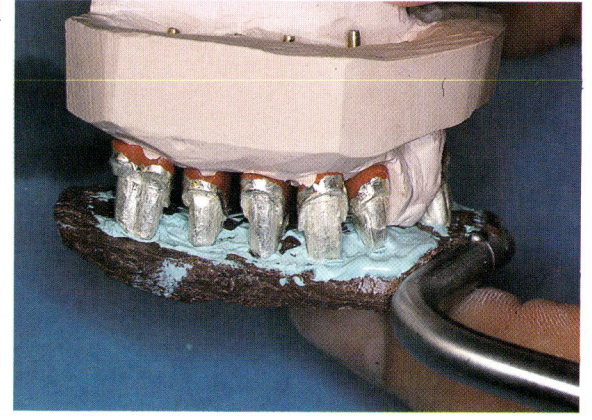

532 Whilst recording the retruded jaw relation, the vertical dimension of occlusion was maintained by the anterior provisional restorations. They acted as an anterior stop or jig, allowing an interocclusal record to be taken between the posterior preparations at the correct VDO.

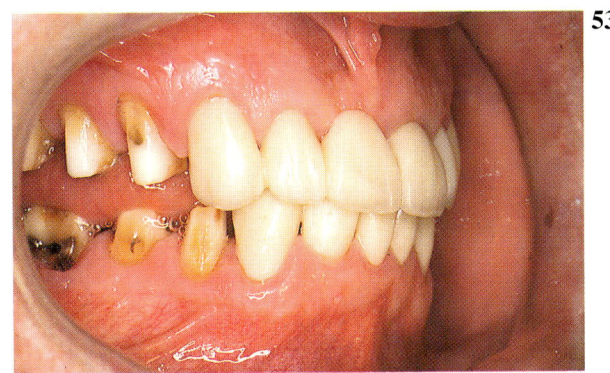

533, 534 The interocclusal record may be taken using a hard wax, or opposing pairs of acrylic resin copings when silver-plated dies are being used. Four pairs of copings were used, on the first premolars and second molars. Cusp cones were added to the four maxillary copings. These were just clear of contact with the occlusal surfaces of the four mandibular copings when the patient closed into contact on the anterior provisionals. Small increments of acrylic resin were added to the lower copings, and the patient's mandible was placed on the retruded axis using bimanual manipulation, and closed until the anterior provisional restorations touched. This position was held until the resin had set.
534 Courtesy of Miss K. Warren.

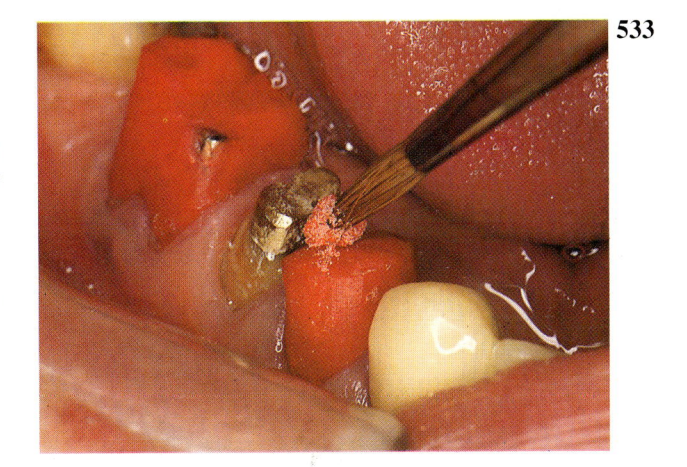

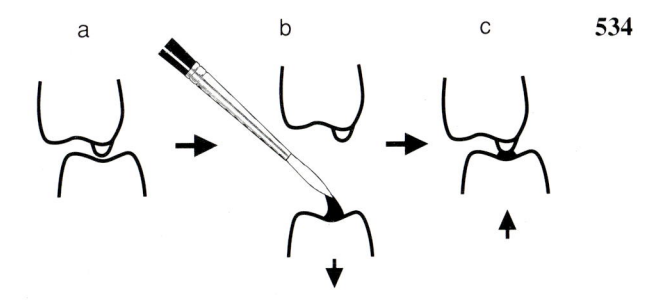

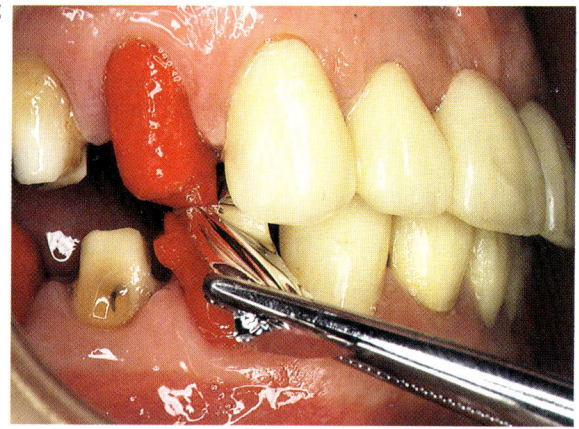

535 The patient was asked to open and the four pairs of copings were removed, separated and replaced on the preparations. The record was checked to see that it was on the retruded axis and all four pairs of copings held shimstock.

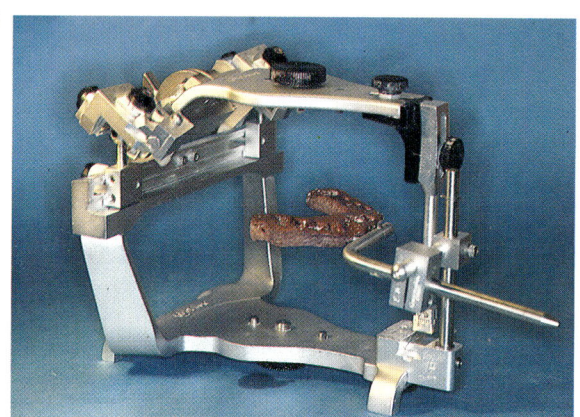

536 The maxillary working cast was mounted on the articulator using an average axis facebow record.

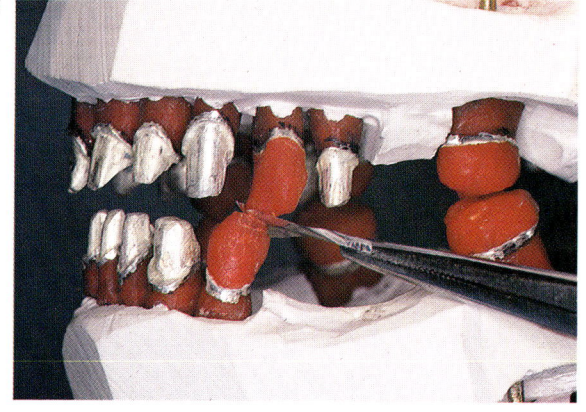

537 It is important to mount the mandibular cast as quickly as possible to reduce the time available for the acrylic resin to distort. The cusp cones should be added to the maxillary copings two days prior to record taking. The increments of resin added to the lower copings should be as small as possible, so that the contraction occurring during polymerization will not produce a significant error.

The mandibular cast was located via the four points of contact between the cusp cones and indentations, and the casts locked together. It was attached to the lower member of the articulator. Once the mounting plaster had fully set, the accuracy of the mounting was verified by checking that all four pairs of copings held shimstock, as they did in the mouth.

538, 539 The restorations were waxed to full-contour, using the shapes of the casts of the provisionals as a guide. The morphology of the articulating surfaces of the anterior and posterior teeth was determined by the incisal guide table and condylar movements.

The wax-ups were cut back, cast and porcelain was applied. These pictures show the finished restorations on the articulator.

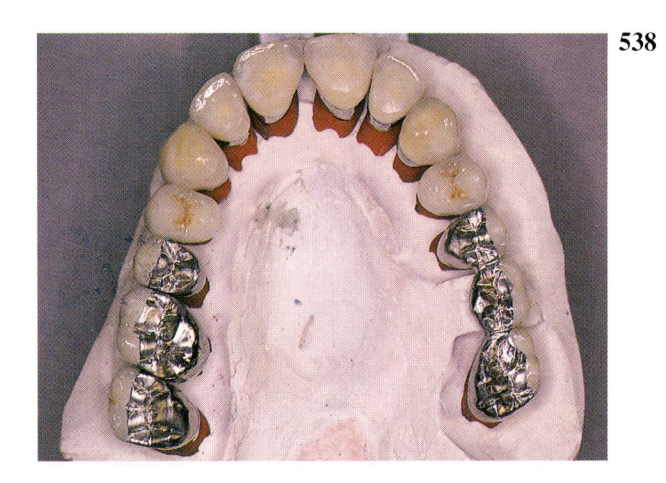

540 The finished restorations in the mouth at the try-in appointment. They were temporarily cemented for about a month to ensure patient acceptance.

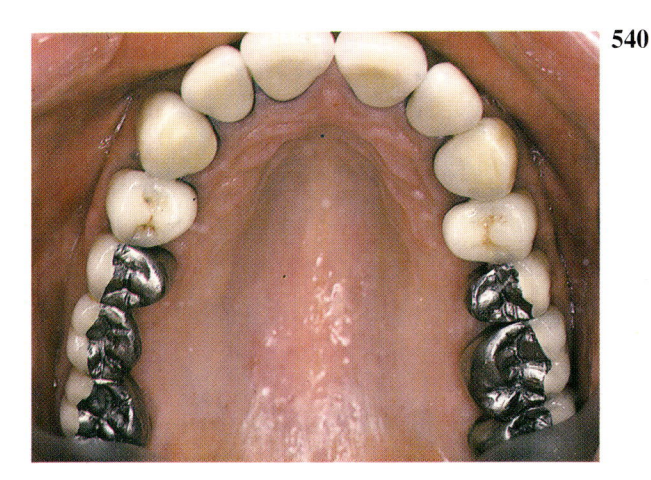

185

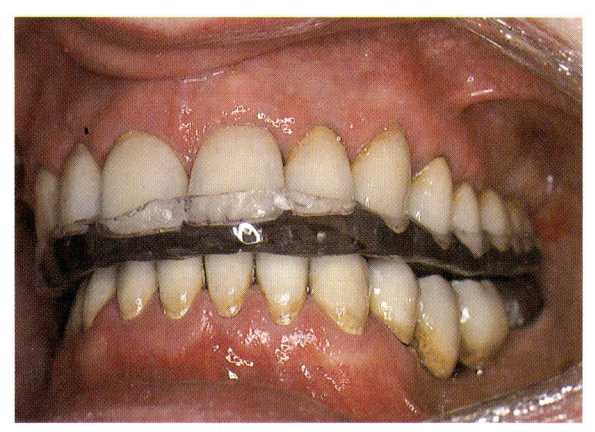

541 A new occlusal splint was made to be worn as a nightguard, as protection against damage caused by continued bruxing.

Conclusion

Reorganizing a patient's occlusion to create a new and stable ICP requires a higher degree of skill and knowledge than conforming to the existing ICP. It is important for the clinician to be able to diagnose when this approach is indicated for a particular patient. He must then decide whether he and his technician possess the knowledge and ability to achieve a satisfactory result.

Chapter 13: Introduction to orthodontic treatment

Following assessment, orthodontic treatment may proceed along the following routes:

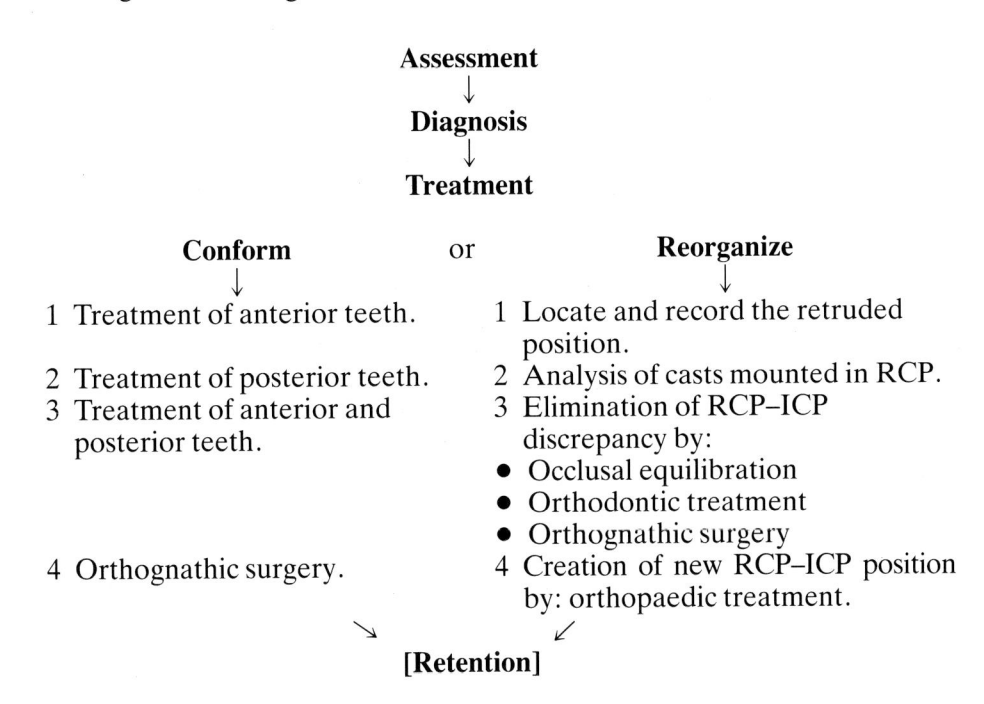

Assessment
↓
Diagnosis
↓
Treatment

Conform or **Reorganize**

1 Treatment of anterior teeth.
2 Treatment of posterior teeth.
3 Treatment of anterior and posterior teeth.

4 Orthognathic surgery.

1 Locate and record the retruded position.
2 Analysis of casts mounted in RCP.
3 Elimination of RCP–ICP discrepancy by:
- Occlusal equilibration
- Orthodontic treatment
- Orthognathic surgery
4 Creation of new RCP–ICP position by: orthopaedic treatment.

[Retention]

Orthodontic treatment is conformative when there is no alteration to the RCP–ICP relationship during treatment. Orthodontic treatment is reorganized when an alteration in the RCP–ICP relationship is one of the main aims of treatment. Treatment may also be **definitive** or **interceptive**. The patient may be at the appropriate age and stage of development to allow treatment of the malocclusion to be definitively completed. Monitoring the dentitions as they develop may establish the presence of conditions that interfere with normal function. If intervention with non-definitive orthodontic treatment can restore normal function, further growth and development in the oro-facial region will be optimized. Appropriate interceptive treatment is therefore undertaken.

A number of orthodontic patients may present with TMJ signs and symptoms and/or difficulty in achieving an accurate retruded position of the mandible. In this group, **occlusal splint therapy** as described in Chapter 9 may be required to facilitate correct analysis of the occlusion, and allow the planning of conformative or reorganized treatment. The occlusal splint is discarded once treatment starts. It has the additional purpose of establishing whether symptoms are relieved by the temporary elimination of RCP–ICP discrepancies.

Orthodontic treatment in the adolescent has traditionally aimed at establishing a static Class 1 occlusion, with improved dentofacial aesthetics, oral health and function. In the adult patient, objectives may be identical or more specific, such as paralleling abutment teeth prior to restorative dentistry. Orthodontists often refer to 'normal' occlusion as a treatment goal. This is based on the work of Andrews (1972) who, during the period 1960–1964, with the help of numerous colleagues built up a collection of 120 study casts of individuals with excellent occlusion. These subjects had never received any orthodontic treatment, and it was considered that orthodontics could not improve their existing occlusion.

Following analysis of these records, 'Six Keys of Normal Occlusion' were proposed as goals for orthodontic treatment; the molar relationship, crown angulation (tip), crown inclination (torque), rotations, contacts and occlusal plane are all specified as **Andrews' Six Keys**. These are related only to static occlusion and do not take into account functional relations. **Roth** (1981) later added **further keys which related to functional occlusion**: coincidence of intercuspal and retruded contact positions, maximum and stable cusp to fossae contacts throughout the buccal segments, disclusion of the posterior teeth in mandibular protrusion by even contacts on the incisors, and lateral movements of the mandible guided by the working side canines, with disclusion of all the other teeth on both working and non-working sides.

Conclusion

A treatment plan that results in optimal facial aesthetics and static and functional occlusion may require orthodontics, orthopaedics and surgery (**542–544**). Acceptability to the patient and availability of health care facilities will, however, dictate what treatment is undertaken. The following conformative or reorganized orthodontic treatments have had the benefit of readily available health care facilities, but are tempered by the consensus of what is acceptable treatment in the United Kingdom. Lack of health care facilities would have limited the **management of some of these patients.**

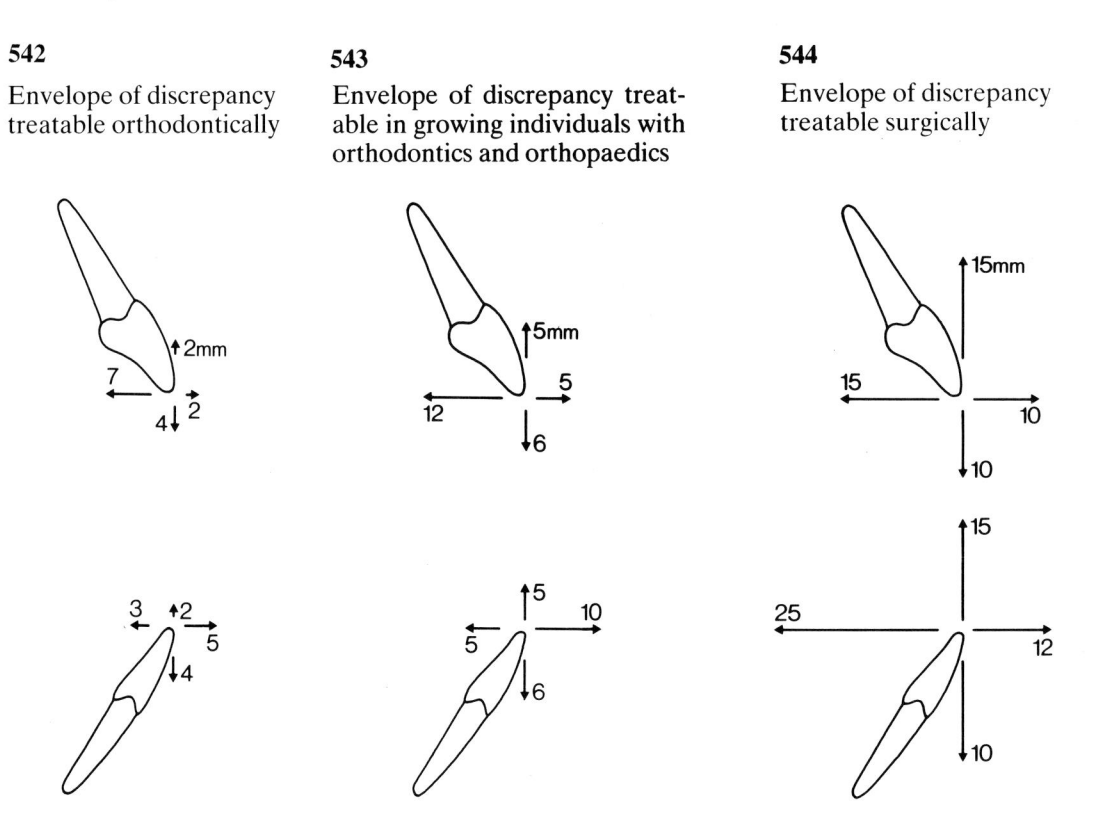

542

Envelope of discrepancy treatable orthodontically

543

Envelope of discrepancy treatable in growing individuals with orthodontics and orthopaedics

544

Envelope of discrepancy treatable surgically

542–544 The limitations of movement achievable in orthodontic therapy, with or without orthopaedics and surgery, are illustrated in the envelopes of Ackerman and Profitt (1985).

Chapter 14: Conformative orthodontic treatment

Orthodontic treatment is conformative when there is no alteration to the RCP–ICP relationship during treatment.

Conformative interceptive treatment

Intervention during the development of the deciduous and permanent dentitions on a conformative basis usually involves treatment for:

- Relief of crowding.
- Abnormal spacing.
- Abnormalities of tooth size.
- Supernumerary teeth.
- Tooth germ malposition.
- Anomalies of tooth structure.

Interceptive conformative orthodontic treatment, as described in detail in orthodontic texts, can be carried out. One example of this interceptive type of treatment is illustrated here.

545 Supernumerary teeth are extra teeth that occur in one per cent of the population. They are more often found in the maxilla than in the mandible. Tuberculate supernumerary teeth overlie the cingulum area of the upper permanent central incisors. They prevent the eruption of the incisors and their presence is suspected when there is an abnormal pattern of incisor eruption.

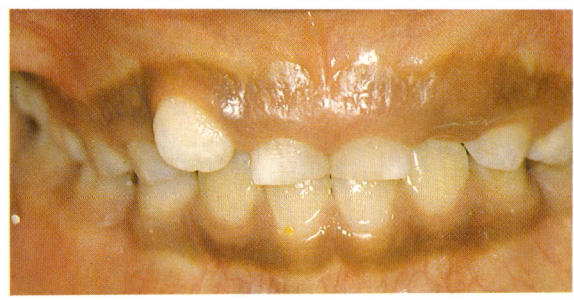

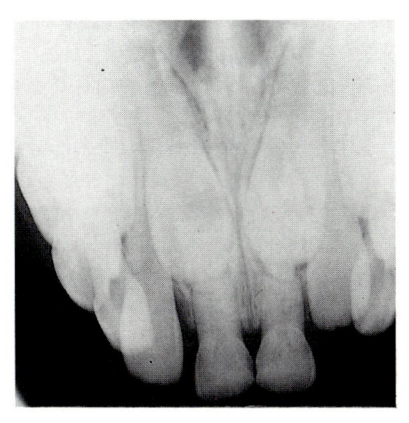

546 The radiographic appearance is typical. The barrel-shaped extra tooth structure is outlined against the crown of the incisor. Tuberculates often occur in pairs, though single ones can also occur.

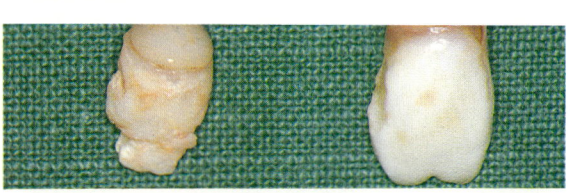

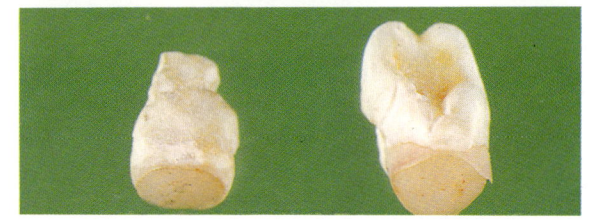

547 Tuberculates must be removed as soon as possible to allow eruption of the permanent incisors. If there is a delay in their removal, space to accommodate the incisors may be lost and the potential for eruption curtailed.

189

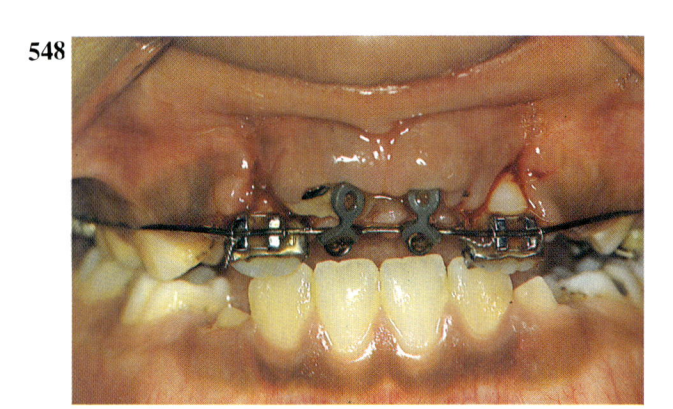

548, 549 Active treatment, when required, involves the recreation of space to accommodate the central incisors, then their exposure and vertical alignment.

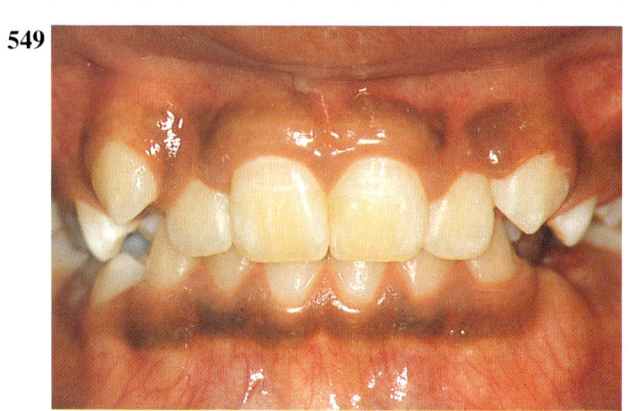

Conformative definitive treatment

Definitive treatment on a conformative basis may undertake adjustment of tooth positions for:

- Anterior malocclusion correction.
- Posterior malocclusion correction.
- Anterior and posterior malocclusion correction.
- Orthognathic surgery correction.

Although in the latter two categories the position of many teeth is being altered when a Class 2 or Class 3 malocclusion is changed to a Class 1, it is conformative, not reorganized management that is occurring, when there is no pre-treatment RCP–ICP discrepancy. At the conclusion of conformative treatment, it is important to check that an RCP–ICP discrepancy has not been introduced by the new tooth positions. Occlusal assessments at the end of active treatment before the removal of appliances, and at the end of the retaining period are as important as at the start of treatment. Similar methods of assessment to those described in Part II are used.

Anterior malocclusion correction

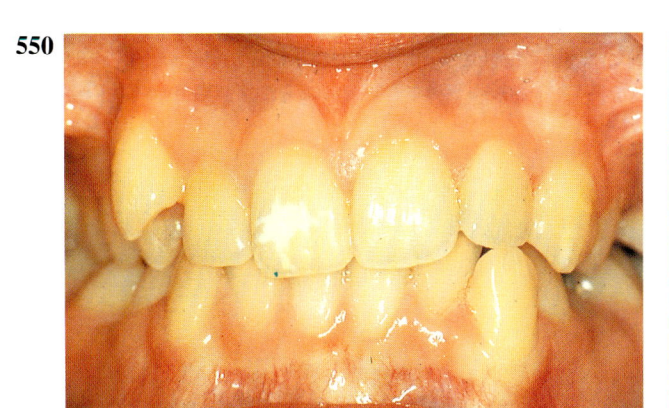

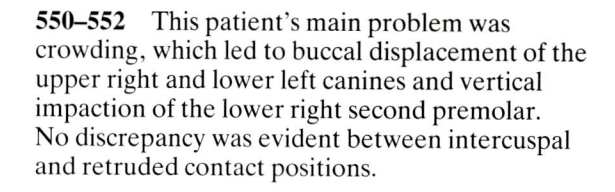

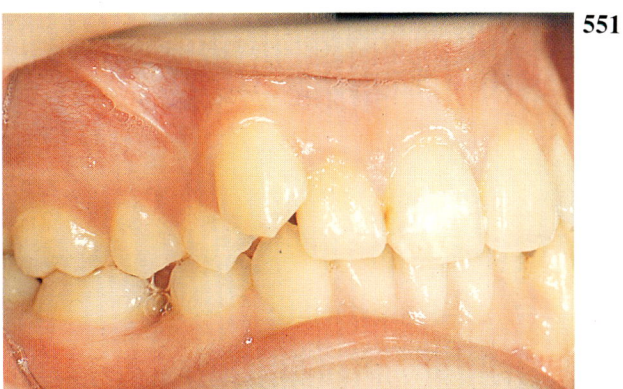

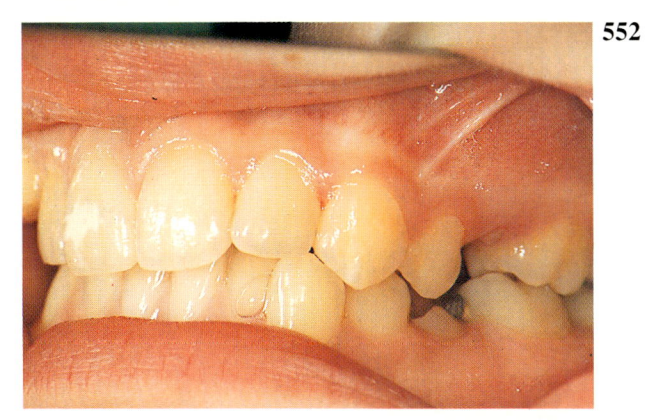

550–552 This patient's main problem was crowding, which led to buccal displacement of the upper right and lower left canines and vertical impaction of the lower right second premolar. No discrepancy was evident between intercuspal and retruded contact positions.

553–555 Extraction of all four first premolars and removable appliance therapy to align the canines to a Class 1 relationship was undertaken. This provides an example of simple orthodontic treatment carried out on a conformative basis.

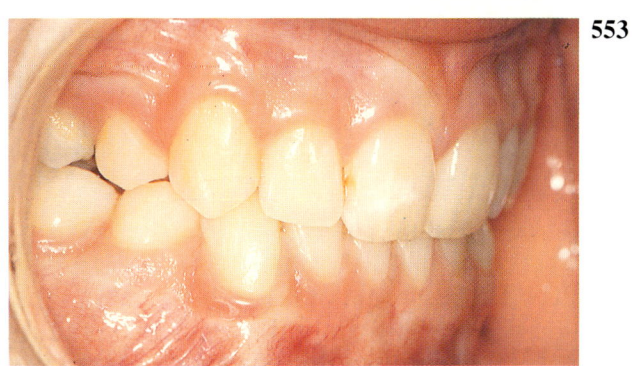

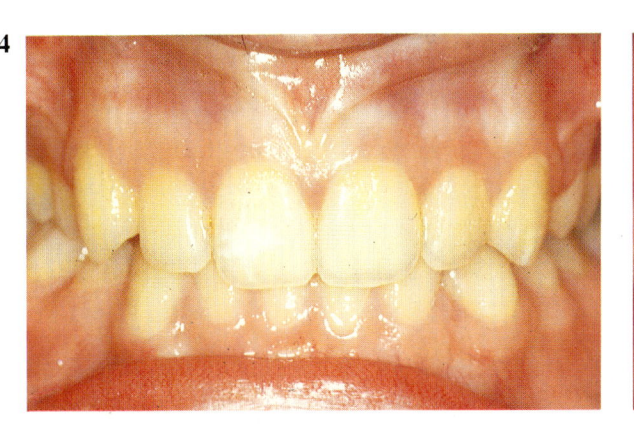

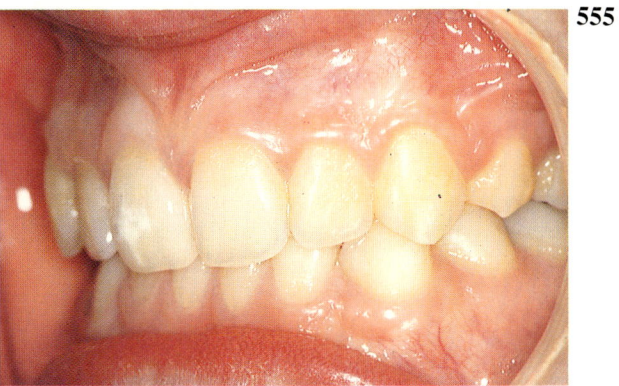

191

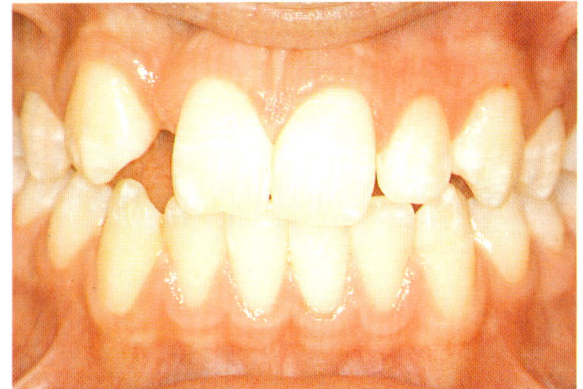

556–558 Creating a space for a replacement of a missing lateral incisor and correcting a centre line discrepancy in this patient provides another example of conformative orthodontics. The relationship between the intercuspal and retruded contact positions was unaffected by the mechanics necessary to accomplish the required result.

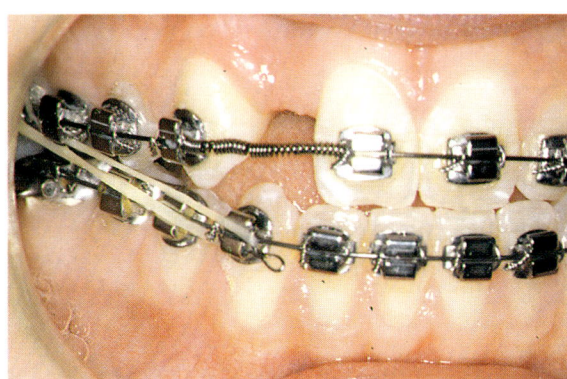

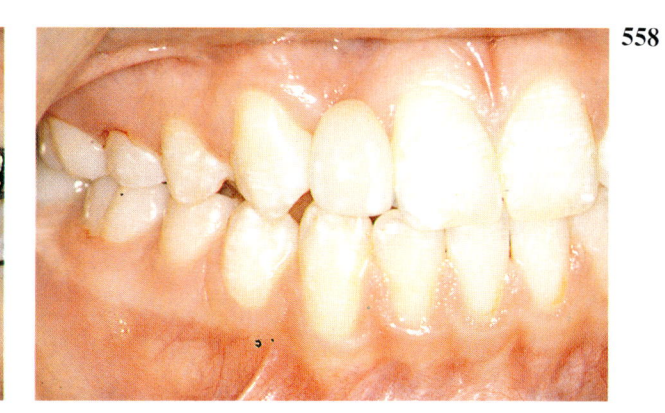

In both these patients, the posterior teeth were in a Class 1 relation pre-treatment. Orthodontics was aimed at adjusting the relationships of the teeth in the anterior segments, while maintaining the posterior relationships.

Posterior malocclusion correction

If the arrangement of the posterior teeth does not allow alignment of the canines to produce a Class 1 relationship, posterior tooth movement may be carried out while maintaining the incisal relationship.

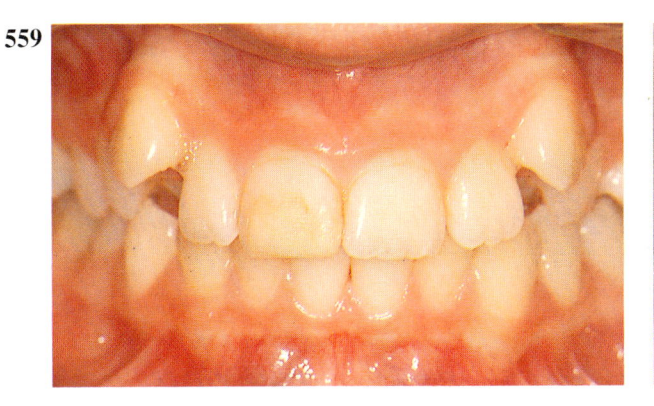

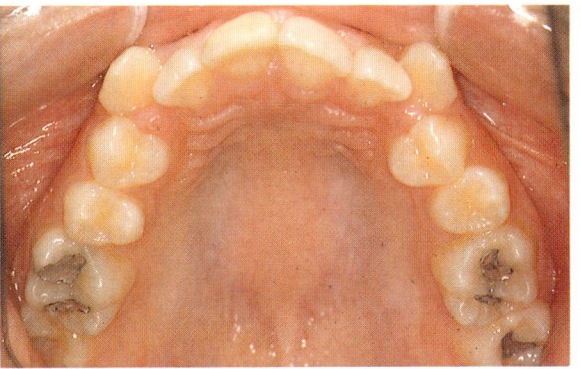

559, 560 In this patient the buccal segment relationship is half a unit Class 2. To align the upper canines, the molars and premolars need to be moved distally to a Class 1 position. This was carried out using extra-oral traction to bands fitted to the first molars.

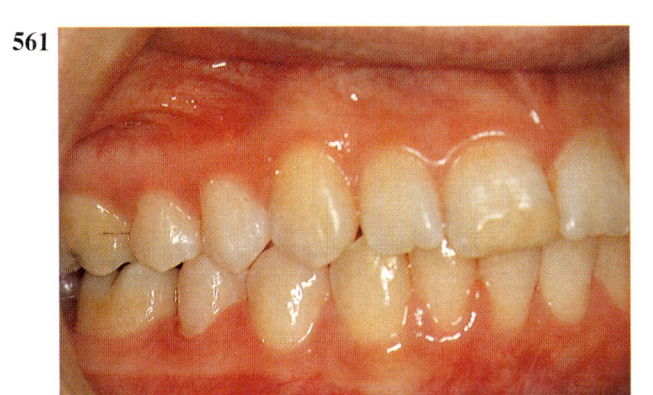

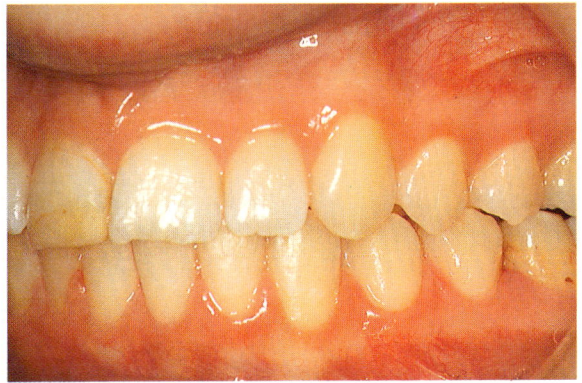

561, 562 At the conclusion of treatment the Class 1 relationship of the posterior segments is well established and has allowed the upper canines to realign. No discrepancy between RCP and ICP was evident pre- and post-treatment; no change was expected as the mechanics were conformative.

Anterior and posterior malocclusion correction

Sometimes both anterior and posterior occlusal relations require correction in patients with no RCP–ICP discrepancy. Overbite and overjet adjustments and coordinated upper and lower arch movements are undertaken. Although the entire occlusion is being changed, the operator works with reference to the existing condylar position.

Orthodontics

563

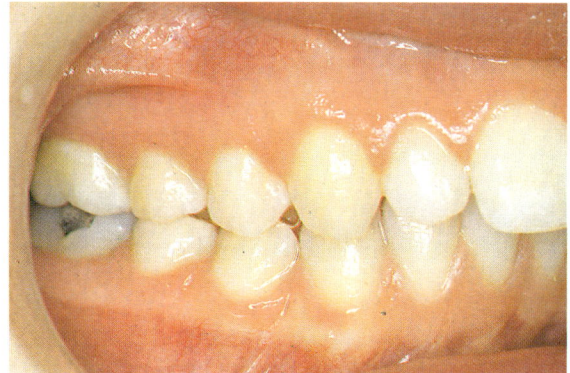

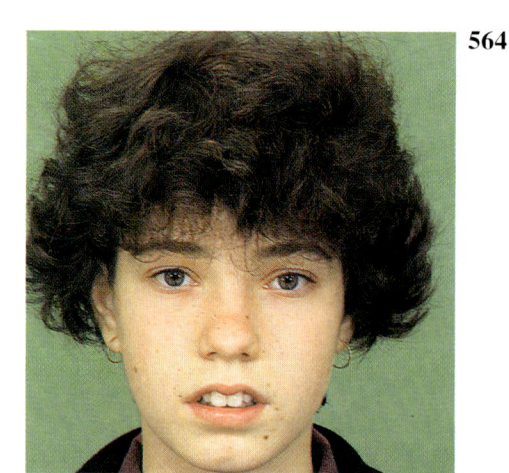

564

565

563–566 This patient required conformative management of her occlusion. No difference between the ICP and RCP of the mandible was evident pre-treatment. Orthodontic correction of the increased overjet of 10mm and the Class 2 relationship of the posterior segments required a complete change of the intercuspal position, so that this reference position was no longer available.

The four first permanent molars were extracted as these had large restorations in an otherwise caries- and restoration-free mouth. Begg multiband treatment was undertaken.

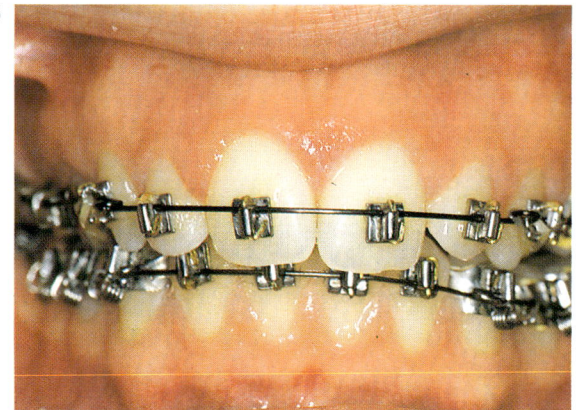

566

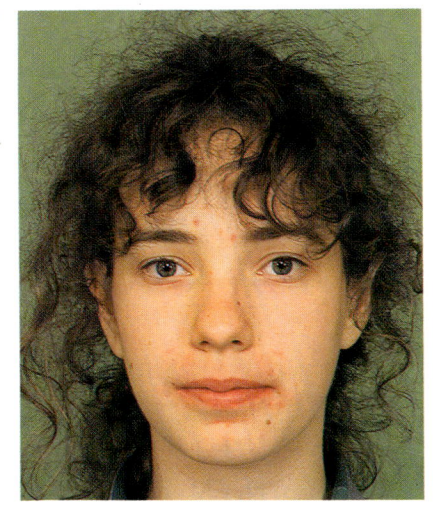

567–570 At the completion of treatment, no discrepancies were evident between the intercuspal and retruded contact position. Treatment progress was checked periodically in the retruded contact position. Particular care was taken while Class 2 elastic traction was being used between the maxillary and mandibular arches.

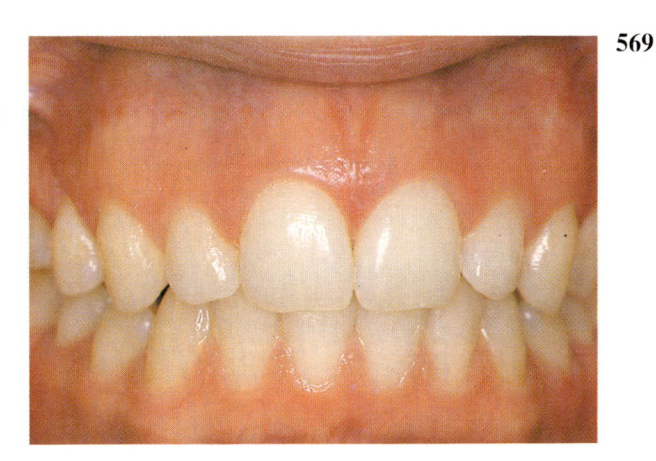

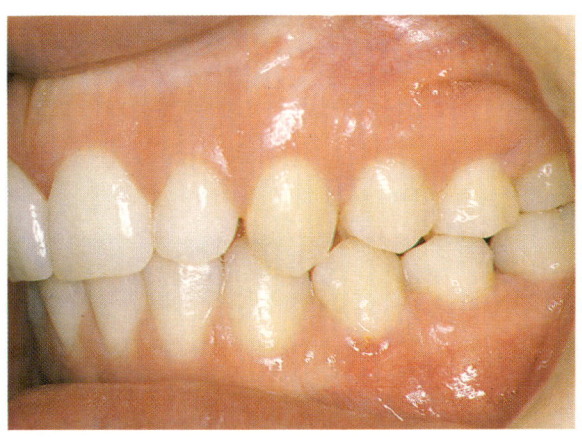

Orthodontics and orthognathic surgery

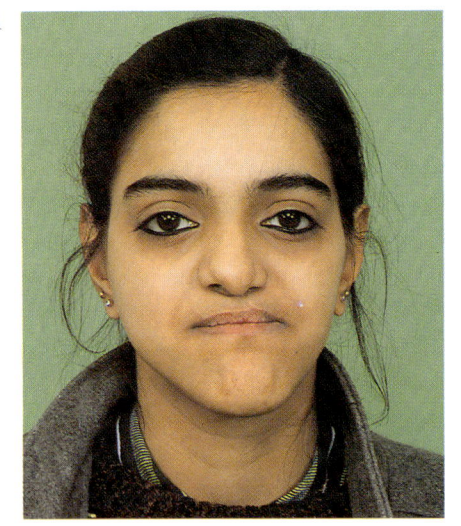

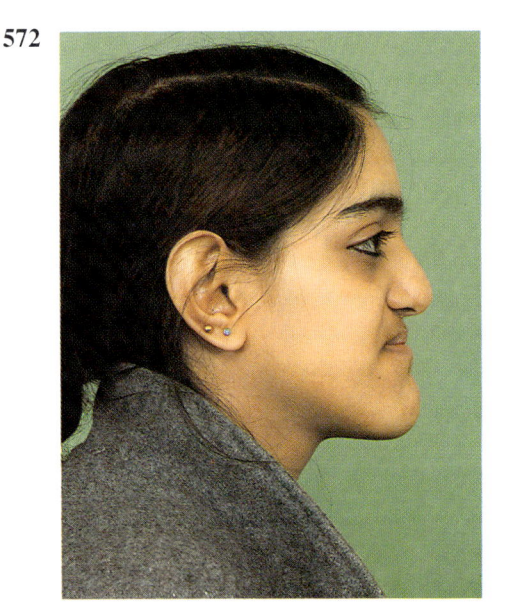

571, 572 Patients with severe mismatch of the jaws may require orthognathic surgery to correct their malocclusion and improve their facial aesthetics and function. Segmental surgery, where a lower labial segment is being moved up or down, maintains the original ICP on the posterior teeth and is similar to conformative orthodontic correction of anterior malocclusion. When full jaw surgery involving a Le Fort 1 pushback or advancement is used, in which the whole of the maxilla is moved, the original ICP is completely changed. The retruded position of the mandible is therefore used for reference. This is similar to conformative orthodontic treatment, during which anterior and posterior teeth are moved simultaneously, provided there is no pre-treatment RCP–ICP discrepancy.

Orthognathic surgery is generally undertaken in the fully grown patient so that the full severity of the malocclusion is established and the result will not be compromised by further growth. An initial period of orthodontic treatment is followed by the surgery, and finally by completion of orthodontic tooth movement.

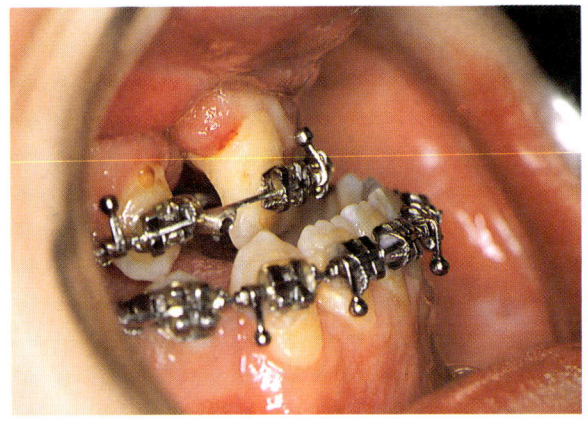

573 The initial orthodontics will result in the original intercuspal position being replaced by a new relationship of the teeth. They are placed in their ideal positions and angulations relative to the skeletal bases. This is called decompensation and it eliminates any soft tissue, tongue and lip effects on the teeth.

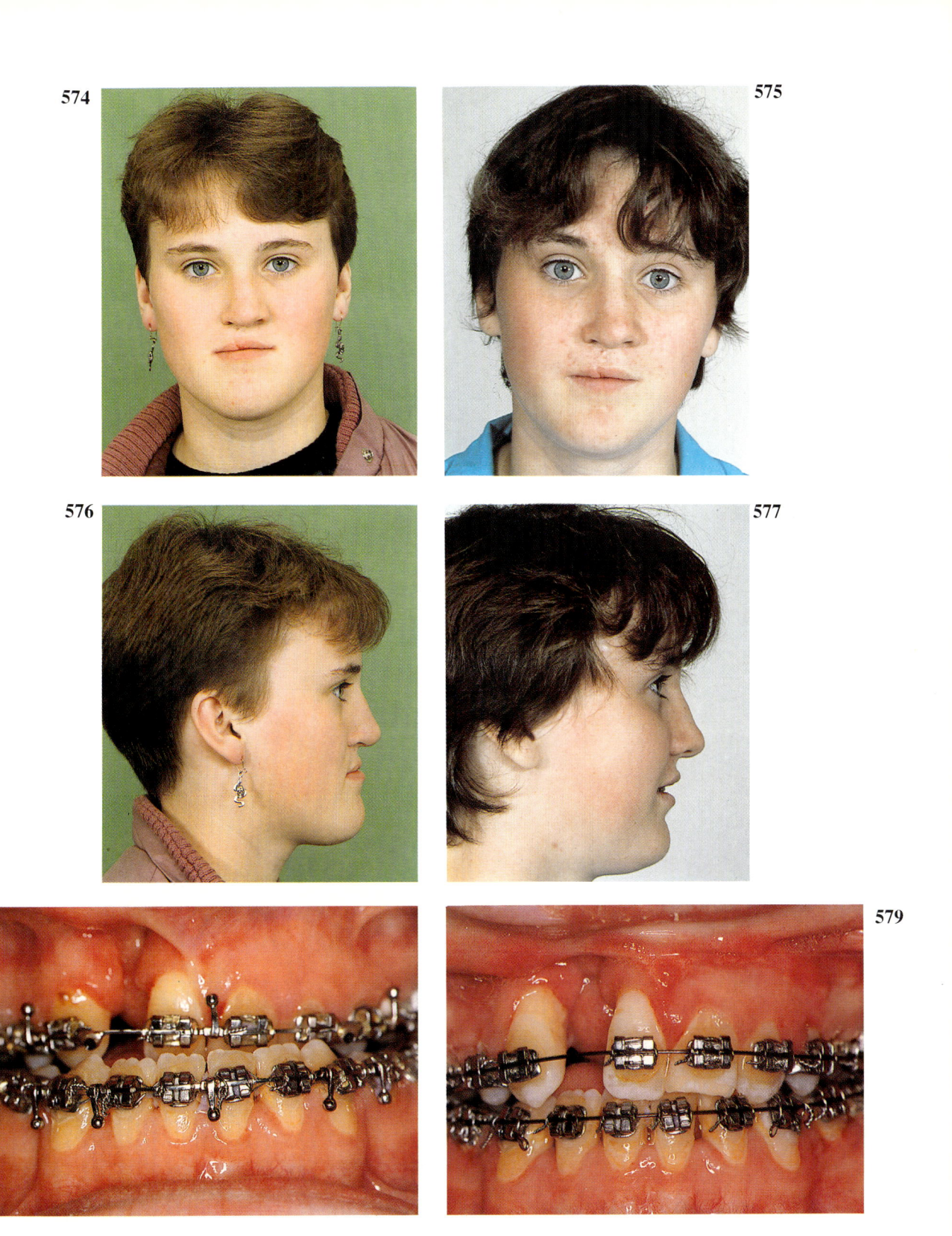

574–579 Surgery then corrects the discrepancy between the jaws in anteroposterior, vertical and lateral directions.

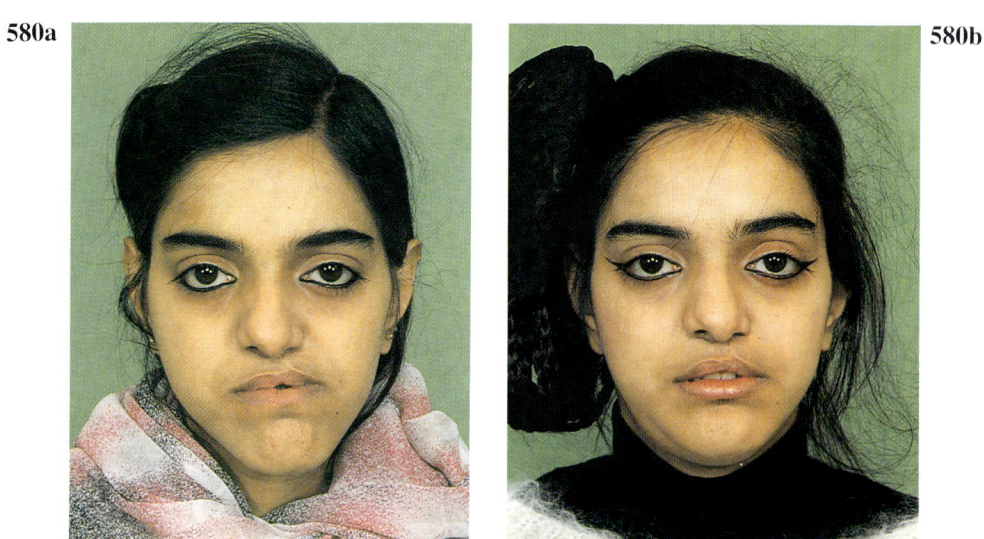

580a–580d Lateral adjustments in the mandible are usually carried out during surgery.

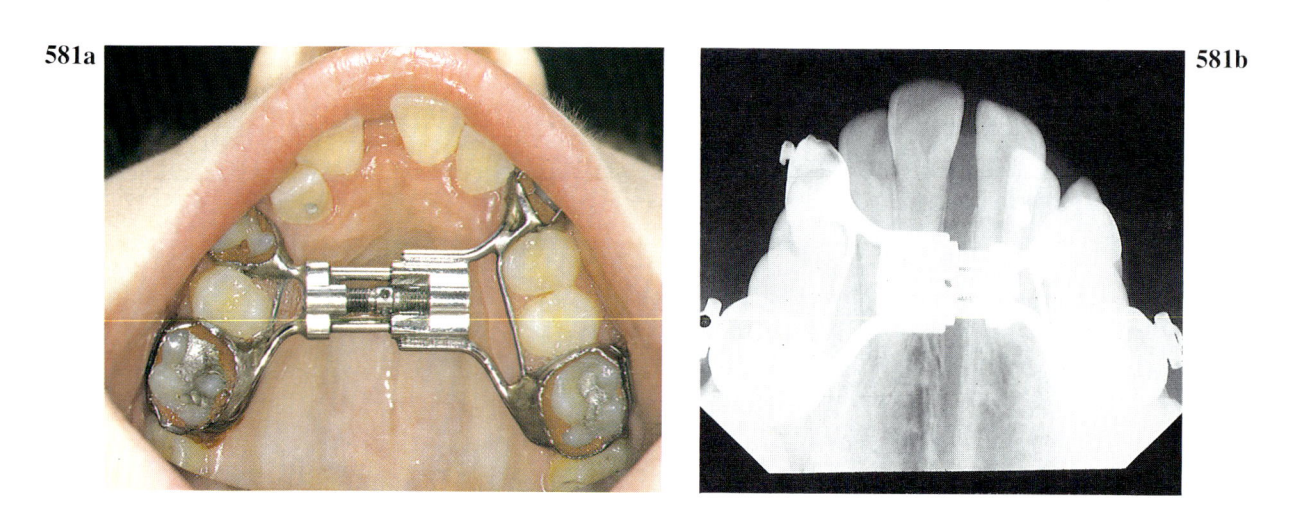

581a, 581b In the maxilla, rapid maxillary expansion using an orthopaedic appliance may be used before surgery to separate the two halves of the maxilla at the mid-palatal suture, and allow bony infilling.

582 During surgery the separated bony segments of the maxilla and/or mandible are repositioned to provide a new intercuspal position of the teeth. The bony segments containing the condyles are carefully maintained in the retruded position in the glenoid fossa. They are reattached to the other mandibular segment(s) during surgery to allow healing whilst being maintained in the retruded position. Conformative management of the occlusion therefore occurs during orthognathic surgery.

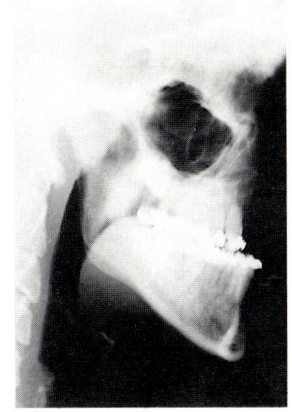

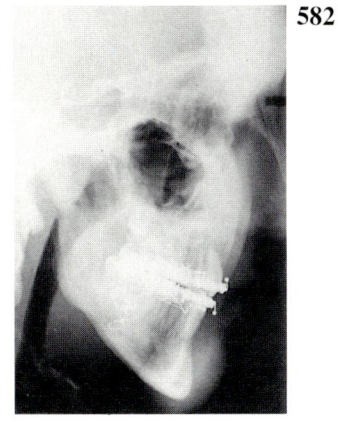

583, 584 When only mandibular surgery is required, a surgical interocclusal wafer is constructed for the post-surgical stabilization of the mandibular dentition on its freed bony segment. The mandibular dentition is held in the new intercuspal position against the maxillary dentition whilst bony healing occurs.

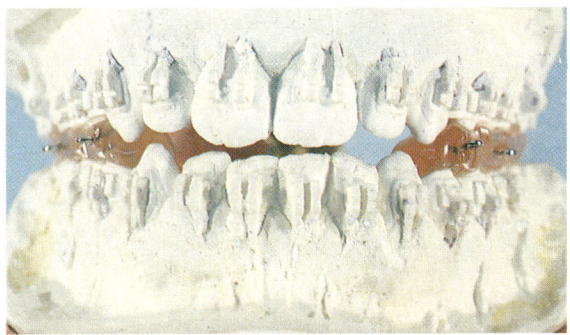

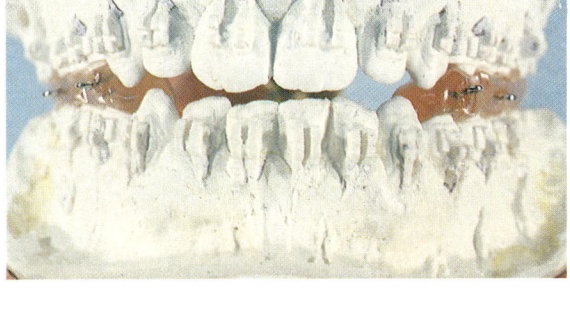

585, 586 Orthognathic surgical planning may indicate the necessity for changes in both maxilla and mandible. First, the maxilla is surgically repositioned and fixed using extra-oral support. There are various types of fixation for the maxilla; supra-orbital pins and a face frame, attached to the maxillary dentition, are illustrated here. The mandibular dentition on its separated bony segment is then positioned in the new intercuspal position, using an interocclusal wafer as before.

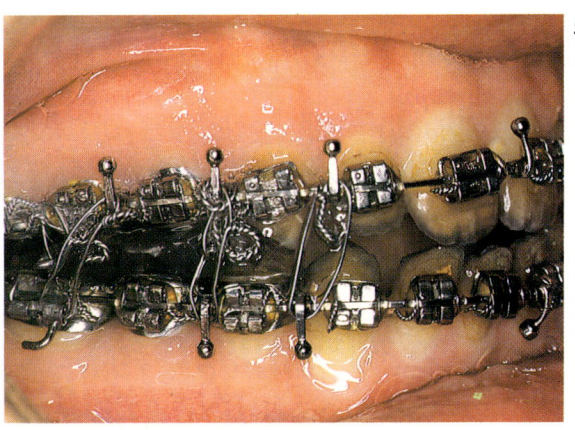

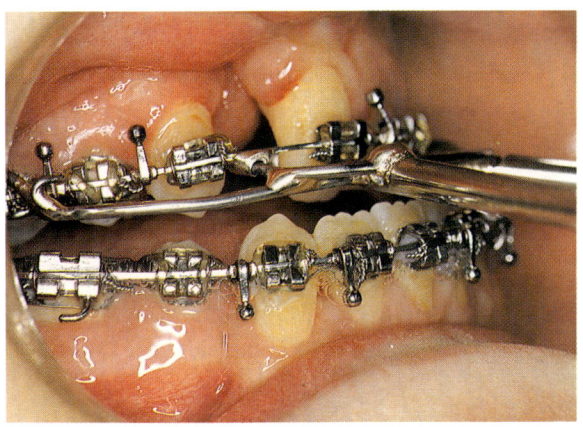

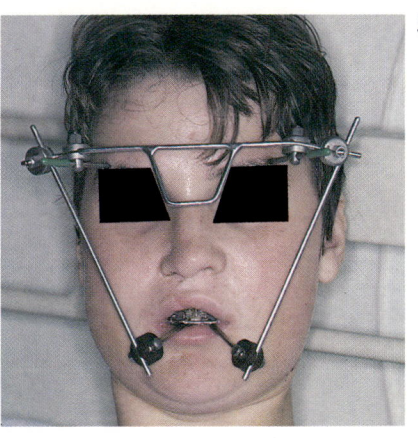

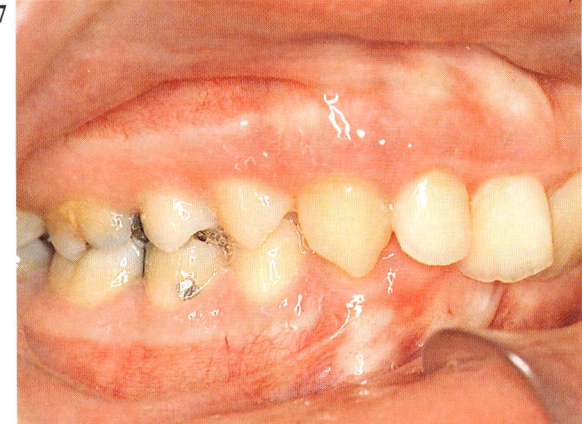

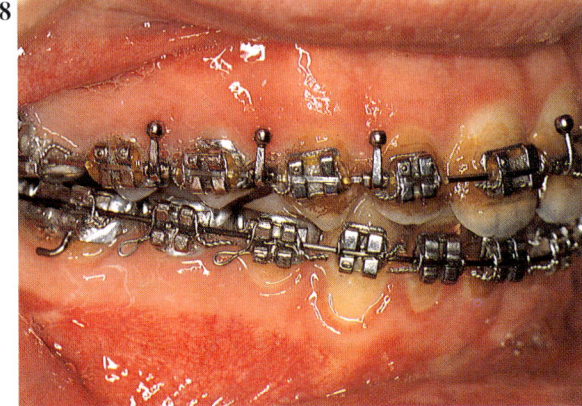

587–589 Post-surgical orthodontics usually undertakes finishing procedures only and is conformative in nature. If there has been incorrect positioning of the condyle in the glenoid fossa during the surgical phase of treatment, reorganized orthodontics may be required post-surgery. This may be needed if a discrepancy between the new intercuspal position and the retruded contact position becomes evident after fixation is removed. If the discrepancy is small and mainly vertical in direction, occlusal equilibration may be undertaken.

This patient had a Class 2, division 2 malocclusion, which required conformative pre-surgical orthodontics, conformative surgical treatment with a bilateral sagittal split and advancement of the mandible, and minimal conformative post-surgical orthodontics, as there were no pre-treatment discrepancies between RCP and ICP.

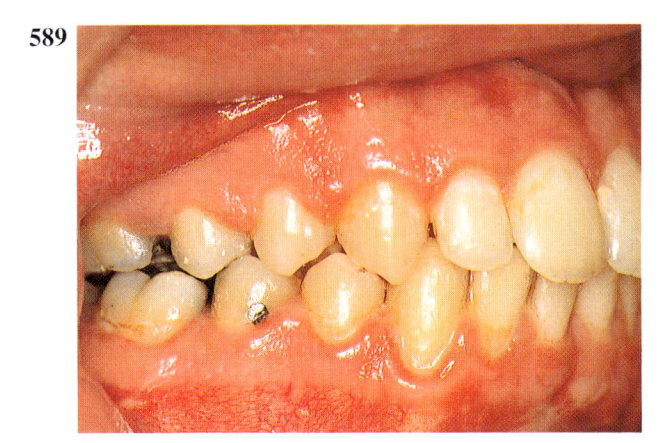

Conclusion

The principle of maintaining the same RCP–ICP relationship in conformative orthodontic treatment has been illustrated. Conformative orthodontic treatment may require the use of a high degree of orthodontic skill and knowledge. It is not synonymous with simpler treatment.

Chapter 15: Reorganized orthodontic treatment

Orthodontic treatment is reorganized when an alteration in the RCP–ICP relationship is one of the main aims of treatment. Reorganized orthodontic treatment is carried out in two main groups of patients:

- Those with a discrepancy between RCP and ICP.
- Those requiring functional appliance therapy.

Interceptive reorganized orthodontic treatment

Occlusal interferences causing discrepancies between RCP and ICP occur in all types of developing malocclusions. Correction of RCP–ICP discrepancies in the deciduous and mixed dentitions eliminates the abnormal mandibular function, may prevent further deterioration in alignment of the teeth, for example centre lines, and, most importantly, allows continued growth and development without abnormal adaptation.

In some patients, assessment may indicate a severe underlying skeletal discrepancy as the main aetiology of the malocclusion. Interceptive reorganization of the occlusion in these patients often corrects a displacement and uses orthopaedic forces to guide the growth potential of the patient, so that bony segments and soft tissues, rather than teeth alone, are moved. There is evidence that functional appliances only produce dentoalveolar changes, and that their effect is enhanced by natural growth changes; many people believe they do not induce extra growth.

The following interceptive treatments illustrate the correction of the RCP–ICP discrepancies at occlusal level. The use of some functional orthopaedic appliances for interceptive treatment is included.

Anterior displacements

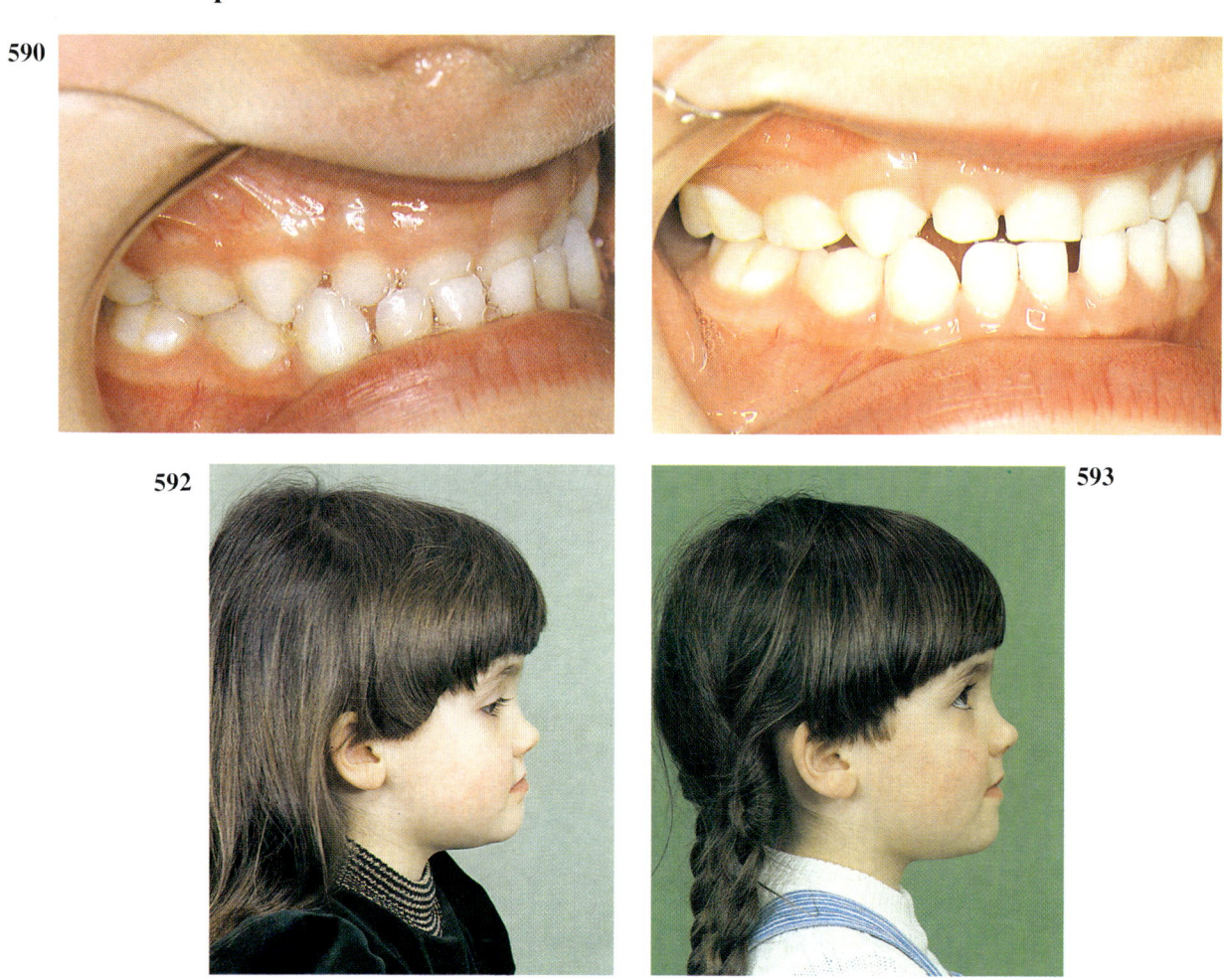

590–593 Anterior crossbites with displacement in the deciduous dentition are corrected by appropriate grinding of the occlusal interference or by upper removable appliance therapy to free the upper incisors and push them forwards.

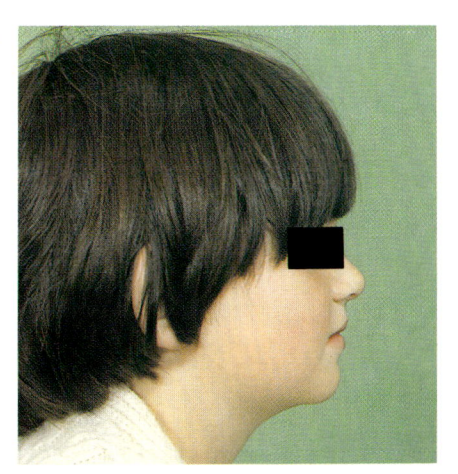

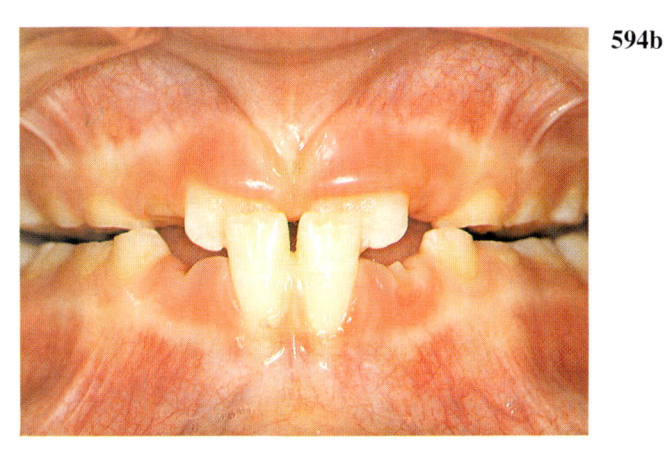

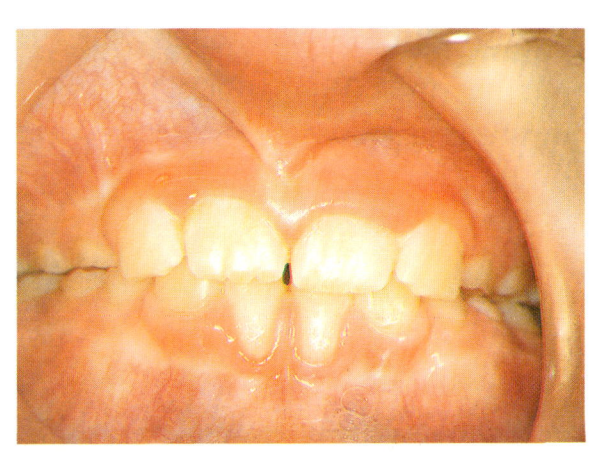

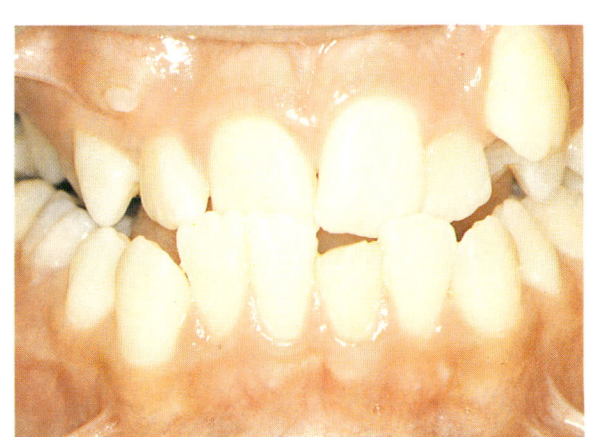

594a–596 Anterior displacements in the mixed dentition are also corrected early. Sufficient overbite to maintain the correction is necessary, as the overbite decreases as the upper incisors are proclined. Benefits are similar to those for the deciduous dentition and include restoration of normal function of the mandible, continued anteroposterior and vertical growth, which is no longer distorted by the abnormal function, and improved aesthetics.

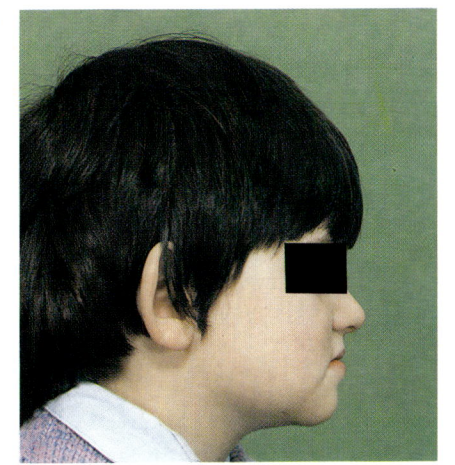

In addition, intervention can prevent further loss of gingival attachment, and the likelihood of trauma to the lower incisors is decreased from both chronic 'jiggling' and from blows or falls, which tend to result in fracture of the most occlusally prominent incisor when the patient closes suddenly into the edge-to-edge retruded contact position.

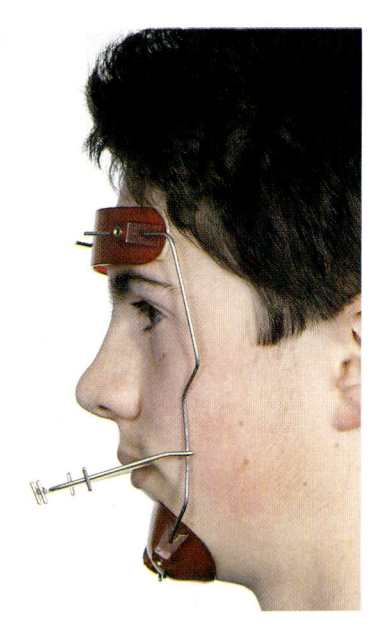

597, 598 The young patient with a large anteroposterior skeletal base discrepancy, resulting in a more severe Class 3 occlusion, with or without displacement, usually has either a retrusive maxilla, a prognathic mandible, or a combination of both. Early treatment of these cases is advocated by some orthodontists, particularly if the parents themselves have a history of a similar problem. Face masks (**597**) using orthopaedic traction to the maxilla in patients aged between five and seven, or early Frankel functional appliance therapy (**598**) are treatments advocated in the established deciduous or early mixed dentition stage. Benefits to the patient are improved anterior guidance, elimination of any abnormal rest position and improved aesthetics; in addition, in the long-term, the necessity for surgical intervention may be eliminated. However, information on the long-term success of these methods in the severe Class 3 patient is limited.

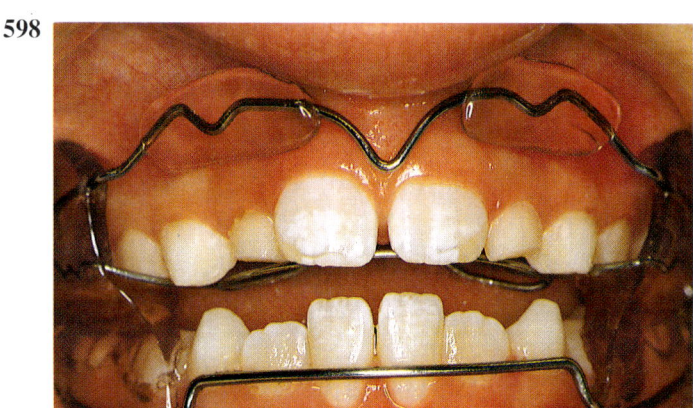

Lateral displacements

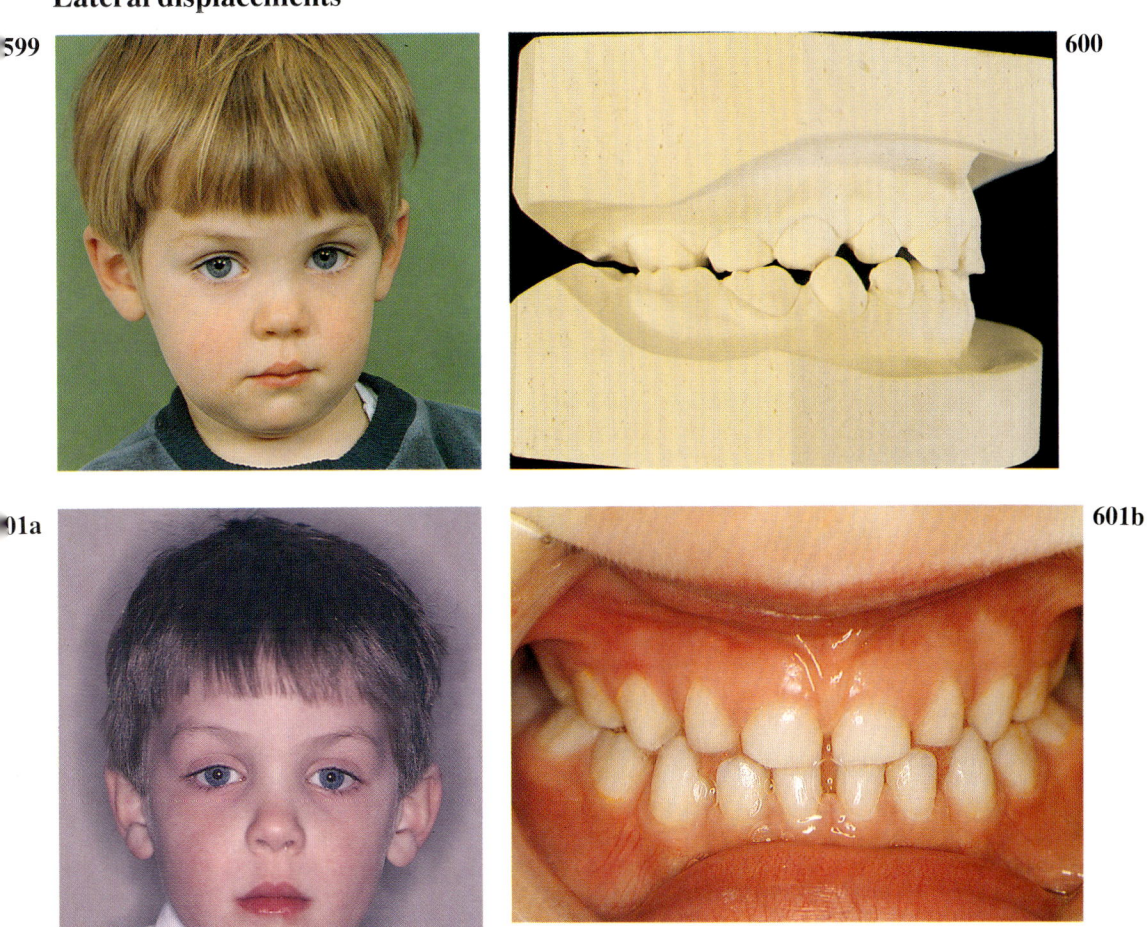

599–601b Interceptive reorganized treatment for lateral crossbites with displacements is undertaken early. Unilateral crossbite in the deciduous dentition, usually accompanied by displacement and asymmetry, is corrected early, either by occlusal adjustment, or active appliance therapy to widen the upper arch.

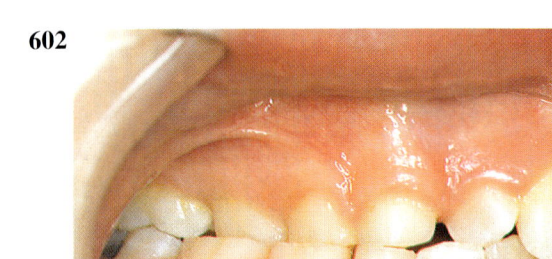

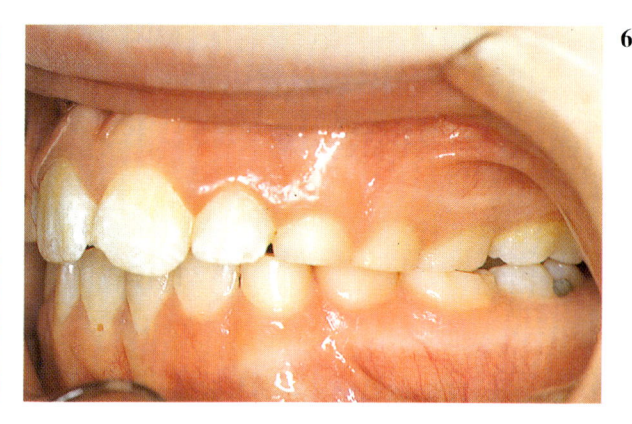

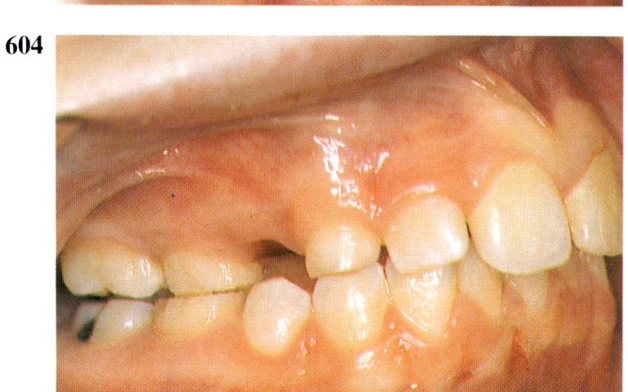

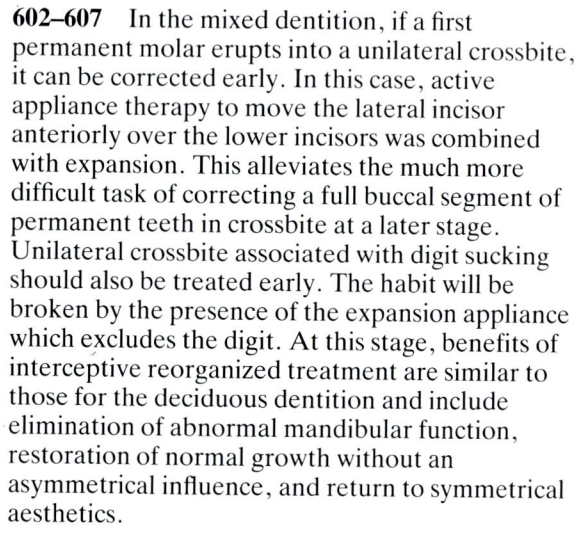

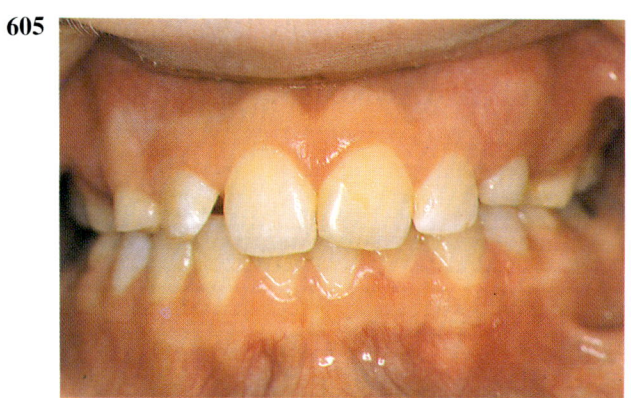

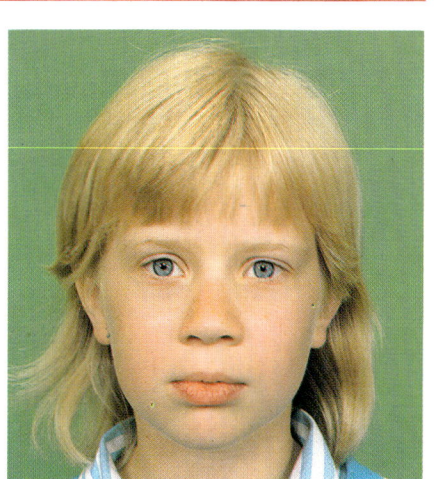

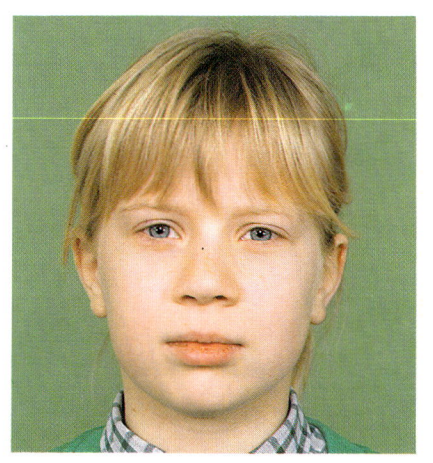

602–607 In the mixed dentition, if a first permanent molar erupts into a unilateral crossbite, it can be corrected early. In this case, active appliance therapy to move the lateral incisor anteriorly over the lower incisors was combined with expansion. This alleviates the much more difficult task of correcting a full buccal segment of permanent teeth in crossbite at a later stage. Unilateral crossbite associated with digit sucking should also be treated early. The habit will be broken by the presence of the expansion appliance which excludes the digit. At this stage, benefits of interceptive reorganized treatment are similar to those for the deciduous dentition and include elimination of abnormal mandibular function, restoration of normal growth without an asymmetrical influence, and return to symmetrical aesthetics.

608, 609 Additional benefit can occur if abnormal loss of gingival attachment is prevented or attenuated. Correction in this case shows that the gingival contour does not recover if treatment is delayed.

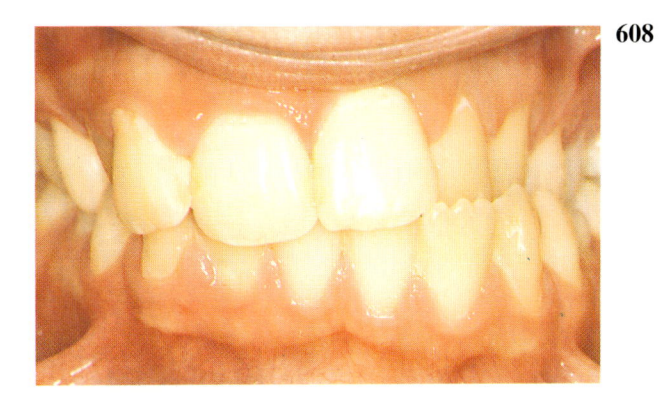

610, 611 If the unilateral crossbite is left, continued growth influenced by the abnormal function and asymmetry of the face may become well established.

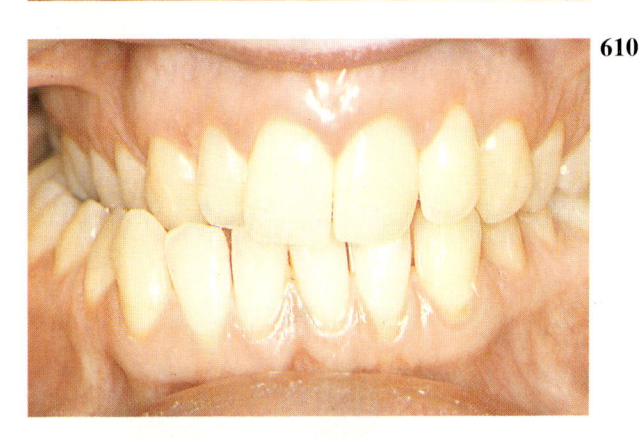

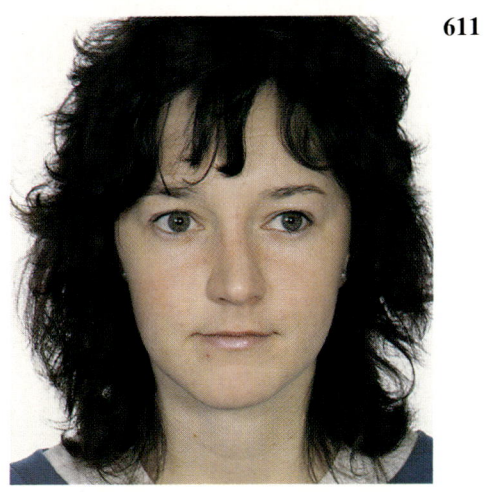

207

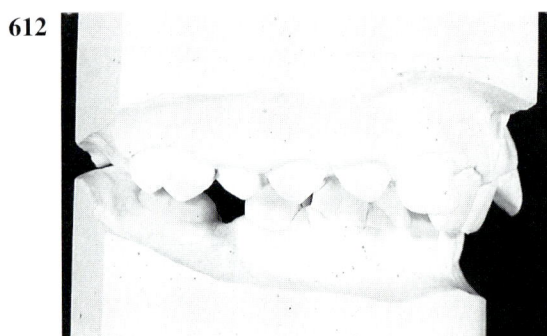

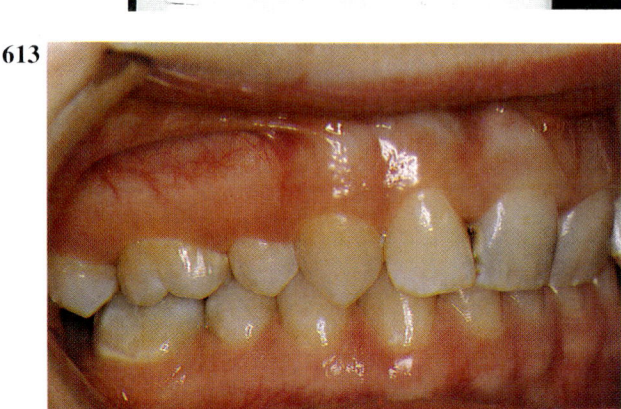

612, 613 Scissor bites of the dento-alveolar type should be treated early. Treatment usually involves narrowing the width of the upper arch combined with any necessary uprighting of the lower buccal segment teeth. Benefits of the interceptive reorganized treatment are the elimination of any mandibular displacement and a return to normal function of the mandible, with further growth occurring without distortion. If the malocclusion is due to lateral jaw discrepancy, surgery is the only option. Single teeth in buccal crossbite are either extracted early as part of relief of crowding, or aligned at a later stage after space is created, usually by distalizing the buccal segments. Any displacement from the tooth is then corrected.

Vertical displacements

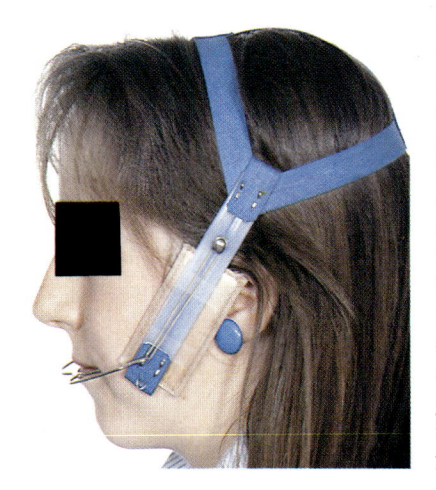

614 Vertical displacements usually require treatment of over-erupted buccal segments by intrusion. The mandible can then return to the retruded position without being deflected by a pivoting occlusal interference. Intrusive forces may be applied extra-orally using head-gear, or intra-orally using palatal arches projecting into the space occupied by the tongue, with most of the intrusive force coming from the tongue. Magnetic forces between the arches have also been used. Vertical displacement may be accompanied by an anterior open bite. Individuals are unable to incise efficiently and excursions of the mandible are guided by the posterior teeth. If treatment results in a positive overbite and overjet, aesthetics and function are both improved.

Posterior displacements

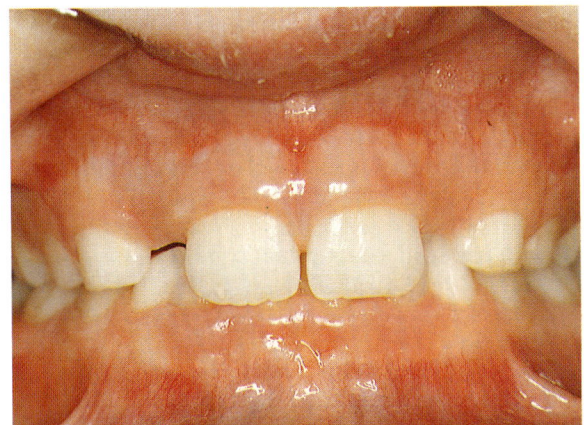

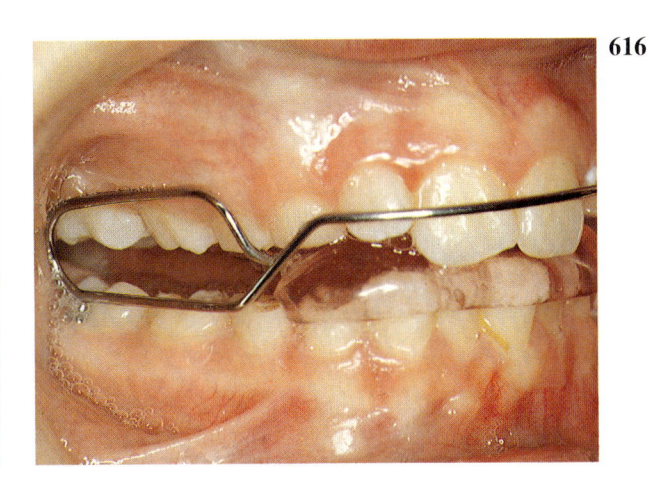

615

616

617

618

615–618 Class 2:2 cases with displacement posteriorly due to very upright or retroclined upper incisors, usually occur in patients with a deep overbite. These are best treated early in the mixed dentition stage by methods which alter the angulation of the upper incisors. This may be achieved by torquing the roots of the upper incisors or by proclining the upper incisors to the ideal angulations to the maxillary plane. This will increase the overjet, and some subsequent use of a functional appliance is necessary. After treatment the mandible is able to close freely into the intercuspal position. The deep overbite is reduced at an early stage and, with a stable inter-incisal angle, allows unimpeded anteroposterior and vertical growth. If trauma to the gingivae is present this would also be eliminated.

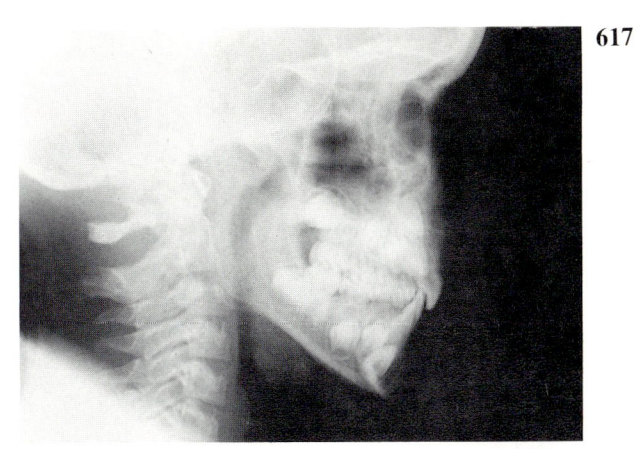

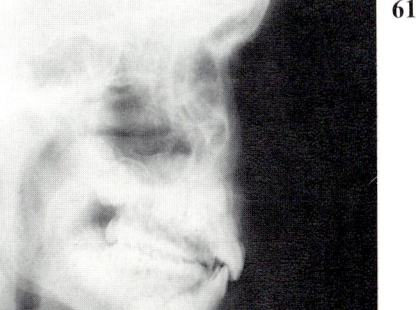

Abnormal rest position

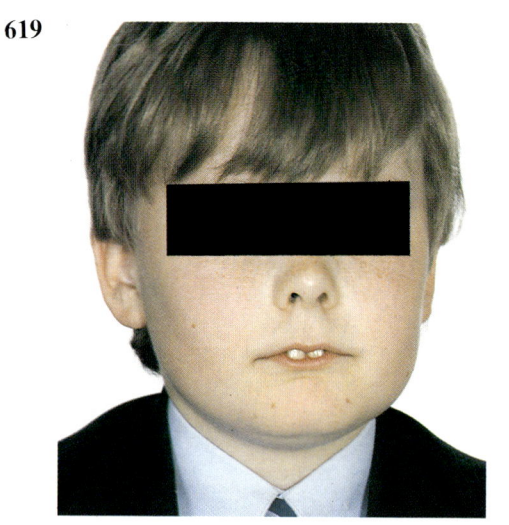

619

620

621

619–621 The Class 2:1 patient with severe arch discrepancy may have an abnormal rest position (Chapter 5). Early treatment of the underlying cause of the habitual rest position is required. Treatment that maximizes the growth potential of the mandible with a functional appliance is often appropriate. The benefits of intervention can include continued vertical and anteroposterior growth, restoration of normal condylar function in the rest position, increased ability to obtain an anterior oral seal by the lips, without deviation of the mandible at rest, and prevention of trauma to the upper incisors. If intervention results in tooth to tooth contact between the incisors in ICP, potential trauma to palatal gingivae will also be eliminated.

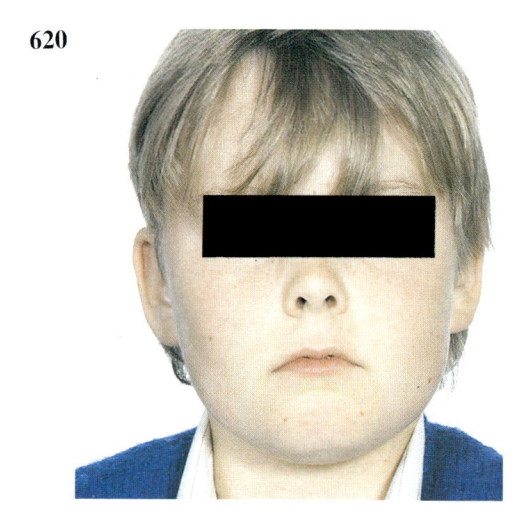

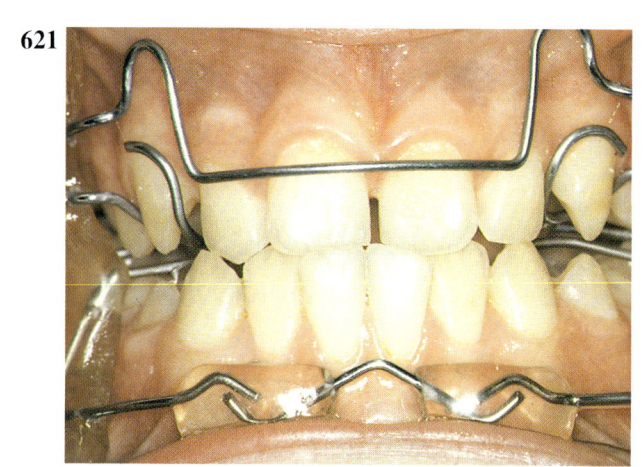

Definitive reorganized orthodontic management

RCP and ICP discrepancies

622, 623 Some orthodontic patients present with a discrepancy between RCP and ICP, which has not been corrected interceptively soon after its development. One aim of the definitive treatment is to establish a new ICP as close to RCP as possible, thus eliminating this discrepancy. In this patient, occlusal interference from the lateral incisor has resulted in palatal positioning of the incisor and anterior displacement of the mandible. The condyle is distracted downwards from its retruded contact position. Reorganization of the occlusion using orthodontic treatment is necessary for these patients, unless the occlusal interference can be eliminated by conservative occlusal equilibration.

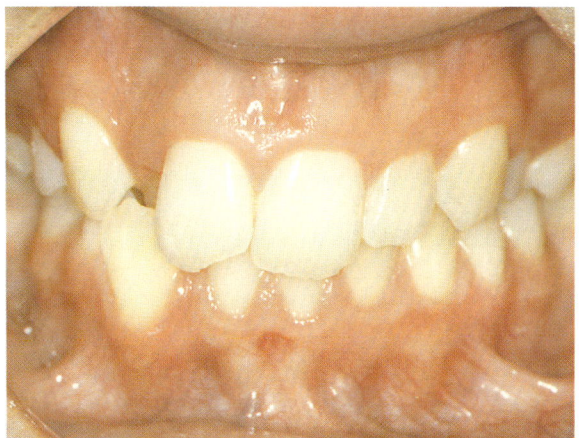

624, 625 In most cases, the deflective contact combined with the malocclusion of the teeth does not permit this simpler treatment option. This patient has an initial contact on the incisors on closing. This has produced an intercuspal position where the mandible is postured forwards, the condyle being displaced in an anterior and downwards direction.

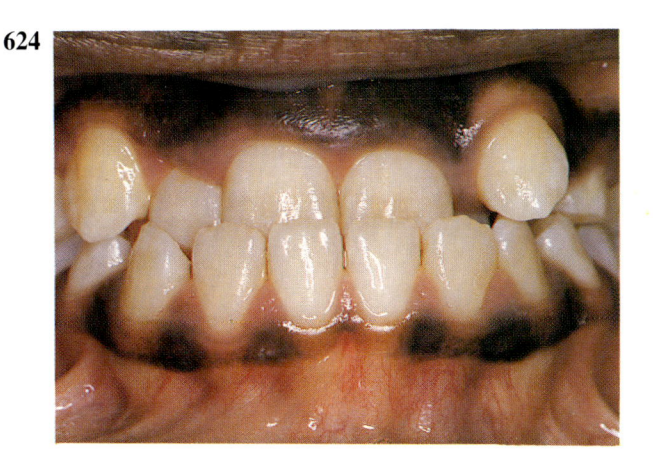

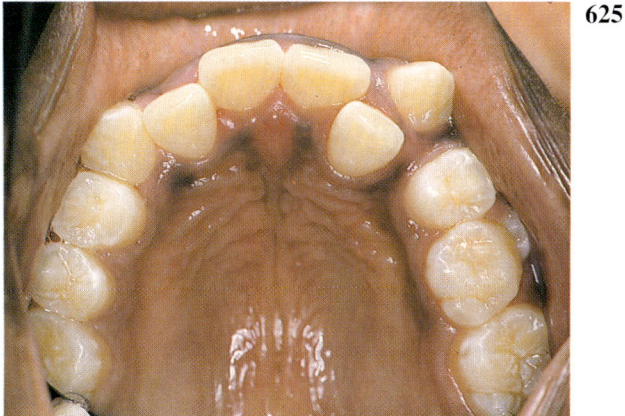

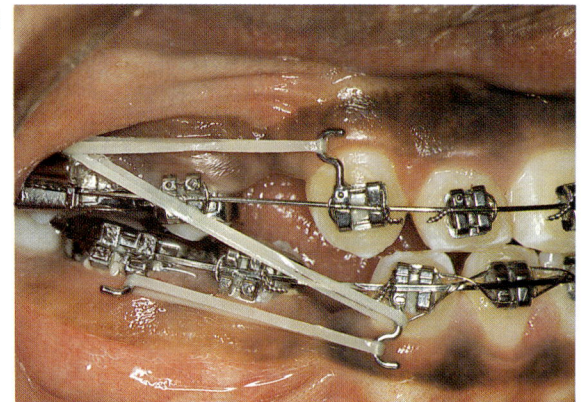

626–628 Multiband straight-wire appliances were used to correct the occlusion after extraction of four first premolars. Class 3 elastic traction was used throughout. At the end of treatment the new intercuspal position was close to the retruded contact position.

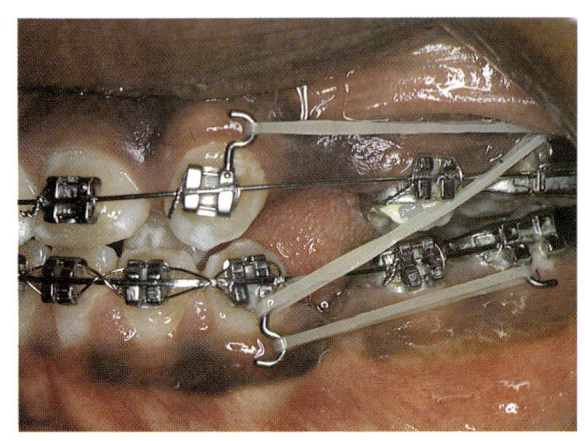

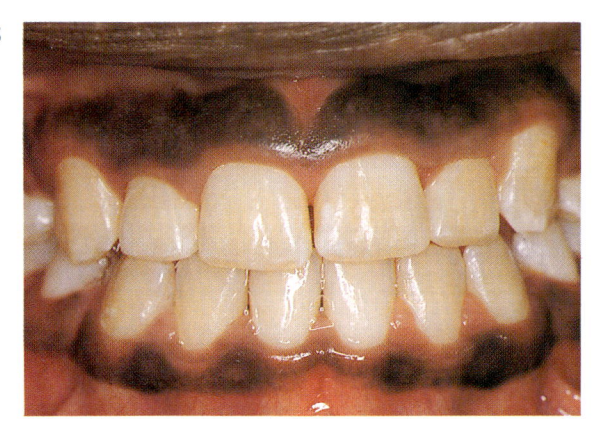

Functional appliance therapy

629–631 The majority of patients treated with functional appliances have a normal sized maxilla and a retrusive mandible. The functional appliance is constructed to a protrusive interocclusal record and mobilizes the forces from the oro-facial muscles. The condyle is pulled downwards and forwards by the appliance, which is only used in a growing individual.

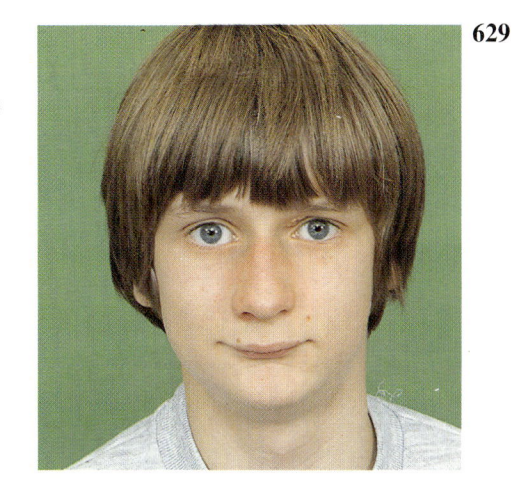

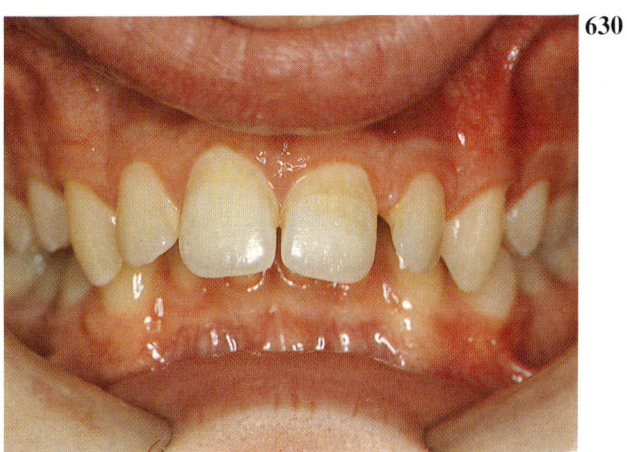

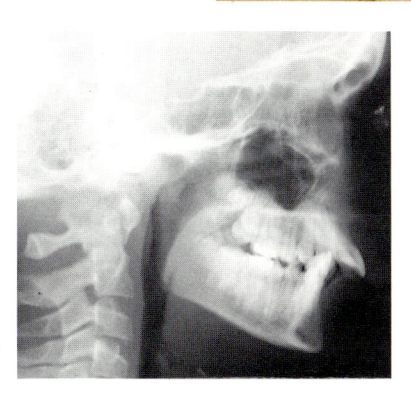

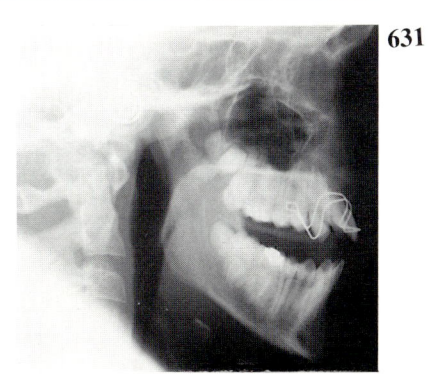

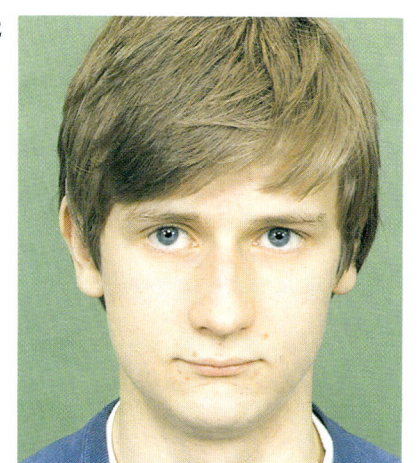

632–634 At the end of the functional treatment phase, eruption of the teeth in an anteroposterior and vertical direction produces a new intercuspal position which, when combined with the growth changes in the glenoid fossa and condyle, results in new and still coincident intercuspal and retruded contact positions. Although anatomical changes have occurred in the joint structures, the relationship of the condyle in its fossa to the other components of the joint is the same in the retruded contact position pre- and post-treatment. This type of reorganized orthodontic treatment aims to produce a new RCP and ICP, taking advantage of growth changes.

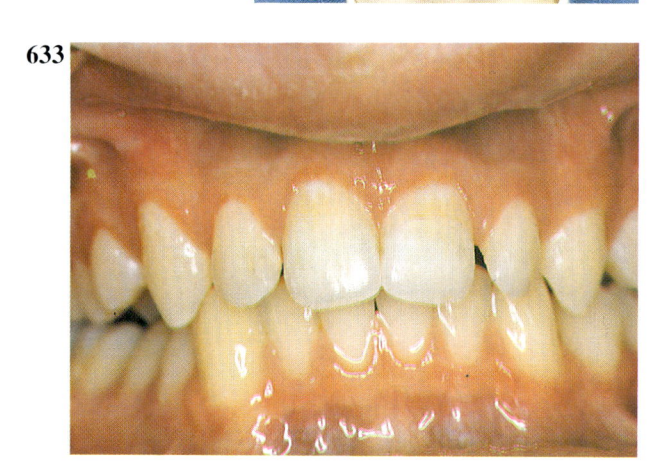

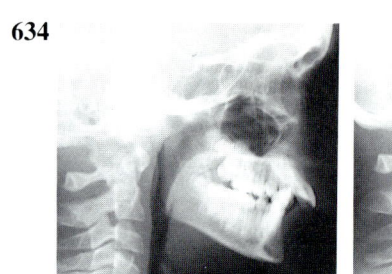

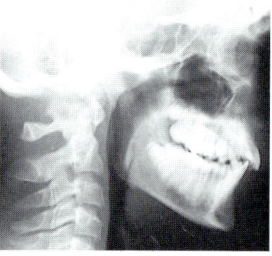

635–637 Further treatment using orthodontic forces only may move individual teeth, as in conformative treatment, by aligning the teeth through closing spaces, derotating and adjusting tooth angulations while the new and coincident intercuspal and retruded jaw positions are maintained.

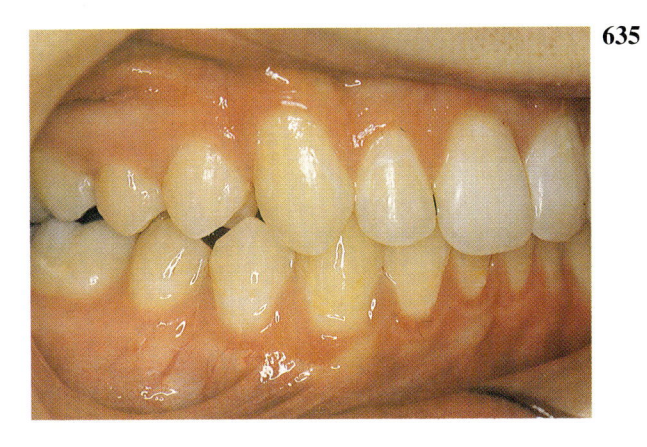

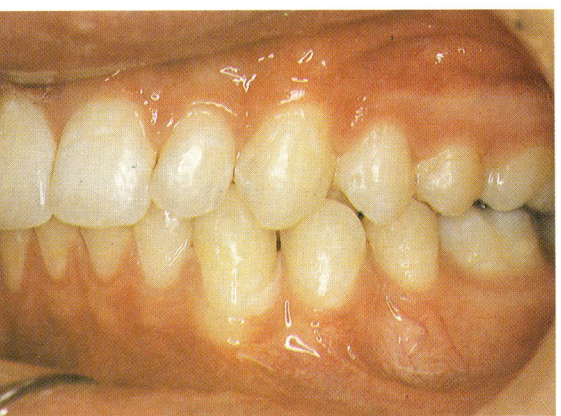

635

636

637a

637b

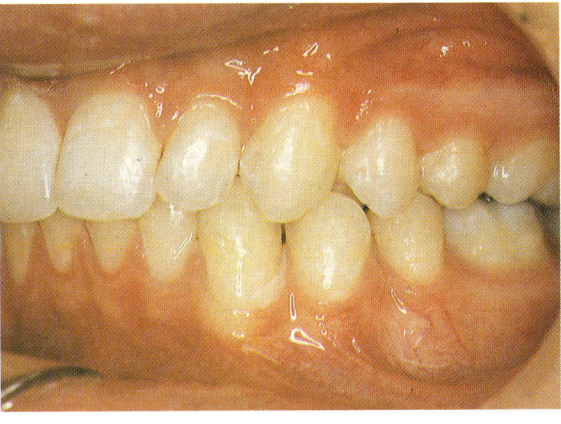

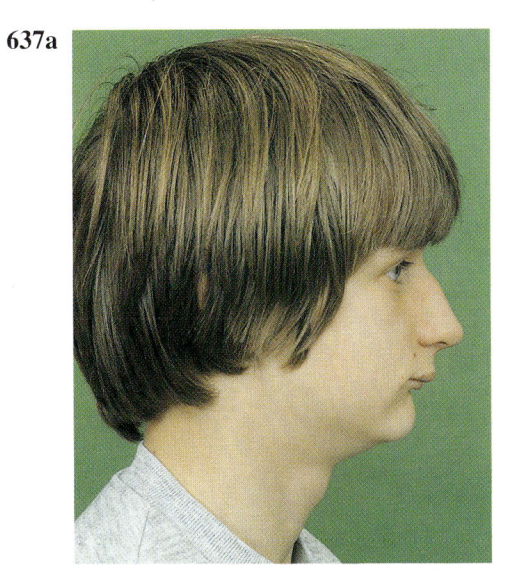

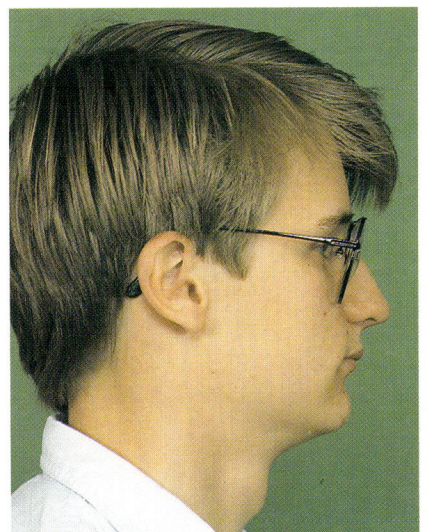

Occlusal assessment at the end of active orthodontic treatment and before removal of appliances is important. It establishes that the RCP–ICP discrepancy initially present has been eliminated or that no new occlusal interferences have been introduced. Following the retention period, during which the new ICP is held with simple fixed or removable passive appliances, an occlusal assessment is also carried out.

Occlusal adjustment using the equilibration techniques described in Chapter 9 may be appropriate if late changes in the occlusion occur, leading to new occlusal interferences after the removal of all appliances. The later developing interferences may be due to:

- Further development of the permanent dentition, for example third molars.
- 'Settling in' of the occlusion.
- Continued vertical alveolar growth.
- Restorative care.

Later developing occlusal interferences not evident at the end of orthodontic treatment may lead to RCP–ICP discrepancies and non-working side contacts during mandibular movements. Although these changes may result in an ideal functional completion becoming less than ideal, the effect of occlusal interferences on the stability of the anatomical occlusion achieved by orthodontic treatment is unknown.

Conclusion

Reorganizing a patient's occlusion to create a new and stable ICP does not require greater skill or more complicated techniques than conformative orthodontic treatment. However, greater skill is required by the clinician in diagnosing a need to alter an RCP–ICP relationship and in monitoring successful achievement of this.

Chapter 16: Complete denture occlusion

The purpose of this chapter is to review the principles in complete denture occlusion. Dental literature describes many different concepts for complete denture occlusion, advocating widely ranging theories of occlusion involving differing posterior tooth forms and a variety of restorative materials. None of the available research supports any one treatment philosophy, and choice of occlusal scheme is based more on experience than scientific evidence. Guides to selection are based on the assessment of the patient and the expertise of clinician and technician.

Certain fundamental principles are, however, generally agreed. These include:

- Even, intercuspal contact of posterior artificial teeth in the retruded position at the established vertical dimension of occlusion.
- Placement of the artificial teeth in a sufficiently close position to the natural teeth to restore appearance and function without compromising the demands of different supporting tissues.
- The arrangement and form of the teeth allows for freedom of movement in eccentric jaw movements.
- Verification and maintenance of occlusal contact at denture delivery and subsequent recall visits.

Consideration is also given to the single complete denture and the hemimandibulectomy patient, because of the particular problems posed by these patients.

Intercuspal position coincident with the retruded position at the established vertical dimension of occlusion

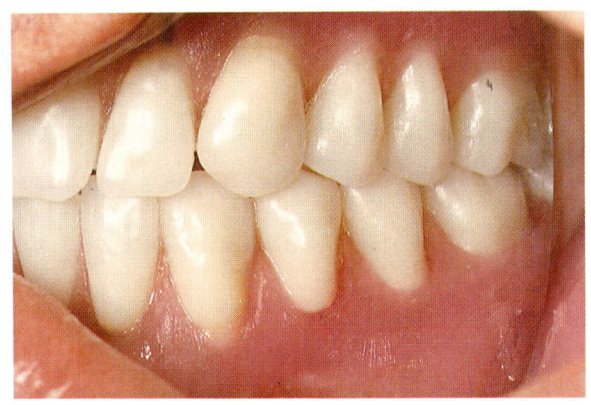

638 One of the most important factors in the stability and comfort of complete dentures is that the opposing teeth should close evenly on both sides of the dental arch, in the retruded position at the established vertical dimension of occlusion.

217

The jaw relationship has two essential components. Firstly, there is the vertical relation, which is considered to be an acceptable height when there is sufficient interocclusal distance between the vertical dimension of rest (VDR) and the vertical dimension of occlusion (VDO). Secondly, there is the horizontal relation, which is the mandible in its most retruded relation to the maxilla. With the loss of periodontal proprioceptors, the retruded position is used as the starting point for establishing intercuspal contact, because it is the only reproducible relation of mandible to maxilla recordable in the edentulous patient.

Clinically, the jaw relations are recorded by the following means:

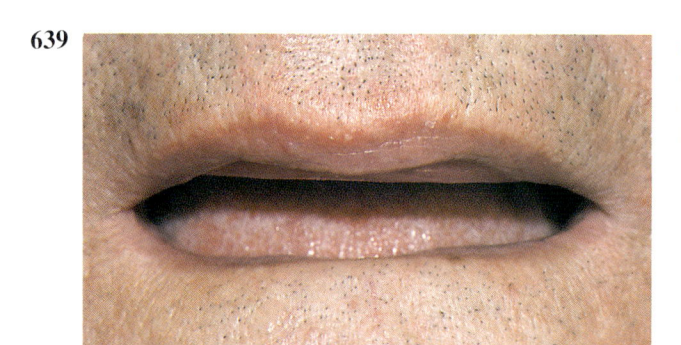

639 Contouring the maxillary rim intra-orally to establish a tentative level of occlusal plane and an arch form which is related to lips, cheeks and tongue.

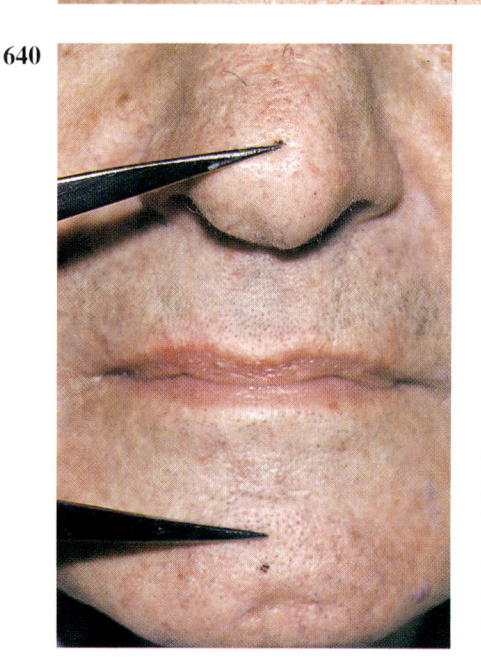

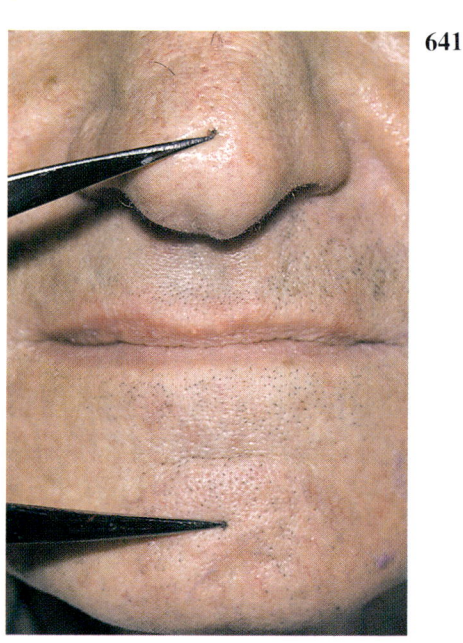

640, 641 Establishing the interocclusal distance by comparing measurements of VDR and VDO. Measurements are made between arbitrary points above and below the lips with dividers, a ruler or a Willis gauge. The patient must be seated in a relaxed but upright position, without head support. The maxillary rim or denture remains in place for the measurement of VDR, which is not accepted until the reading is consistent. The mandibular occlusion rim is then trimmed to provide a measurement for VDO, which should be 2–4mm smaller than VDR.

642 Insufficient interocclusal distance may cause generalized soreness of the tissues beneath the dentures, clicking teeth, and unclear speech. Sibilant speech sounds provide a guide to establishing the correct vertical relation. A space between the premolars of about 1 mm should be present when pronouncing sounds such as 'S', 'SH' and 'Z'. The comment that patients often make when there is a lack of interocclusal distance is that they have 'too many teeth'. Excessive interocclusal distance creates a poor facial profile, the teeth appear to be absent, and patients complain that they are unable to chew effectively.

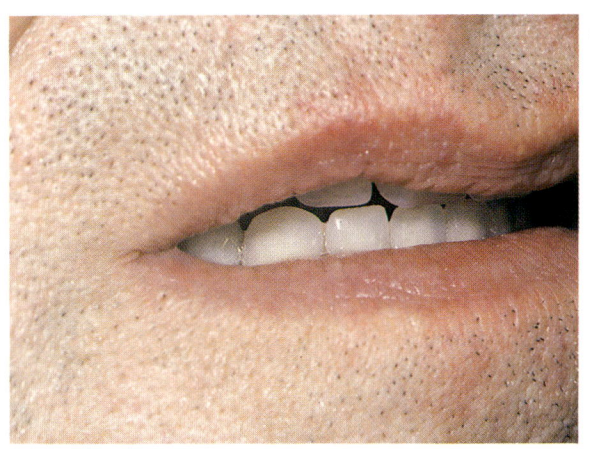

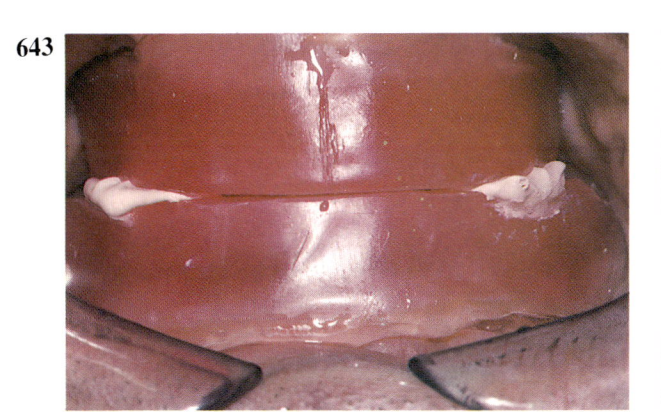

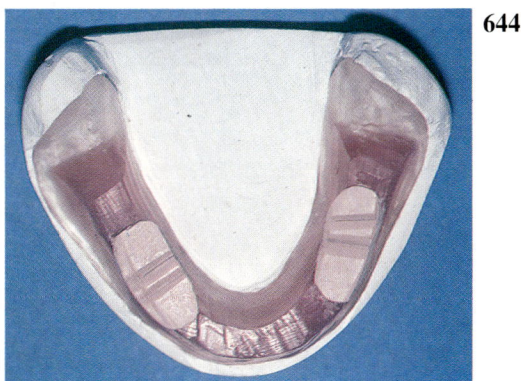

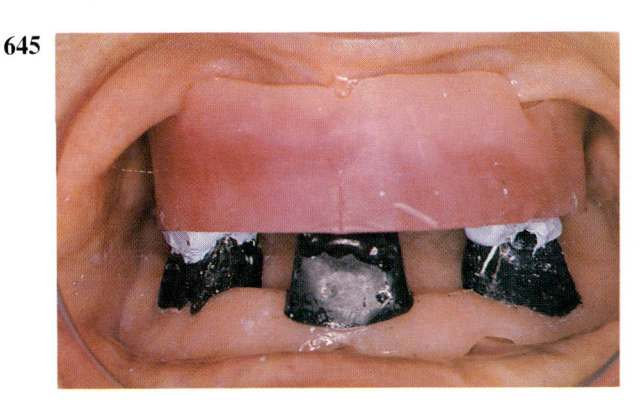

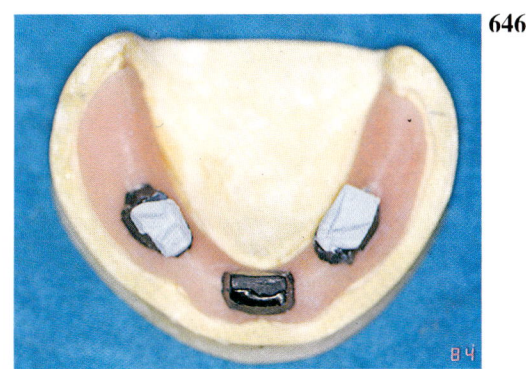

643–646 Making a record of the retruded position at the established vertical dimension of occlusion.

There are a number of methods to record the horizontal relation, the most popular of which are the interocclusal records. The most important feature of the record is that there is repeatable, uniform contact of the recording medium on the occlusion rims, made under minimal closing pressure. It is essential that the occlusion rims remain stable and correctly seated during record making.

The ideal recording medium is one which is soft during record making, but rigid once set. Quick-setting plaster and zinc oxide-eugenol are the materials of choice, but wax, if handled correctly, may be used successfully. Whichever material is used, the record should be checked before it is considered acceptable. **643 & 644**: An interocclusal record made in quick-setting plaster; **645 & 646**: an interocclusal record made in zinc oxide/Eugenol paste.

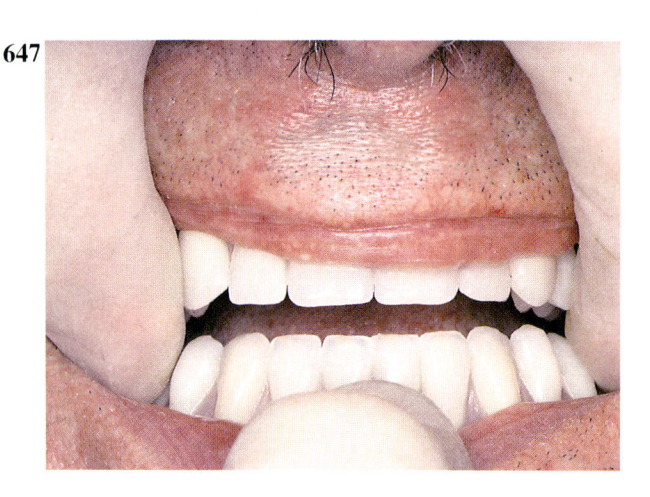

647, 648 One technique is to place the thumb and index finger of one hand (the left hand of the right-handed clinician) on the buccal surface of the maxillary and mandibular occlusion rims, while the thumbnail of the other hand, lightly touching the mandibular teeth, feels for movement of the base during closure into the recording medium.

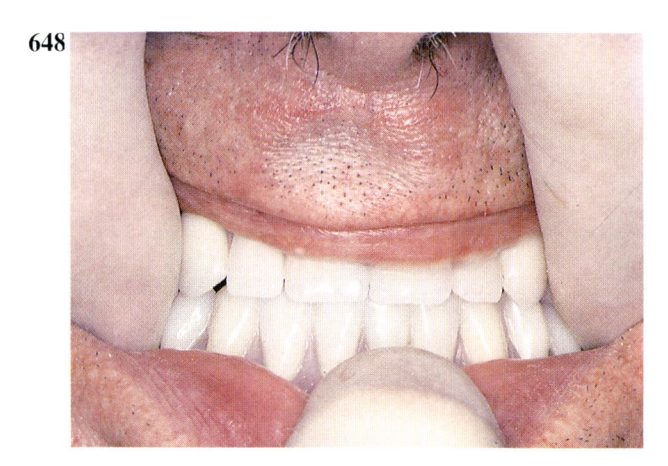

649 The maxillary cast is mounted in a semi-adjustable articulator with facebow transfer, using average retruded axis location. The mandibular cast is then related to the maxillary cast with the interocclusal record. The facebow transfer orientates the casts in the articulator so that they adopt the same relationship as that of the jaws to the retruded axis. If non-anatomic teeth are set up in monoplane occlusion with records made exactly at the vertical dimension of occlusion, the facebow is not essential. Its importance in limiting occlusal errors only becomes significant when interocclusal records are made with the teeth out of contact, or if a balanced, anatomical occlusal scheme is used.

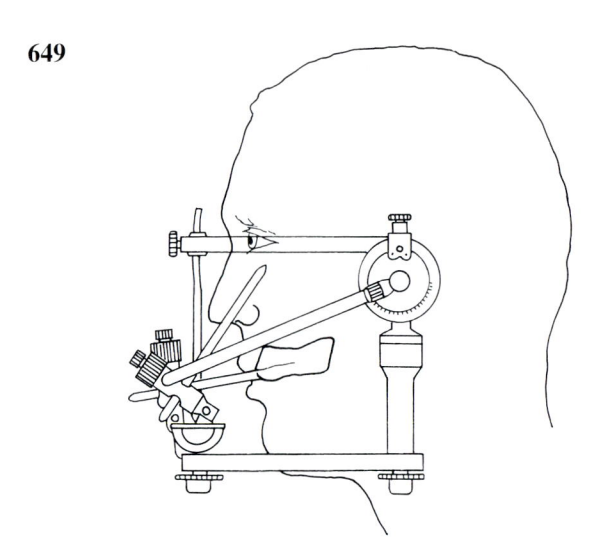

Reproduced with permission, McGraw-Hill, Inc. ©. Adapted from *Complete Denture Prosthodontics*, J.J. Sharry, 1974.

Arrangement of artificial teeth

The aim in setting artificial teeth is to place the teeth in as close a position to the natural teeth as possible. Not only are correctly positioned teeth attractive to look at, but the patient invariably experiences fewer difficulties with speech, chewing and post-insertion discomfort. The rationale for setting teeth over the residual ridge is that occlusal forces are then directly over the remaining bone support. However, no consideration is made for the significant influence that the oral musculature plays in denture stability.

Arrangement of artificial teeth may be considered under the following headings:

- Tooth position
- Tooth form
- Occlusal scheme
- Material selection.

Tooth position

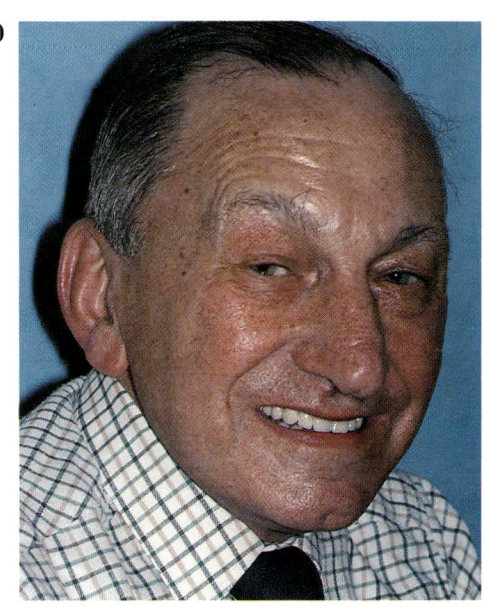

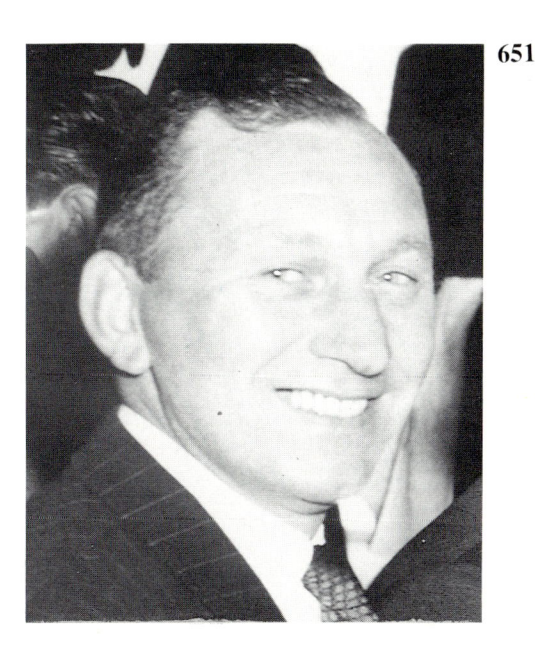

650, 651 In the absence of pre-extraction information, anatomical and phonetic guides have been suggested to help position the artificial teeth. Selected anterior teeth are arranged to satisfy the patient's demands for appearance. In function, there should be clear speech, no anterior tooth contact in the retruded position and large vertical overlap is compensated for with sufficient horizontal overlap. Old photographs (**651**) may be helpful in anterior tooth positioning.

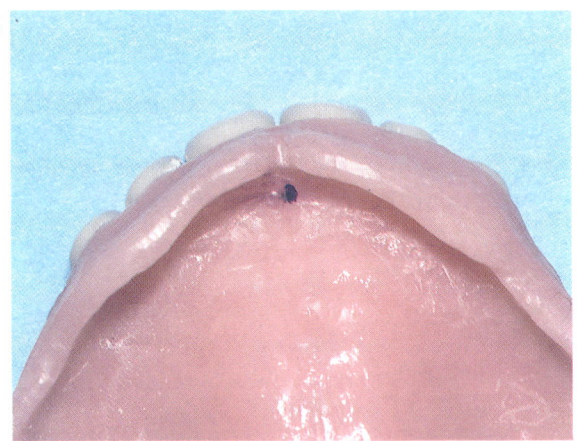

652 The position of the labial surfaces of the central incisors is approximately 8–10 mm anterior to the centre of the incisal papilla.

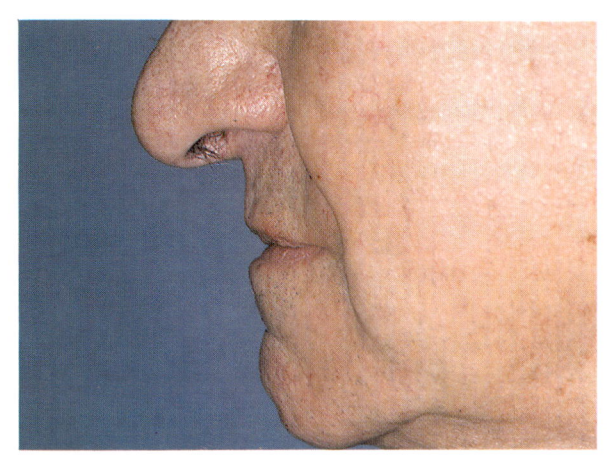

653 Lip contour should be evaluated for adequate support.

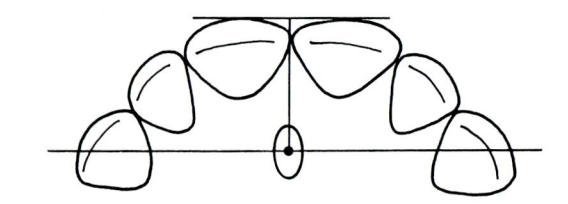

654 Large deviations of the central incisor midline from the centre of the incisal papilla are unusual, and the incisal papilla may be used to determine the midline between central incisor teeth. A line perpendicular to the midline through the incisal papilla passes close to the tips of the maxillary canines, and provides a guide to their position.

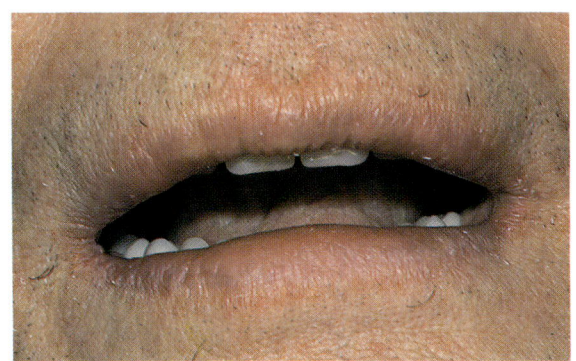

655 The height of the maxillary incisors below the upper lip varies depending on lip activity and length, but is usually 1–2 mm below the upper lip at rest. The mandibular incisal edges and tips of canines and premolars are visible at the corner of the mouth, with the lips slightly parted.

656 Fricative sounds, 'F' and 'V', cause the maxillary incisors to rest at the junction between the 'dry' transitional epithelium and the 'wet' oral mucosa of the lower lip. This phonetic test may provide a useful guide to the correct portion of maxillary incisors.

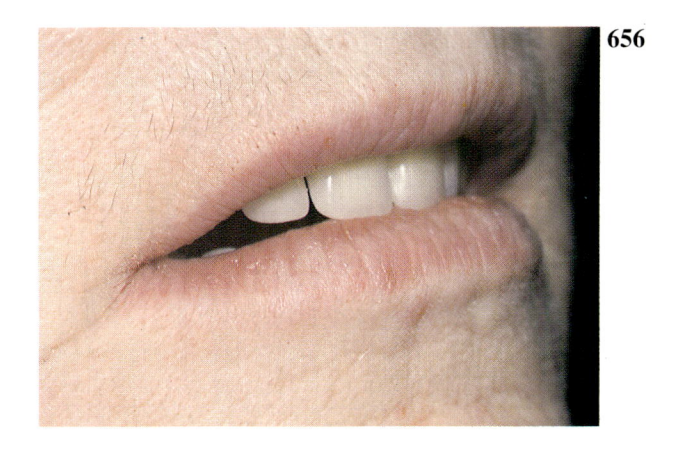

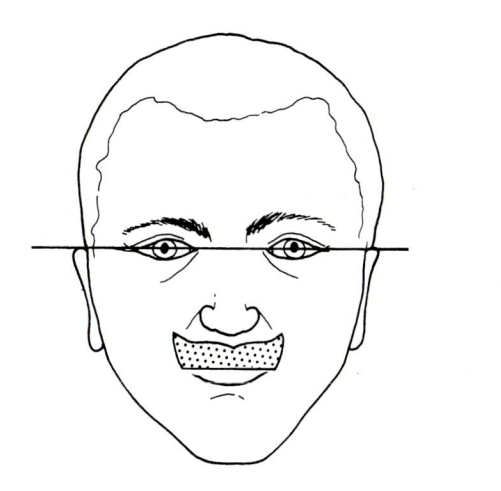

657a, 657b The occlusal plane should be parallel to the interpupillary line when viewed from the front.

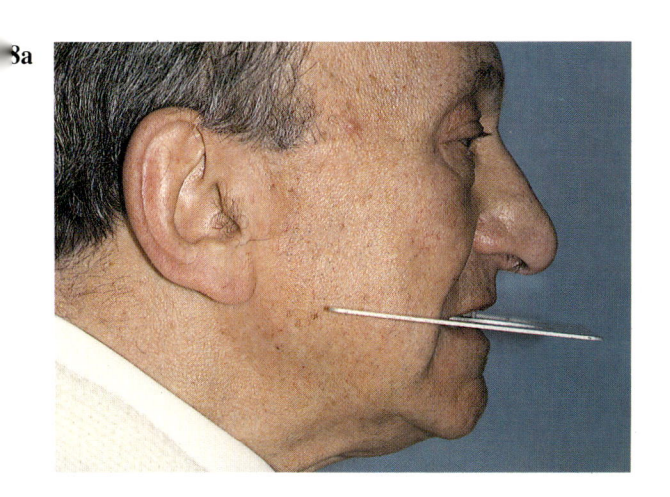

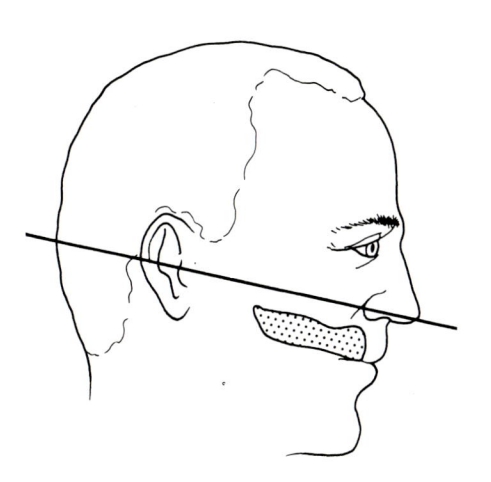

658a, 658b The alatragal line provides a tentative guide to parallelism of the occlusal plane from the lateral view.

223

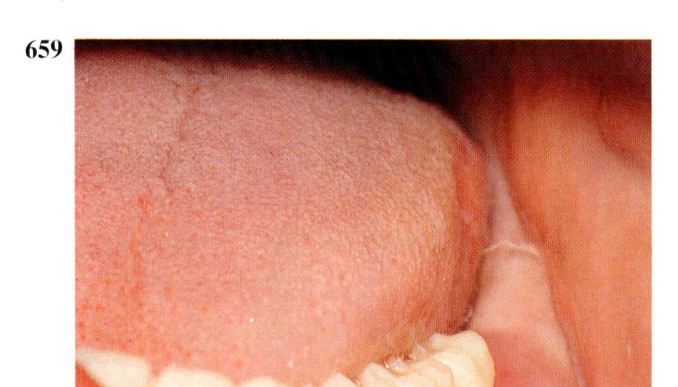

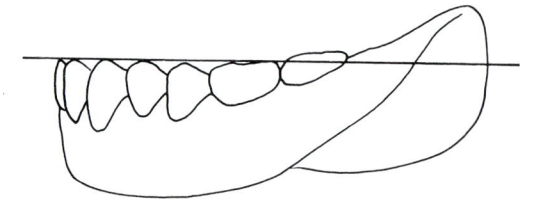

659, 660 Once the anterior teeth have been set, the definitive occlusal plane is determined by extending an imaginary line from the tips of the mandibular canines to ½–⅔ the distance up the retromolar pads.

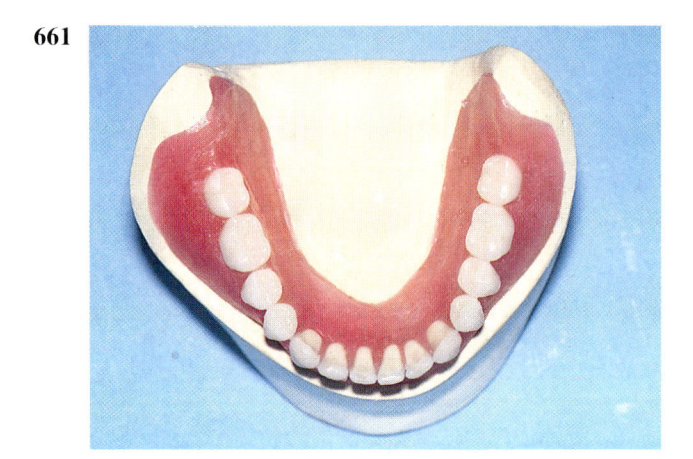

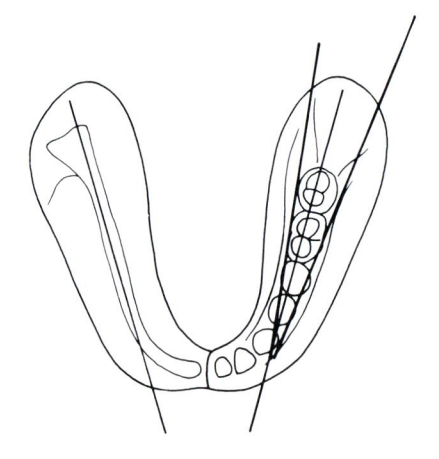

661, 662 Viewed occlusally, the mandibular posterior teeth are set within an area bounded by a line from the mandibular canine tip to the buccal and lingual borders of the retromolar pad.

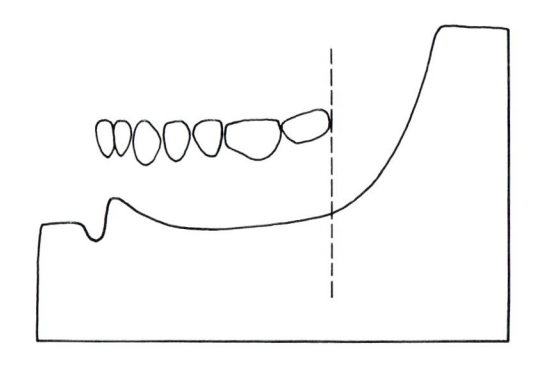

663 Mandibular posterior teeth should not be set on the upward curve of the mandibular ramus. Occlusal forces on this inclined plane will cause the denture base to shift forward.

Tooth form

664 Posterior tooth form is divided into two categories: anatomic and non-anatomic. These describe their resemblance to natural tooth form. While non-anatomic teeth are flat (0°), anatomic teeth range in cusp angle from 33° to 20°, imitating occlusal wear patterns.

Both posterior tooth forms may be used in various permutations of occlusal schemes, in an attempt to provide effective mastication, whilst minimizing force on the residual ridges. It has been suggested that anatomic teeth improve masticatory efficiency but place more horizontal force on the residual ridge. Non-anatomic teeth may not penetrate food as effectively as anatomic tooth forms, but may direct occlusal forces axially, stabilizing the position of the denture bases.

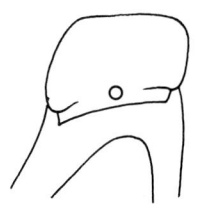

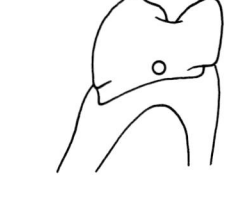

Non-anatomical   Anatomical

665 Ridge morphology may be one guideline for the selection of posterior tooth form. Anatomic teeth are recommended for well formed residual ridges with their potential to resist lateral forces, and non-anatomical tooth forms are recommended when there has been marked bone resorption leaving a flat residual ridge.

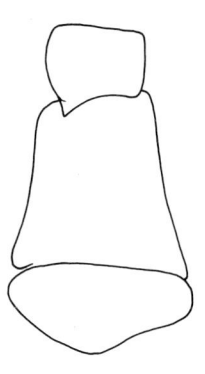

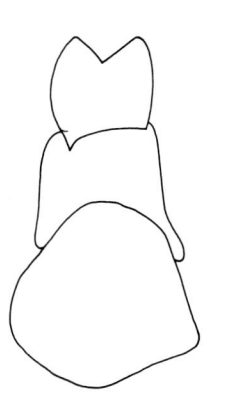

Occlusal scheme

Artificial tooth arrangement may be divided into two groups: balanced occlusion and non-balanced occlusion. Both occlusal arrangements require even, bilateral posterior contact, but in balanced occlusion there is eccentric occlusal balance to maintain the contact in eccentric mandibular positions.

Various tooth arrangements have been described, with differing posterior tooth forms. Two of the most commonly used occlusal schemes are discussed below: balanced occlusion with anatomic teeth, and non-balanced, non-anatomic occlusion.

Balanced occlusion with anatomic teeth. A facebow transfer is used to mount the maxillary cast in a semi-adjustable articulator.

The trial set-up is checked in the mouth to verify that intercuspal contact coincides with the retruded position, at the established vertical dimension of occlusion.

666, 667 A protrusive record is made to set the condylar angles in the articulator. This accommodates the posterior separation of the jaws due to condylar inclination (Christensen's phenomenon).

Lateral guides are adjusted on the articulator by using Hanau's formula:

$$\text{Lateral shift} = \frac{\text{condylar angle}}{8} + 12$$

Alternatively, left and right lateral interocclusal records are made to represent static eccentric jaw position, to which lateral excessive contacts are adjusted.

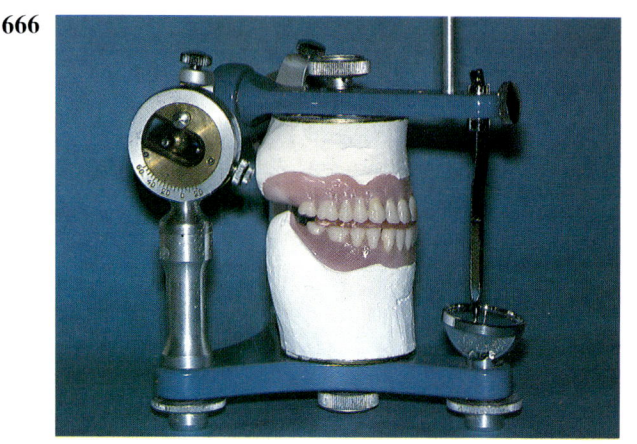

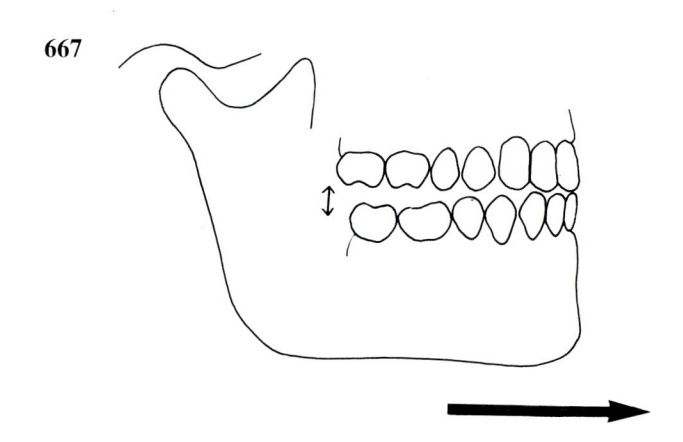

668–672 Balanced occlusion is then perfected in the articulator. Five main factors control balanced occlusion:

- Condylar guidance (**668**) is determined by the movement of condyles on the articulor eminence and cannot be altered by the clinician; this is recorded by the protrusive record.
- Incisal guidance (**669**) is determined by the position of anterior teeth, as decided by the demands of appearance and phonetics.
- Orientation of occlusal plane (**670**).
- Cusp angle (**671**).
- Compensating curve (**672**).

The latter three factors are adjusted to achieve balance. A correctly balanced occlusion will allow for freedom of movement in excursions.

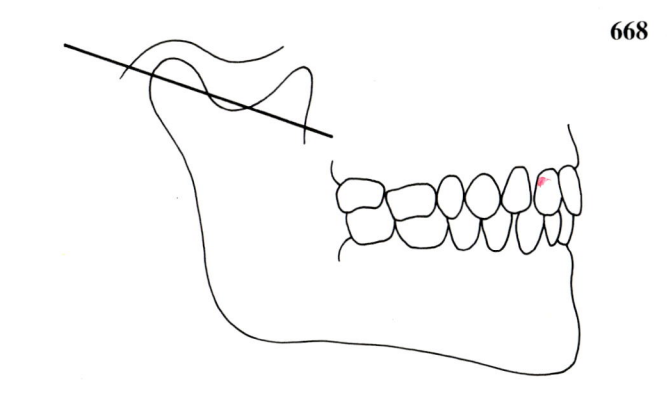

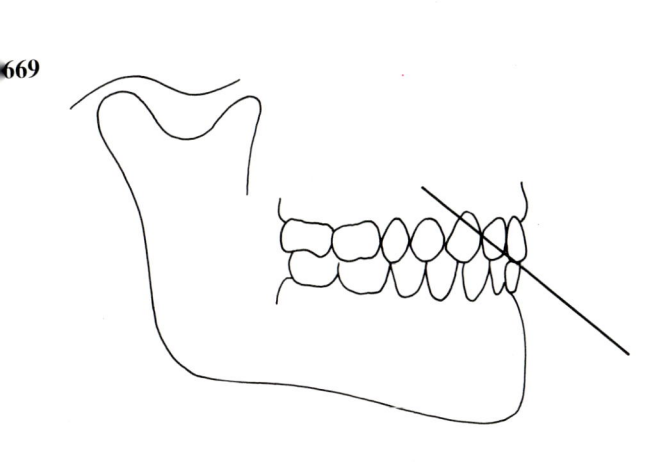

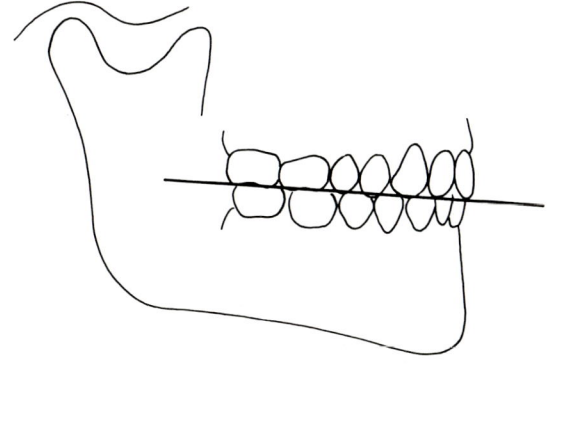

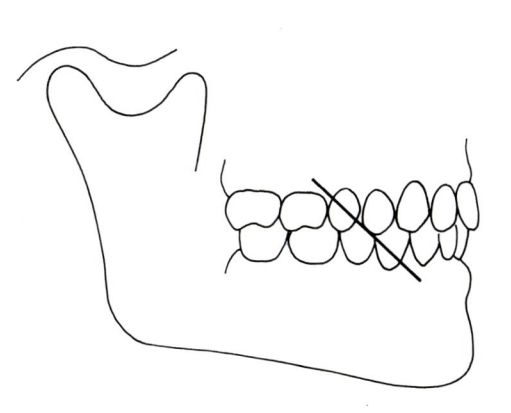

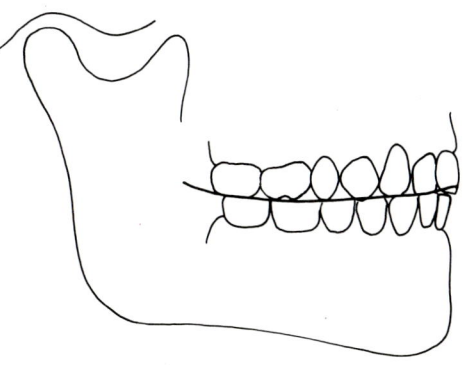

The advantages of an anatomic balanced occlusion are easier penetration of food, improved aesthetics and that para-functional forces are not as disruptive to denture stability.

Non-balanced, non-anatomic occlusion. No facebow transfer is needed, provided the occlusal plane is set exactly to the interocclusal record (the retruded position at the established vertical dimension of occlusion). Any change in vertical relation, occlusal plane or compensating curve requires orientation of the casts to the retruded axis in the articulator.

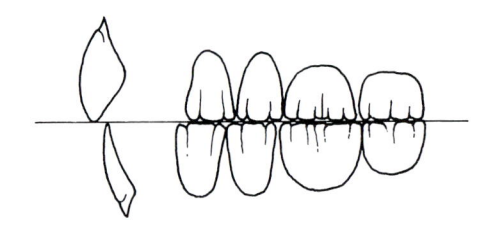

673 In a non-balanced, non-anatomical occlusion, there is usually no vertical overlap of the anterior teeth, but any amount of horizontal overlap, consistent with the relationship of the ridges, the appearance and phonetics. Vertical overlap may be considered only when the anterior teeth are outside the functional range of jaw movements, as in skeletal Class 2 jaw relationships. Freedom of movement in excursions is therefore ensured.

Non-anatomic, non-balanced occlusal schemes are considered an advantage when residual ridges are flat, in posterior crossbites and in skeletal Class 2 and 3 relationships.

Material selection

There are no definite rules for selecting the material for artificial teeth. Acrylic resins are the most commonly available. Porcelain teeth may also be used. Gold, cobalt chromium metal blades, or amalgam imbedded in acrylic resin have also been suggested.

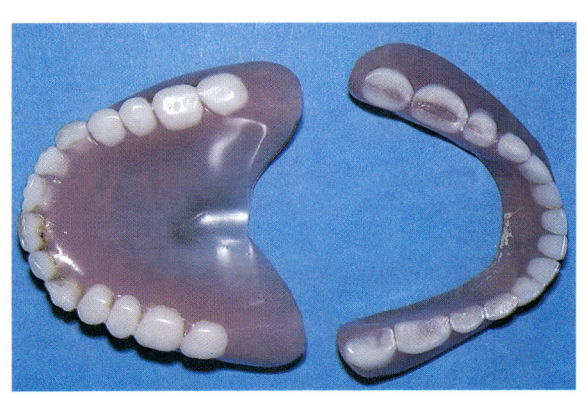

674 The advantage of acrylic resin is its versatility. Easily adjusted and polished, resin teeth bond well to the denture base. However, occlusal surfaces wear considerably, resulting in loss in occlusal vertical dimension and consequent anterior shift of mandibular jaw position. Occlusal contacts are altered and, if left unchecked, lead to potentially harmful forces on the supporting tissues.

Porcelain teeth wear much more slowly than resin and, as a result, occlusal vertical dimension and chewing effectiveness are maintained. However, they do not bond to resin denture bases and need mechanical retention. This may be lost following grinding of the ridge lap when interarch space is restricted. It is important that once occlusal surfaces are ground, they are highly polished to reduce friction and prevent chipping.

Combinations of porcelain and resin teeth in opposing dentures have been used, but occlusal wear of resin teeth remains a problem. Porcelain posterior teeth with resin anterior teeth are acceptable. Resin posterior and porcelain anterior teeth should never be considered because of the traumatic effect on the supporting tissues of anterior interferences occurring, following wear of the resin posterior teeth.

Verification and maintenance of occlusal contacts

Verification and maintenance of occlusal contacts should be achieved at initial delivery, and then maintained at subsequent recall appointments.

675 Initial placement of the dentures includes adjustment to base adaptation and extension to ensure comfort, stability and retention. Indicator paste may be used to help locate pressure areas more precisely, rather than relying on patient direction.

676 An interocclusal jaw registration, at a slightly increased vertical dimension of occlusion on the retruded axis, is then made with a suitable recording medium.

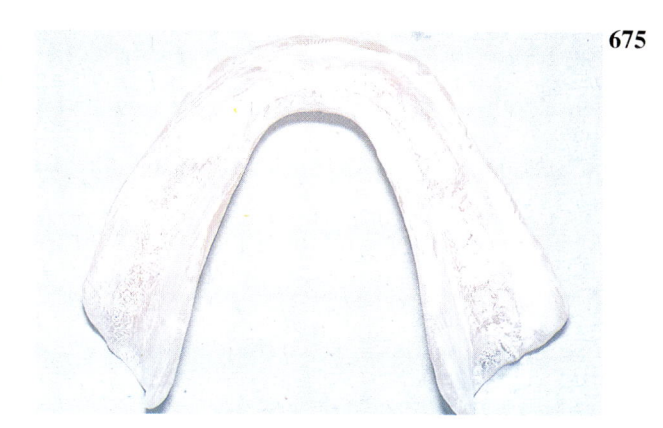

677 The dentures are then remounted in the articulator. A facebow transfer is required, whichever occlusal scheme is used, because of the increase in the occlusal vertical relation of the interocclusal record.

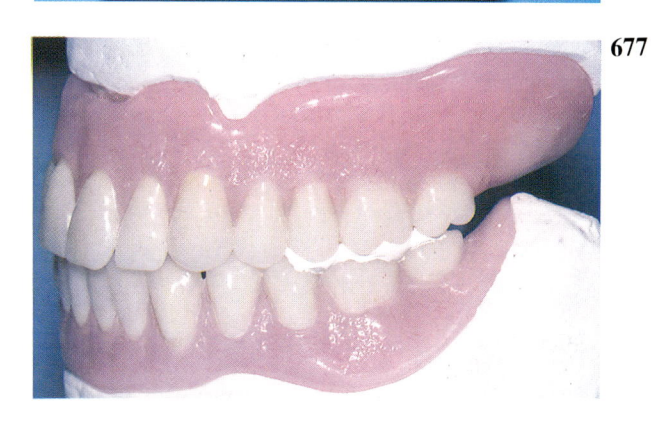

678 Before any occlusal adjustments are made, the interocclusal record should be checked. Another intra-oral interocclusal record is made and the dentures are reseated on the remounted casts. The condylar locking screws are loosened and, with the interocclusal record in place, the condylar ball should be in contact with the condylar adjustment nut. If it is not, further interocclusal records are made to produce a repeatable registration of the retruded position.

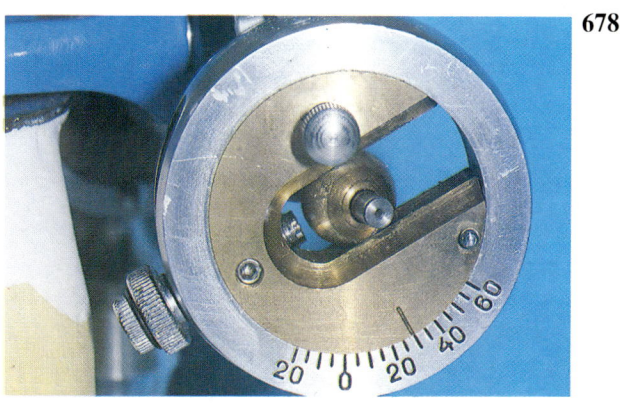

679

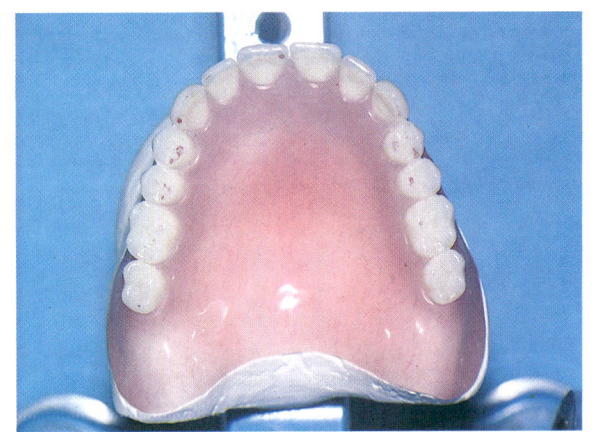

679–681 Occlusal contact may then be refined with selective grinding before denture delivery.

At subsequent recall visits, further remount procedures may be necessary to account for changes in occlusion due to tissue displacement and bone resorption.

The patient is shown before (**679**) and after (**680**, **681**) completion of occlusal adjustment.

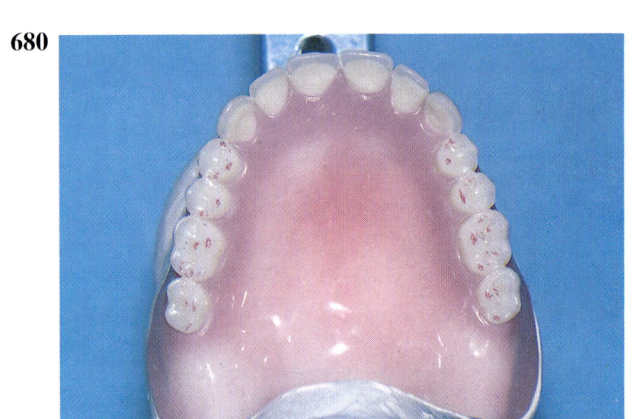

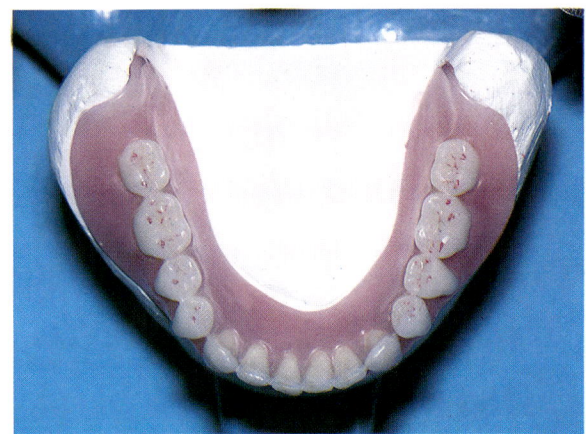

680

681

Alteration in denture base adaptation is often noted following insertion of immediate replacement dentures, or after an extended period of denture use. Relining or rebasing may then be used to refit the tissue surface of the denture while conforming to the occlusal relationship.

A successful reline impression must not only satisfy all the requirements for a working impression, but also maintain intercuspal position coincident with the retruded position at the established vertical dimension of occlusion. However, if there is a discrepancy in vertical relation of more than 2–3 mm, or a large difference between the intercuspal and retruded positions, relining alone will be insufficient and new dentures should be considered.

Insertion of the relined denture should always include a clinical remount procedure to verify jaw relation records.

Denture copying techniques are used to replicate acceptable features of existing dentures, while improving inadequate aspects of denture design. Immediate replacement dentures, which have preserved the natural tooth position, may demonstrate evidence of poor base adaptation following alveolar ridge resorption, as well as wear of the occlusal surfaces of the teeth. The aim in making a copy denture is to restore base adaptation and vertical relation.

The technique is also of value in duplicating dentures worn successfully for many years, usually by elderly patients who may not tolerate changes in tooth positions and vertical relation. Worn occlusal surfaces and base adaptation may be improved without altering the fundamental tooth arrangement and polished contours.

Special considerations

Single dentures

A single denture, usually a complete maxillary denture opposing remaining mandibular natural teeth, presents difficulties in developing an occlusal scheme. Tilting and drifting of natural teeth results in an alteration in the level of the occlusal plane, against which the artificial teeth are set. If occlusal adjustment of the natural teeth is not carried out, artificial tooth contacts on natural tooth inclines may dislodge even the best fitting denture base. Mounted diagnostic casts enable the clinician to plan corrections to the occlusal plane. Adjustments can then be made to improve the occlusal plane either by restoration or reduction of tooth surfaces.

682–684 In this clinical situation, where the occlusal plane had previously been restored and was not easily altered, a functionally generated path technique was used to develop an acceptable occlusal scheme in harmony with the existing restoration.

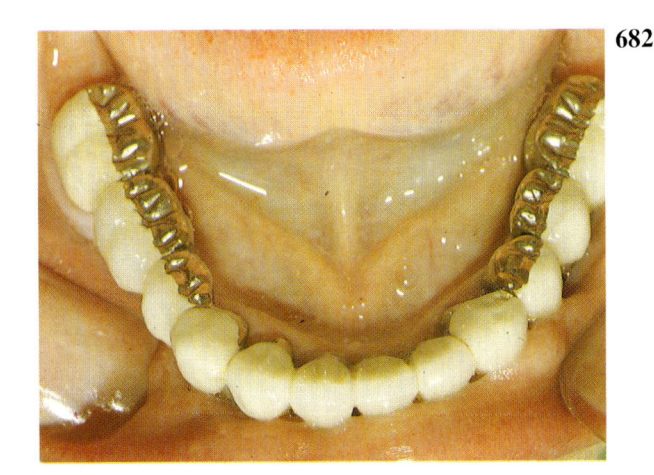

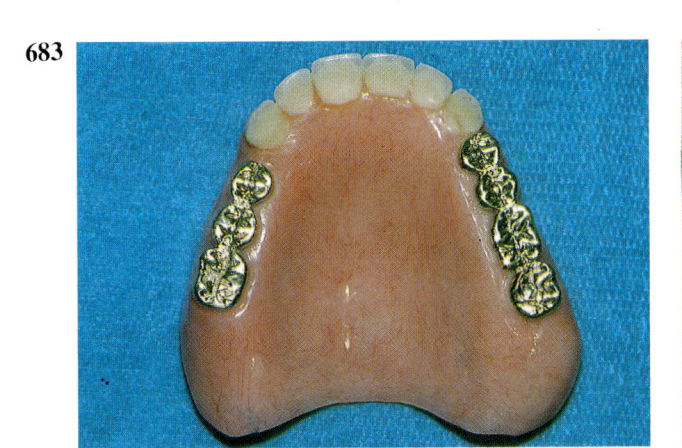

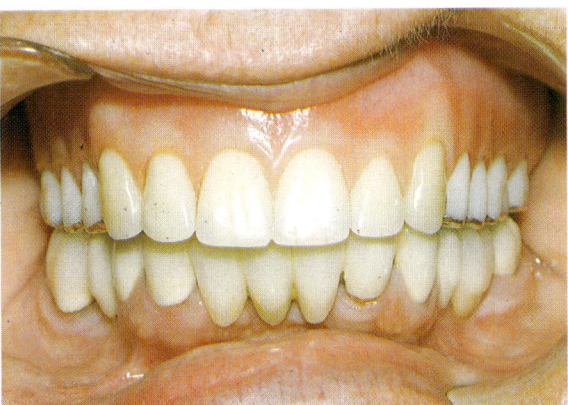

Hemimandibulectomy

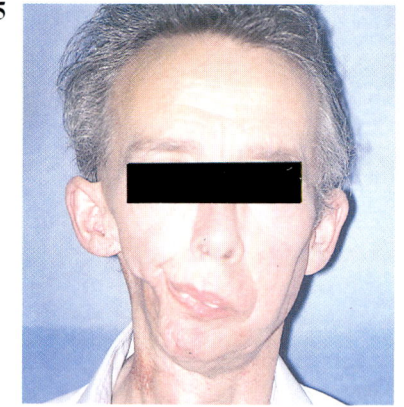

685–687 When the continuity of the mandibular bone is disrupted, as might follow surgical management of a neoplastic lesion, there is a deviation and retrusion towards the unoperated side due to the pull of the remaining muscles and tissue attachments. The effect is to alter facial appearance, and effective chewing becomes difficult because of the change in occlusal relations.

Techniques to reduce the deviation include intermaxillary fixation and the use of either maxillary- or mandibular-based guiding restorations, combined with jaw exercises that involve manipulating the remaining mandible towards the unaffected side. Success in limiting the deviation is variable and depends on numerous factors, of which the extent of the primary lesion and its surgical treatment are the most important. The presence of teeth improves the stability of prostheses and invariably, the deviation is accepted and occlusal contact established at the altered jaw position.

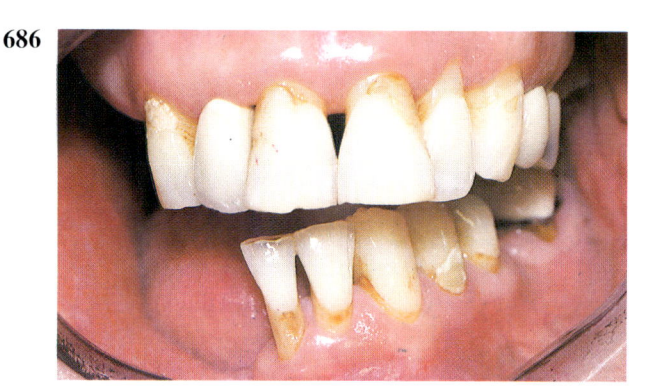

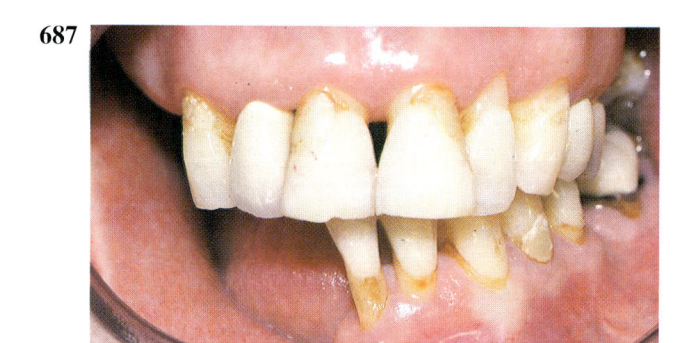

Conclusion

The basic principles of complete denture occlusion have been discussed. There is no scientific evidence to support which occlusal scheme is chosen and the clinician relies on guides in selecting and arranging the complete denture occlusion. The ultimate success of complete denture treatment lies in its ability to fulfill the goals of restoring appearance, comfort and function, while maintaining the health of the remaining tissues.

Further Reading

CHAPTER 1

Clayton, J.A. (1971) 'Border positions and restoring the occlusion', *Dent. Clin. N. Am.*, **15**, (July), 525.

De Pietro, A.J. (1963) 'A system based on rotational centres of the mandible', *Dent. Clin. N. Am.*, (Nov.), 607.

Posselt, U. (1957) 'Terminal hinge movement of the mandible', *J. Prosthet. Dent.*, **7**, 787.

CHAPTER 2

Hobo, S., Shillingburg, H.T. and Whitsett, L.D. (1976) 'Articulator selection for restorative dentistry', *J. Prosthet. Dent.*, **36**, 35.

Mohamed, S.E., Schmidt, J.R. and Harrison, J.D. (1976) 'Articulators in dental education and practice', *J. Prosthet. Dent.*, **36**, 319.

Posselt, U. 'Registration of the condylar path inclination by intra-oral wax records. Variation in three instruments', *J. Prosthet. Dent.*, **10**, 441.

Teteruck, W.R. and Lundeen, H.C. (1966) 'The accuracy of the ear face-bow', *J. Prosthet. Dent.*, **16**, 1039.

Weinberg, L.A. (1963) 'An evaluation of basic articulators and their concepts. Part II. Arbitrary, positional, semi-adjustable articulators', *J. Prosthet. Dent.*, **13**, 645.

Weinberg, L.A. (1963) 'An evaluation of basic articulators and their concepts. Part IV. Fully-adjustable articulators', *J. Prosthet. Dent.*, **13**, 1038.

CHAPTERS 3 & 4

Beard, C.C. and Clayton, J.A. (1980) 'Effects of occlusal splint therapy on TMJ dysfunction', *J. Prosthet. Dent.*, **44**, 324.

Butler, J. and Stallard, R. (1969) 'Effect of occlusal relationships on neurophysiological pathways', *J. Periodont. Res.*, **4**, 141.

Capp, N.J. (1986) 'Temporomandibular joint dysfunction – its relevance to restorative dentistry. Part I', *Rest. Dent. Vol. 2*, **2**, 36.

Crum, R.J. and Loiselle, R.J. (1972) 'Oral perception and proprioception. A review of the literature and its significance to prosthodontics', *J. Prosthet. Dent.*, **28**, 215.

Furstman, L. (1965) 'The effect of loss of occlusion upon the temporomandibular joint', *Am. J. Orthod.*, **51**, 1245.

Helkimo, M. (1979) 'Epidemiological surveys of dysfunction of the masticatory system' in G.A. Zarb and G.E. Carlsson, *Temporomandibular joint function and dysfunction*, Munksgaard Copenhagen, p. 182.

Kantor, M.E., Silverman, S.I. and Garfinkel, L. (1972) 'Centric relation recording techniques. A comparative investigation', *J. Prosthet. Dent.*, **28**, 593.

Morgan, D.W., Cornella, M.C. and Staffanou, R.S. (1975) 'A diagnostic wax-up technique', *J. Prosthet. Dent.*, **33**, 169.

Ramjford, S.P., Walden, J.M. and Enlow, R.D. (1971) 'Unilateral function and the temporomandibular joint in Rhesus monkeys', *Oral Surgery*, **32**, 257.

Robinson, H.B.G. (1963) 'The nature of the diagnostic process', *Dent. Clin. N. Am.*, (March), 3.

Shields, J.M., Clayton, J.A. and Sindledecker, L.D. (1978) 'Using pantographic tracings to detect TMJ and muscle dysfunctions', *J. Prosthet. Dent.*, **39**, 80.

Teo, C.S. and Wise, M.D. (1981) 'Comparison of retruded axis articulator mountings with and without applied muscle force', *J. Oral Rehabil.*, **8**, 363.

Weinberg, L.A. (1973) 'What do we really see in a TMJ radiograph?', *J. Prosthet. Dent.*, **30**, 898.

CHAPTERS 5 & 6

Ash, M. and Ramjford, S.P. (1982) *An introduction to functional occlusion*, W.B. Saunders, Philadelphia.

Carlson, D.S., McNamara Jnr, J.A. and Ribbens, K.A. (1985) 'Developmental aspects of temporomandibular joint disorders', *Monograph 16, Craniofacial Growth Series*, Center for Human Growth and Development, University of Michigan.

Graber, T.M. and Swain, B.F. (1985) *Orthodontics. Current principles and techniques*, C.V. Mosby Co.

Foster, T.D. (1982) *A textbook of orthodontics*, 2nd edition, Blackwell.

Houston, W.J.B. (1982) *Orthodontic diagnosis. A dental practitioner handbook: No. 4*, 3rd edition. Wright, PSG.

Johnstone Jnr, L.E. (1985) *New vistas in orthodontics*, Lea and Febiger, Philadelphia.

Mills, J.R.E. (1982) *Principles and practice of orthodontics*, Churchill Livingstone.

Moyers, R.E. (1988) *Handbook of orthodontics*, Year Book Medical Publishers Inc.

Rakosi, T. (1982) *An atlas and manual of cephalometric radiography*, Wolfe Medical Publications Ltd.

Slavicek, R. (1988) 'Clinical and instrumental functional analysis for diagnosis and treatment planning. Part 4: Instrumental analysis of mandibular casts using the mandibular position indicator', *J. Clinical Orthodont.*, **22**, 566–575.
'Part 5: Computer-aided diagnosis and treatment planning system', *J. Clinical Orthodont.*, **22**, 718–729.

Thilander, B. and Ronning, O. (1985) *Introduction to orthodontics*, 5th edition, Tandläkarförlaget, Stockholm.

Van der Linden, F.P.G.M. (1984) *Development of the dentition*, Quintessence Publishing Co.

CHAPTER 7

Hickey, J., Zarb, G. and Bolender, C. (1986) *Boucher's prosthodontic treatment for endtulous patients*, 9th edition, C.V. Mosby Co., St. Louis.

Heartwell, C.M. and Rahn, A.O. (1981) *Syllabus of complete dentures*, Lea & Febiger, Philadelphia.

Laney, W.R. and Gibilisco, J.A. (1983) *Diagnosis and treatment in prosthodontics*, Lea & Febiger, Philadelphia.

Watt, D.M. and Macgregor, A.R. (1986) *Designing complete dentures*, 2nd edition, John Wright, Bristol.

CHAPTER 9

Capp, N.J. (1986) 'Temporomandibular joint dysfunction. Its relevance to restorative dentistry. Part II', *Rest. Dent.*, Vol. 2, **3**, 62.

Dawson, P.E. (1974) *Evaluation, diagnosis and treatment of occlusal problems*, C.V. Mosby Co., St. Louis, chapter 5.

King, C.J., Richardson, J.T. and Cleveland, J.L. (1976) 'The technician as part of the team', *J. Am. Dent. Assoc.*, **92**, 374.

Ramjford, S.P. and Ash, M.M. (1983) *Occlusion*, 3rd edition, W.B. Saunders Co., Philadelphia, chapter 3.

CHAPTER 10

Capp, N.J. (1985) 'The diagnostic use of provisional restorations', *Rest. Dent.*, **4**, 92.

Dawson, P.E. (1974) *Diagnosis and treatment of occlusal problems*, C.V. Mosby Co., St. Louis, chapters 23, 24.

Schyler, C.H. (1963) 'The function and importance of incisal guidance in oral rehabilitation', *J. Prosthet. Dent.*, **13**, 1011.

CHAPTER 11

Clayton, J.A. (1980) 'A stable base precision attachment removable partial denture. Theories and principals', *Dent. Clin. N. Am.*, **24**, 3.

Nagasawa, T. and Tsuru, H. (1973) 'A comparative evaluation of masticatory efficiency of fixed and removable restorations replacing mandibular first molars', *J. Prosthet. Dent.* **30**, 263.

Shillingburg, H.T., Wilson, E.L. and Morrison, J.T. (1984) Guide to occlusal waxing, 2nd edition, Quintessence Publishing Co.

CHAPTER 12

Carlsson, G.E., Ingervall, B. and Kocak, G. (1979) 'Effect of increasing vertical dimension on the masticatory system in subjects with natural teeth', *J. Prosthet. Dent.*, **41**, 284.

Garnick, J.J. and Ramjford, S.P. (1962) 'Rest position: an electromyographic and clinical investigation', *J. Prosthet. Dent.*, **12**, 895.

Lucia, V.O. (1962) 'The gnathological concept of articulation', *Dent. Clin. N. Am.*, (March), 183.

Mann, A.W. and Pankey, L.D. (1963) 'The P–M philosophy of occlusal rehabilitation', *Dent. Clin. N. Am.*, (March), 621.

Storey, A.T. (1962) 'Physiology of changing vertical dimension', *J. Prosthet. Dent.*, **12**, 912.

CHAPTERS 13, 14 and 15

Andrews, L.F. (1972) 'The six keys to normal occlusion', *Amer. J. Orthodontics*, **62**, 296–309.

Begg, P.R. and Kesling, P.C. (1977) *Begg orthodontic theory and technique*, 3rd edition, W.B. Saunders Co.

Bell, W.H., Profitt, W.R. and White, R.P. (1980) *Surgical correction of dentofacial deformaties*, W.B. Saunders Co.

Foster, T.D. (1982) *A textbook of orthodontics*, 2nd edition, Blackwell Scientific Publications.

Graber, T.M. and Swain, B.F. (1985) *Orthodontics current principles and techniques*, C.V. Mosby Co.

Graber, T.M., Rakosi, T. and Petrovic, A.G. (1985) *Dentofacial orthopedics with functional appliances*, C.V. Mosby Co.

Graber, T.M. and Neumann, B. (1984) *Removable orthodontic appliances*, 2nd edition, W.B. Saunders Co.

Houston, W.J.B. and Isaacson, K.G. (1980) *Orthodontic treatment with removable appliances. A dental practitioner handbook: No. 25*, 2nd edition, Wright, PSG.

Isaacson, K.G. and Williams, J.K. (1984) *An introduction to fixed appliances. A dental practitioner handbook: No. 17*, 3rd edition, Wright, PSG.

Moyers, R.E. (1988) *Handbook of orthodontics*, Year Book Medical Publishers Inc.

Profitt, W.R. and Ackerman (1985) *Orthodontics: current principles and techniques*, T.M. Graber and B.F. Swain (eds.), C.V. Mosby Co.

Richardson, A. (1982) 'Interceptive orthodontics in general dental practice', *Brit. Dent. J.*, **152**, 85–89, 123–7, 166–70.

Roth, R.H. (1981) 'Functional occlusion for the orthodontist. Part 1', *J. Clinical Orthodontics*, 15, 32–51. 'Part 3', **15**, 174–198.

Roth, R.H. and Rolfs, D.A. (1981) 'Functional occlusion for the orthodontist. Part 2', *J. Clinical Orthodontics*, **15**, 100–123.

Roth, R.H. and Woodford W.G. (1981) 'Functional occlusion for the orthodontist. Part 4', *J. Clinical Orthodontics*, **15**, 246–265.

Roth, R.H. (1987) 'The straight-wire appliance – 17 years later', *J. Clinical Orthodontics*, **21**.

Van der Linden, F.P.G.M. (1986) *Facial growth and facial orthopedics*, Quintessence Publishing Co.

CHAPTER 16

Academy of Denture Prosthetics (1989) 'Principles concepts and practices in prosthodontics 1989', *J. Prosthet. Dent.*, **61**, 88.

Beck, H.O. (1972) 'Occlusion as related to complete removable prosthodontics', *J. Prosthet. Dent.*, **27**, 246.

Beumer, J., Curtis, T.A. and Firtell, D.N. (1979) *Maxillofacial rehabilitation: prosthodontic and surgical considerations*, C.V. Mosby Co., St. Louis, chapter 4.

Devan, M.M. (1954) 'The concept of neutrocentric occlusion as related to denture stability', *J. Am. Dent. Assoc.*, **48**, 165.

Jordan, L.G. (1978) 'Arrangement of anatomic-type artificial teeth into balanced occlusion', *J. Prosthet. Dent.*, **39**, 484.

Lang, B.R. and Kelsey, C.C. (1973) *International prosthodontic workshop on complete denture occlusion*, University of Michigan Press, Ann Arbor.

Morrow, R.M., Rudd, K.D. and Eissmann, H.F. (1981) *Dental laboratory procedures; complete dentures*, Vol. 1, C.V. Mosby Co., St. Louis.

Neill, D.J. and Nairn, R. (1982) *Complete denture prosthetics*, 2nd edition, John Wright, Bristol.

Ortman, H.R. (1977) 'Complete denture occlusion', *Dent. Clin. N. Am.*, (April), 299.

Renner, R.P. (1981) *Complete dentures*, Masson Publishing USA Inc., New York, chapter 4.

Index

All references are to page numbers

A
Abnormal swallowing, 9
Acid etch-retained bridges, 147–8
   failures, 150
   hypodontia treatment, 147
   periodontal retainer, 150
   post-orthodontic retainer, 150
   replacement of teeth lost through trauma or resorption, 148–9
Adjustable intercondylar distance, 29
Amalgam, 156
Andrew's Six Keys, 188
Angular chelitis, 114
Anterior guidance, 12, 47–51
Anterior malocclusion correction, 191–2
Anterior open bite, 89
Anterior-posterior malocclusion correction, 193–5
Anterior region, reorganization to create space in, 65
Anterior teeth restoration, 129–50
   achieving stable ICP contacts, 132–3
   acid etch-retained bridges, *see* acid etch-retained bridges
   altering existing guidance, 137–9
   cantilevered pontics, 139–40
   choice of type of guidance, 132–3
   class 2 jaw relation, 142–5
   deep overbites, 88, 140–1
   malaligned guidance teeth, 146
   metal coping design, 131–2
   partial denture occlusion, 150
   reproducing correct maxillary lingual concavity, 129–30
   restoring anterior guidance, 133–6
   short clinical crowns, 145–6
Anterior-posterior teeth replacement, 179–86
Anteroposterior buccal segment relationships, 90
Anteroposterior incisal relationship, 85–7
Arthrography, 54
Articulated diagnostic casts, 55
Articulators, 17–32
   average-value, 18
   cast relators, 17–18
      simple hinges, 17
      verticulator, 18
   classification, 17
   fully-adjustable, 28–32
      applications, 32
      condylar adjustment, 29–31
   semi-adjustable, 18–23
      anterior guidance table, 23
      applications, 28
      arcon, 19
      condylar adjustment, 19–23
      limitations, 28
      non-arcon, 19

B
Bennett angle, 15, 22
Bennett movement, 13
Border movements, *see* mandibular movements
Bruxing (tooth grinding), 9, 44, 83
Buccal crossbite, 92
Buccal segment relationships, 91–4

C
Canine guidance, 13
Cantilevered pontics, 139–40
Cast relators, 17–18
Cephalometry, 75, 110
   RCP–ICP conversion, 112
Christensen's phenomenon, 226
Class 2 jaw relation, 142–5
Cleft lip and palate, 75
Complete denture assessment, 113–20
   examination, 114–20
      existing dentures, 118
      extra-oral, 114
      factors influencing retention and stability of dentures, 117–18
      intra-oral, 115–18
      supporting tissues, 115–16
      temporomandibular joint, 114
   history, 113
   mounted diagnostic casts, 120
   radiographs, 120
Complete denture occlusion, 217–32
   artificial teeth arrangement, 221–8
      balanced occlusion with anatomic teeth, 226–7
      material selection, 228
      non-balanced, non-anatomic occlusion, 228
      occlusal scheme, 226–8
      tooth form, 225
      tooth position, 221–4
   intercuspal position coincident with retruded position at established vertical dimension of occlusion, 217–20

occlusal contact, verification and maintenance, 229–30
single dentures, 231
Complete overbite, 88
Condyle, 40
non-working (balancing) side, 13
working side, 13
Conformative definitive treatment, 190–200
anterior malocclusion correction, 191–2
anterior-posterior malocclusion correction, 183–5
orthodontics, 196–200
orthognathic surgery, 196–200
posterior malocclusion correction, 192–3
Conformative interceptive treatment, 189–90
Conformative–reorganized equation, 121–2
Cranio Mandibular Positioner (CMP), 111
Crossbite
buccal, 92
lingual, 92
Cusps
non-supporting, 12
supporting, 12

D
Deep overbites, 140–1
Definitive reorganized orthodontic management, 211–16
functional appliance therapy, 213–16
RCP–ICP discrepancies, 211–12
Denar system, 25
5A, 28
MKII, 19–22
pantograph, 29
Vericheck, 27
Dentatus, 19–21
Development, general, 109–10
Deviation, 95–6
Diagnostic casts, 66
instrumental analysis, 111
RP mounted, analysis of, 124
Displacement, 96–101

E
Extra-oral forces, 204, 208

F
Facebow, 23–5
average, 24–5
kinematic (hinge axis), 24
Facial microsomia, 78
Fixed appliance therapy, 147, 190, 192–200, 212
Four-unit bridge, 166–70
Freeway space (interocclusal distance), 10
Functional appliance therapy, 213–16

G
Gold, 131
type 3, 157
Gothic arch, 15
Group function, 13
Growth, general, 109–10

H
Hanau's formula, 226
Hemimandibulectomy, 232
Hypodontia treatment, 147–8

I
Incisal relationship, 85–90
Interceptive reorganized orthodontic treatment, 201–10
abnormal rest position, 210
lateral displacements, 205–8
posterior displacements, 209
Intercuspal position (ICP), 7, 10, 38–9
abnormality in rest position, 94–5
conforming to existing, 55–9
RCP–ICP conversion on lateral cephalometric radiograph, 112
large horizontal, small vertical RCP–ICP discrepancy, 63–4
large vertical, small horizontal RCP–ICP discrepancy, 60–3
maximal and stable occlusal contacts, 85–92
anteroposterior buccal segment relationships, 90
anteroposterior incisal relationships, 85–7
lateral buccal segment relationships, 92
lateral incisal relationships, 90
maximal and stable occlusal contacts, variation in, 92–4
vertical buccal segment relationships, 91
vertical incisal relationships, 88–9
reorganizing so that RCP=ICP, 125–6
Interocclusal distance (freeway space), 10
Interocclusal records, 26–7

J
Jaw posturing, 9

L
Lateral buccal segment relationships, 92
Lateral incisal relationships, 90
Lingual crossbite, 92

M
Malaligned guidance teeth, 146
Mandible
anterior deviation, 96
rest position, 94
vertical deviation, 96

Mandibular dysfunction, acute, 66
Mandibular movements, 9–16, 102–8
　border movements in coronal plane, 12–13
　border movements in horizontal plane, 15
　border movements in sagittal plane, 10–12
　control of, 15
　dysfunctional, 9
　excessive occlusal wear, 102
　functional, 9
　lateral, 102, 104–7
　protrusive, 102–3
Mandibular position
　border, 9
　intercuspal, 10
　retruded, 11
　retruded contact, 11
Mandibular Position Indicator (MPI), 111
Masticatory muscle assessment, 36
Mesencephalic nucleus, 15
Muscle palpation, 36
　lateral pterygoid, 36
　medial pterygoid, 36

N
Neuromuscular system, 40
Non-working contacts, 14
Non-working side interferences, 14

O
Occlusal analysis, 55
Occlusal contacts, marking, 37–8
Occlusal equilibration, 125
Occlusal plane irregularities, 52
Occlusal splint therapy, 69–72, 124, 187
Occlusal wear, excessive, 102
Occlusion assessment, 33, 52
　restorative, *see* restorative assessment
Occlusion reorganization, 65–6
　space creation in anterior region, 65
Occlusion restoration, 123–8
　additions to existing dentures, 128
　analysis of diagnostic casts mounted in RP, 124
　elimination of RCP–ICP discrepancy, 125–8
　　occlusal equilibration, 125
　　orthognathic surgery, 128
　　provisional restorations to re-establish anterior guidance and posterior stability, 126–7
　　reorganized orthodontics, 128
　occlusal splint therapy, 124
Orthodontic assessment, 73–108
　extra-oral examination, 74–9
　　aesthetics, 74–9
　　cephalometrics, 75
　　dentofacial proportions, 74–9
　　full face, 77–88
　　lips position, 79
　　nasal air passages, 79
　　orofacial muscle balance and function, 78
　　photographic, 74–5
　　profile, 75–6
　　radiographic, 74–5
　　temporomandibular joint, 79
　　tongue position, 79
　history, 73
　intra-oral examination, 80–108
　　dentitions, 82–108
　　orthodontic records, 80–1
　　soft tissues, 81–2
Orthodontic treatment, 187–200
Orthognathic surgery, 128, 196–200
Overbite, complete, 88

P
Pantograph, 28–9, 67–8
Parafunctional activity, 199
Partial coverage occlusal splint, prolonged use, 44
Partial denture occlusion when posterior teeth require replacement, 178
Pencil biting, 9
Periodontal membrane, 40
Periodontal retainer, 150
Plagiocephaly, 78
Porcelain, 131
Porcelain-fused-to-metal crowns, 157
Posterior lateral arch relationships, 92
Posterior malocclusion correction, 192–3
Posterior occlusal stability, 38–9
Posterior stability loss, 41–4
Posterior teeth restoration, 151–78
　anterior and posterior determinants, 151–2
　four-unit bridge, 166–70
　gold v. porcelain occlusal surfaces, 157–9
　maintenance and reproduction of stable ICP contacts, 153–5
　materials for restoring occlusal surfaces, 156–7
　no anterior tooth contact in ICP, 155
　occlusal aspects of tooth preparation, 160
　opposing quadrants, 171–7
　partial denture occlusion when posterior teeth require replacement, 178
　single unit porcelain-fused-to-metal crown, 161–5
　three-unit bridge with cantilevered pontic, 165–6
　working casts, mounting, 161
Post-orthodontic retainer, 150

R
Radiographs, 53–4, 74–5
Removable appliance therapy, 191, 202–3, 205–6
Resins, 156

239

Restorative assessment, 33–52
　aims of occlusal examination, 33
　examination, 34–52
　　anterior guidance, 47–51
　　discrepancy between RCP and ICP, 45–6
　　extra-oral, 35–6
　　intercuspal position, 38–9
　　intra-oral, 36–52
　　muscles, 36
　　occlusal contacts, marking, 37–8
　　occlusal plane irregularities, 52
　　periodontal membrane, 40
　　posterior occlusal stability, 38–9
　　posterior stability loss, 41–4
　　temporomandibular joints, 35
　　vertical dimension, 52
　history, 34
Retruded axis (terminal hinge axis), 11
Retruded contact position (RCP), 7
　RCP–ICP discrepancies, 96–101
　　anterior displacements, 97–8
　　elimination, *see under* occlusion restoration
　　large horizontal, small vertical RCP–ICP discrepancy, 63–4
　　large vertical, small horizontal RCP–ICP discrepancy, 60–3
　　lateral displacement, 99–101
　　posterior displacement, 99
　　vertical displacement, 101

S
Sam system, 26
Scissor bite, 92
Sensory receptors, 15
Short clinical crowns, 145–6
Sideshift
　immediate (early), 13
　progressive, 13

Simple hinges, 17
Single unit porcelain-fused-to-metal crown, 161–5
Soft tissue examination, 81

T
Teeth
　absence of, 82–3, 147–8, 192
　acid erosion, 45
　clenching, 1
　grinding (bruxing), 9, 44, 83
　severely worn anterior, 41
　supernumeraries, 189
Temporomandibular joint
　adaptive capacity, 15
　articulator surface degeneration, 35
　assessment, 35, 79, 114
　closed lock, 35
　mandibular excursions, 10–15, 102–8
　mandibular movement control, 97
　radiographs, 54
Terminal hinge axis (retruded axis), 11
Thumb sucking, 9
Trigeminal nerve nucleus, 15
Tripodization, 153

V
Vertical buccal segment relationship, 91
Vertical dimension of occlusion, 10
　assessment, 52, 118
Vertical dimension of rest, 10, 118
Vertical incisal relationship, 88–9
Verticulator, 18

W
Whipmix, 19–22, 26